Health, disease and society in Europe
1800–1930

Health, disease and society in Europe 1800–1930

A source book

edited by
Deborah Brunton

Manchester University Press
Manchester and New York
distributed exclusively in the USA by Palgrave
Published in association with

The Open
University

Published by Manchester University Press
Oxford Road, Manchester M13 9NR, UK
and Room 400, 175 Fifth Avenue, New York, NY 10010, USA
www.manchesteruniversitypress.co.uk

Distributed exclusively in the USA by
Palgrave Macmillan, 175 Fifth Avenue, New York, NY 10010, USA

Distributed exclusively in Canada by
UBC Press, University of British Columbia,
2029 West Mall, Vancouver, BC, Canada V6T 1Z2

British Library Cataloguing-in-Publication Data
A catalogue record for this book is available from the British Library

Library of Congress Cataloging-in-Publication Data applied for

978 0 7190 6739 6 paperback

First published 2004

First reprinted 2009

This publication forms part of an Open University course: A218 *Medicine and Society in
Europe, 1500–1930*. Details of this and other Open University courses can be obtained
from the Course Information and Advice Centre, PO Box 724, The Open University, Milton
Keynes MK7 6ZS, United Kingdom: tel. +44 (0)1908 653231, e-mail general-enquiries@open.
ac.uk. Alternatively, you may visit the Open University website at http://www.open.ac.uk
where you can learn more about the wide range of courses and packs offered at all levels
by The Open University.

Printed by the MPG Books Group in the UK

Contents

Acknowledgements

The editor and publisher would like to thank all the contributors to *Medicine Transformed*: Jonathon Andrews, Roger Cooter, L.S. Jacyna, Hilary Marland, James Moore, Maxine Rhodes, Thomas Schlich, Paul Weindling and Michael Worboys for selecting the readings reproduced here. The editor would also like to thank Colin Chant, Peter Elmer, Gill Hudson and Gerrylynn Roberts for their help in preparing this book.

The editor and publisher would also like to thank the following for permission to publish the enclosed documents: N.D. Jewson, 'The disappearance of the sick-man from medical cosmology, 1770–1870' *Sociology* 10 (1976), reprinted by permission of Sage Publications Ltd © BSA Publications Limited, 1974. Mary E. Fissell, *Patients, Power and the Poor in Eighteenth-century Bristol* (Cambridge, Cambridge University Press, 1991), reprinted with permission of the publisher and author. Stephen Jacyna, 'Mr. Scott's case: A view of London medicine in 1825' in Roy Porter (ed.), *The Popularization of Medicine 1650–1850* (London and New York, Routledge, 1992), reprinted with permission. Dora B. Weiner, *The Citizen-Patient in Revolutionary and Imperial Paris*, pp. 177–83. © 1993 Dora B. Weiner. Reprinted with the permission of The Johns Hopkins University Press. *Rules and Regulations of the Huddersfield and Upper Abrigg Infirmary, 1834*, Huddersfield Public Library (Kirklees District Archives and Local studies department) B.362. Reproduced with permission from Huddersfield Public Library. [W. Turnbull], *An Appeal on Behalf of the Intended Hospital at Huddersfield*, (Huddersfield, n.p [c.1825]), Kirklees Central Library, Local History (Tomlinson Collection). Reproduced with permission from Huddersfield Public Library. John Woodward, *To Do the Sick No Harm. A Study of the British Voluntary Hospital System to 1875* (London and New York, Routledge, 1974), reprinted with permission. Christopher Lawrence, 'Democratic, divine and heroic: the history and historiography of surgery', from *Medical Theory, Surgical Practice: Studies in the History of Surgery*, ed. Christopher Lawrence (London, Routledge, 1992), reprinted with permission. Martin S. Pernick, *A Calculus of Suffering. Pain, Professionalism and Anesthesia in Nineteenth-century America* (New York, Columbia University Press, 1985), copyright © Martin S. Pernick. Reprinted with permission from author.

Claude Bernard, *An Introduction to the Study of Experimental Medicine*, trans. H.C. Greene (New York, Dover Publications, 1957 (originally 1865)), reprinted with permission from publisher. Andrew Cunningham, 'Transforming Plague. The Laboratory and the Identity of Infectious Disease', *The Laboratory Revolution in Medicine* (Cambridge, Cambridge University Press, 1992), reprinted with permission of the publisher and author. Richard L. Kremer, 'Building Institutes for Physiology in Prussia, 1836–1846. Contexts, Interests and Rhetoric', *The Laboratory Revolution in Medicine* (Cambridge, Cambridge University Press, 1992), reprinted with permission of the publisher and author. L.S. Jacyna, 'The Laboratory and the Clinic: The Impact of Pathology on Surgical Diagnosis in the Glasgow Western Infirmary, 1875–1910', *Bulletin of the History of Medicine*, 62 (1988) 389–90, 391–4. © The Johns Hopkins University Press. Reprinted with permission of The Johns Hopkins University Press. Michael Worboys, 'Vaccine Therapy and Laboratory Medicine in Edwardian Britain', in John Pickstone (ed.), *Medical Innovations in Historical Perspective* (Basingstoke, Macmillan, 1992), reproduced with permission of Palgrave Macmillan. Ivan Waddington, *The Medical Profession in the Industrial Revolution*, (Dublin, Gill and Macmillan Ltd, 1984), reprinted with permission from the publisher. Irvine Loudon, *Medical Care and the General Practitioner 1750–1850* (Oxford, Clarendon Press, 1986), reprinted with permission from Oxford University Press. Alison Winter, 'Ethereal epidemic: Mesmerism and the Introduction of Inhalation Anaesthesia to early Victorian London' *Social History of Medicine*, vol. 4 (1991), reprinted with permission from Oxford University Press. Anthony Trollope, *Dr Thorne* (London, Wordsworth Classics, 1996 (originally published 1859)), reproduced by kind permission of Wordsworth Editions Ltd. Margaret Forster, *Significant Sisters: The Grassroots of Active Feminism 1839–1939* (London, Penguin, 1984). Copyright © 1984 by Margaret Forster, by kind permission of the author and The Sayle Literary Agency. Robert Dingwall, Anne Marie Rafferty and Charles Webster, *An Introduction to the Social History of Nursing* (London, Routledge, 1988), reprinted with permission from the publisher. Erwin H. Ackerknecht, *A Short History of Medicine*, pp. 210–17. © 1982 Erwin H. Ackerknecht. Reprinted with permission of The Johns Hopkins University Press. Christopher Hamlin, 'Edwin Chadwick, "Mutton medicine", and the Fever Question', *Bulletin of the History of Medicine*, 70 (1996), 237–42, 244–5, 248, 250, 255–6, 260. © The Johns Hopkins University Press. Reprinted with permission of The Johns Hopkins University Press. Gerry Kearns, 'Cholera, nuisances, and Environmental Management in Islington 1830–1855 in W.F. Bynum and Roy Porter (eds), *Living and Dying in London*, London: Wellcome Institute for the History of Medicine, 1991. © The Trustee of the Wellcome Trust, reproduced with permission. David Arnold, *Colonizing the Body. State Medicine and Epidemic Disease in Nineteenth-century India*, (London and Berkeley, University of California Press, 1993). Copyright © 1993 The Regents of the University of California. Reprinted with permission from the publisher and Oxford University Press, India. Maryinez Lyons, 'Sleeping Sickness

Epidemics and Public Health in the Belgian Congo' in David Arnold (ed.), *Imperial Medicine and Indigenous Societies: Disease, Medicine and Empire in the Nineteenth and Twentieth Centuries* (Manchester, Manchester University Press, 1988). Reprinted with the kind permission of the author. Reprinted by permission of the publisher from *The pasteurization of France* by Bruno Latour, translated by Alan Sheridan and John Law (Cambridge, Mass., Harvard University Press), copyright © 1988 by the President and Fellows of Harvard College. John Andrew Mendelsohn, 'Cultures of Bacteriology: Formation and Transformation of a Science in France and Germany, 1870–1914' (Ph.D. dissertation, Princeton University, 1996) vol. I, reprinted with the permission of the author. Maria Sophia Quine, *Population Politics in Twentieth-century Europe* (London, Routledge, 1996). Reprinted with permission from the publisher. Susan Gross Solomon, 'Social Hygiene in Soviet Medical Education', *Journal of the History of Medicine and Allied Sciences*, 45 (1990), reproduced with permission from Oxford University Press. Lutz D. H. Sauerteig, 'Sex education in Germany from the eighteenth to the twentieth centuries', in Franz X. Eder, Lesley A. Hall and Gert Hekma (eds), *Sexual Cultures in Europe: Themes in Sexuality*, Manchester, Manchester University Press, 1999. Reprinted with the kind permission of the author. Jean-François Picard and William H. Schneider, 'The Rockefeller Foundation and the Development of Biomedical Research in Europe', in Giulana Gemelli, Jean-François Picard and William H. Schneider (eds), *Managing Medical Research in Europe: The Role of the Rockefeller Foundation 1920s–1950s* (Bologna, CLUEB, 1999). Reprinted with permission from the publisher. M. Burleigh and W. Wippermann, *The Racial State: Germany, 1933–1945* (Cambridge, Cambridge University Press, 1991), reprinted with permission of the publisher and author. M. Burleigh, *Death and Deliverance: 'Euthanasia' in Germany, c. 1900–1945* (London, Pan Books, 1994). Reprinted with permission from Pan Macmillan and David Godwin Associates. Dorothy Porter, 'Enemies of the Race: Biologism, Environmentalism, and Public Health in Edwardian England' *Victorian Studies* vol. 34, 1991, reprinted with permission from Indiana University Press. F.A.E. Crew et al., 'Social Biology and Population Improvement', reprinted by permission from *Nature* vol. 14 1939 (16 Sept), Macmillan Publishers Ltd. Andrew Scull, *The Most Solitary of Afflictions. Madness and Society in Britain, 1700–1900* (New Haven and London, Yale University Press, 1993). Reprinted with permission from the publisher. J.K. Walton, 'Casting out and bringing back in Victorian England: pauper lunatics 1840–70', in W. F. Bynum, Roy Porter and Michael Shepherd (eds) *The Anatomy of Madness: Essays in the History of Psychiatry, vol. II, Institutions and Society* (London, Tavistock Press, Routledge, 1985), reprinted with permission from publisher. J. Winter, *The Great War and the British People* (London, Macmillan, 1985), reproduced with permission of Palgrave Macmillan. Linda Bryder, 'The First World War: healthy or hungry?', *History Workshop Journal* 24 (1987), reprinted with permission from Oxford University Press. Joanna Bourke (ed.), *'The Misfit Soldier' Edward Casey's War story, 1914–1918* (Cork, Cork University Press, 1999) © Joanna Bourke 1999 by permission of Cork University Press Ltd, Crawford Business Park, Crosses Green, Cork, Ireland. Anne Digby, *The Evolution of British General Practice 1850–1948* (Oxford, Oxford University Press, 1999), reprinted with permission from Oxford University Press. Linda Bryder, *Below the Magic Mountain. A Social History of Tuberculosis in Twentieth-century Britain* (Oxford, Clarendon Press, 1988), reprinted with permission from Oxford University Press. Margery Spring Rice, *Working Class Wives. Their Health and Conditions* (London, Virago Ltd, 1981), reprinted with permission from Time Warner Books UK.

Introduction

The nineteenth and early twentieth centuries have long been identified as a crucial period in the development of medicine. At this time, medicine became recognisably modern. At the beginning of the nineteenth century practitioners finally abandoned a heritage of medical theory dating back to Classical times which saw the body as a holistic entity of fluids and energies, in favour of a reductionist model which placed disease in organs, tissues and finally cells. By 1930 therapeutics were based on the rationale we use today, with drugs to target specific physiological functions, vaccines based on the body's responses to bacteria, and, perhaps most successfully, highly complex surgical interventions to deal with a wide range of conditions. Preventative medicine acquired a new priority. Infectious disease was no longer a temporary problem, requiring action only during severe epidemics. Instead, all sorts of health problems were subjected to constant monitoring and control by a whole new infrastructure of medical officers, laboratories, and isolation procedures. Medical institutions, too, took on a modern cast between 1800 and 1930. Medicine was transformed from a divided occupation into a unified profession, in which practitioners strictly regulated standards of education and behaviour, and rigorously excluded those who did not conform to those standards (although without ever preventing alternative healers from selling their services). Hospitals moved from the margins to the centre of medicine. In 1800 they offered fairly basic care to the sick poor: by 1930 they provided specialised therapy to all social classes and had become centres for the training of new practitioners and in the production of new medical knowledge. Asylums became the accepted place for the care of the mentally ill and laboratories acquired established functions in research, teaching and diagnostics. Perhaps most importantly, the period between 1800 and 1930 saw the expectation – if not the realisation – that medical services should be available to all. The voluntary sector remained an important means of providing health care to those too poor to purchase the services of doctors and nurses, and charities took on a new role in health education. However, by the 1930s, the health of the public became an accepted responsibility of states in Europe and in her colonies, in peacetime and in war. From the nineteenth century central governments all over Europe regularly passed legislation on health matters and set up administrative departments to oversee its implementation. Local government became an important provider of care through clinics and hospitals. The role of the state should not be exaggerated – through insurance schemes and nursing homes, the private sector also played a part in opening up health care to all classes.

This book aims to capture some of the major features of these changes. It has its origins in an Open University course *Medicine and Society in Europe, 1500–1930* (A218). The extracts reproduced here are chosen to accompany the topics explored in the course textbook *Medicine Transformed: Health, Disease and Society in Europe, 1800–1930* (Manchester University Press in association with the Open University, 2004). However, this book is also designed to be used independently, with brief introductions setting each reading in its historical or historiographical content. The secondary sources are reproduced without their original footnotes except when necessary to locate a substantive quotation. A full reference is provided for readers who wish to consult the original source. Notes have been added to gloss some of the more obscure terms and to identify some of the more important figures.

Both *Medicine Transformed* and this volume aim to provide a broad survey of some of the major developments in medicine between 1800 and 1930 and to reflect the current state of scholarship in this area within the history of medicine. The topics covered by these books therefore include well-established areas of historical interest such as the medical profession, hospitals, surgery, public health and welfare. They also reflect those topics of interest where research has flourished only in the last twenty or so years – colonial medicine, asylums, laboratories, war medicine and gender. However, given limitations of space, it is impossible to include every area of interest, and sadly there is little in this work on childhood, old age or unorthodox medicine for example. It has also proved very difficult to present a genuinely European coverage of these topics. Despite the recent interest among historians of medicine in comparative studies of medical experiences in different countries, the subject continues to be dominated by British and American researchers who retain a strong focus on medicine in Britain (which, in practice, often means medicine in England and Wales).

The extracts consist of a mix of primary and secondary materials, and are chosen to help students to understand some of the important themes and issues within the history of medicine in the nineteenth and twentieth centuries. There is no rigid balance between primary and secondary sources – some parts of the book have no contemporary accounts, others give almost equal space to primary and secondary materials. Since the individual extracts were chosen to exemplify a specific teaching point, this book is not, in any sense, a survey of either contemporary or historical writing on the subject. (Such a survey would have undoubtedly contained extracts from founders of the field such as Henry Sigerist and George Rosen, and from Michel Foucault.) The extracts from primary sources encapsulate contemporary thinking about some topic of concern and debate. The secondary sources are selected to give an insight into how historians, past and present, have interpreted historical events. They therefore also give a sense of historiographical developments within the field. A few sources exemplify the approach of the first generation of historians of medicine, many of whom were medical professionals, with accounts focusing on great men and great ideas (see for example the extract on public health by Erwin Ackerknecht). Since then, historians of medicine have reflected a more critical view of medicine. In the 1970s, commentators wondered if medical technology was swamping the patient and doing more harm than good. The AIDS epidemics of the 1980s proved beyond all doubt that medicine was not all-powerful. A new generation of academically-trained historians argued that the history of medicine was not a story of constant progress, from useless or even dangerous treatments to highly effective therapies, and from wholly inadequate provision of medical services to comprehensive 'cradle to grave' care. Rather, medicine was a social phenomenon, in which the production and application of knowledge had been shaped by a multitude of factors, including culture, politics, class and gender.

Most of the extracts reproduced here are taken from work published in the last twenty years, and reflect this new social history of medicine. The sources include selections from articles which have become classics in the field (such as N.D. Jewson's article on how changes in medical theory led to the disappearance of the sick-man or Christopher Hamlin's account of the circumstances shaping Edwin Chadwick's *Sanitary Report*). The bulk of the extracts are from works that were novel at their time of publication, and have since found an established place in the literature. They show how historians of medicine have moved away from examining the work of elite researchers to explore the experiences of ordinary practitioners and their patients (see for example the extracts by Mary Fissell, Stephen Jacyna on 'Mr Scott's case' and Martin Pernick). Historians have also questioned why and how new ideas and practices were adopted (or not) by practitioners. These complex processes are analysed by Bruno Latour and Alison Winter, and the difficulties of implementing health policies are demonstrated in extracts from the work of Gerry Kearns and Anthony Wohl. The reader can also get a sense of how historical knowledge progresses, through debates among historians. (For example, see Linda Bryder's response to J. Winter's analysis of the impact of the First World War on civilian health.) It also gives some examples of the reinterpretation of accepted ideas in the light of detailed local studies or case studies of particular institutions, such as John Walton and David Wright's work on asylum admissions. Some extracts are chosen to illustrate particular genres of writing – for example Margaret Forster's biography of one of the first women doctors.

The extracts also give a flavour of the interdisciplinary character of the history of medicine – the wide range of approaches adopted by historians of medicine being one of the features of the field. They show the use of an anthropological approach – for example in Megan Vaughan's account of the clash between Western and non-Western understandings of madness – and the influence of sociologists (see the extracts from N.D. Jewson and Ivan Waddington on medical knowledge and the medical profession). Historians of medicine have also made use of techniques adopted from demography as in J. Winter's article on the health of wartime populations. The influence of the sociology of knowledge, and ideas about the social construction of medical knowledge, are exemplified by the extract from Andrew Cunningham's account of the identification of the plague bacillus. The extracts also show how history of medicine has reflected developments within the broader field of history. This has helped to generate interest in specific topics, such as colonial medicine and gender, and has also inspired historians of medicine to look at well-researched areas in a new way, such as Anne Digby's research into medical practice as an economic activity.

Medical historians' continuing interest in 'medicine from below' is also reflected in the choice of primary sources. There are very few sources exemplifying 'great leaps forward' in medical knowledge. Only the extracts by Claude Bernard and Emil Kocher on the value of experimental physiology to medicine and, perhaps, Florence Nightingale's prescriptions on hospital design fit into that category. Far more authors chose to include readings on the experience of ordinary people – of patients in hospital (see the extracts from Bella Aronovitch, Martin Goldman and the Rules of Huddersfield Infirmary), of unhealthy environments (described by Henry Mayhew, Charles Dickens, and the editor of *The Times*) and of the medical marketplace (see for example Robert Roberts' account of sales of patent medicine). The primary sources reproduced here also encapsulate some of the concerns of nineteenth-century rank and file practitioners – over the status of their occupation (especially the impact of the entry of women practitioners – seen in the extracts from *The Lancet*), the rise in asylum populations (see the sources written by John Carswell, James Coxe and Ethelinda Hawden) and the need to reform military medical services (described by Edward Wrench).

The first four parts of this book explore some of the most fundamental changes in nineteenth and twentieth century medicine – in theory and practice and in institutions. Part one re-examines N.D. Jewson's description of early nineteenth-century 'hospital medicine' and explores issues of patient/practitioner power: how hospital patients became passive subjects for teaching and research, while private patients, with their financial lever continued to exert control over the medical encounter. Part two surveys the design and function of late nineteenth-century hospitals – how these institutions were reshaped to take account of new sanitary standards (and their success in curing patients) and the relationships between patients, staff and donors. Part three explores the interrelations between new medical theories and professional and technical changes in surgery, re-examining the impact of anaesthesia on surgical practice. The complex and contested functions of late nineteenth-century laboratories are explored through the series of extracts in Part four which look at how laboratories shaped knowledge and practice, and functioned in diagnostics and teaching.

The development of medicine from a fragmented occupation to a unified profession is examined in Parts five and six. Part five explores a range of issues within professionalisation – the relationships between different groups of practitioners, the rise of ethics, the creation of a professional boundary and the methods used to exclude 'unorthodox' practitioners or 'inappropriate' behaviour. Part six re-examines these issues in a different context – the motives for and attempts to exclude women from the medical profession, and the evolution of nursing into a profession.

Parts seven, eight, nine and ten are linked by a common focus on the application of medicine to protect or improve health within populations. Part seven surveys past and present understandings of nineteenth-century public health through extracts ranging from contemporary understandings of the causes of ill-health, to an early historical interpretation of sanitary reform as an unproblematic 'good thing' to modern accounts of the political shaping of public health problems and the difficulties of implementing solutions. Part eight looks at public health in colonial contexts and how Western medicine was applied in occasionally draconian fashion to African problems with little sympathy for native customs or understandings of health problems. Part nine explores the shift from public health practices based around a germ theory to social medicine, in which disease was seen to be rooted in a living conditions. They show how the acceptance of the germ theory and its associated health strategies reflected professional interests, and how aspects of social medicine such as sex education were shaped by wider political ends. Part ten examines the use of eugenics in different contexts, and how a body of ideas about inheritance were turned into a range of policies applied to social problems in various ways in different countries.

Parts eleven and twelve explore historiographical debates in two particular areas of medical history – the growth of asylums in nineteenth-century Britain and the relationship between war and medicine. Part eleven explores the broad range of contemporary and historical interpretations of the growth in the numbers of patients in asylums in the late nineteenth century – public demand, the supply of asylum places, the power of medical profession and claims to be able to successfully treat insanity. Part twelve surveys how authors have seen the relationship between war and medicine, from contemporary accounts of individual heroic struggle to debates over shell-shock – a medical condition apparently peculiar to the battlefield – to the impact of war on civilian health, and medicine from the soldier's perspective. Part thirteen addresses issues around the growth of access to medical services at the end of the nineteenth and in the early twentieth centuries. The extracts here survey the medical services available at this time, from improving health to self-treatment with patent medicines to primary care through general practitioners to hospital care. The extracts also question whether the expansion of services meant equal quality of care for all, and whether patients always used the medical services on offer.

Deborah Brunton

Part one

The rise of hospital medicine

1.1

Hospital and laboratory medicine

N.D. Jewson, 'The Disappearance of the Sick-Man from
Medical Cosmology, 1770–1870', *Sociology* 10 (1976), pp. 228,
235–8 [pp. 225–44].

In the 1970s, Nicholas Jewson, a sociologist, published two highly
influential articles on how medical knowledge mediated the relationship between patient and practitioner. These articles proved
tremendously influential, coinciding with the new thrust to study
'medicine from below', and inspiring historians of medicine to
explore the thinking of patients and practitioners, especially in
the eighteenth century. This extract explores the shift from a
'person-oriented' cosmology – a form of medical thinking centred
on the patient's body, lifestyle and symptoms – to an 'object-
oriented' cosmology, in which disease was seen as dysfunction in
organs or cells.

Hospital Medicine was based upon a new type of relation between the
sick-man and the medical investigator. Interaction between clinicians
and hospital patients was organized around a nexus[1] of formally
defined statuses and strictly prescribed patterns of deference. Henceforth the medical investigator was accorded respect on the basis of the
authority inherent in his occupational role rather than on the basis of
his individually proven worth. The public guarantee of the safety and
efficacy of theories and therapies no longer rested upon the patient's
approval of their contents, but upon the social status of their authors
and advocates. The new occupational standing of the clinician was

---

[1] *nexus*: connections.

Diagram 1: Three Modes of Production of Medical Knowledge

	Patron	Occupational Role of Medical Investigator	Source of Patronage	Perception of Sick-man	Occupational Task of Medical Investigator	Conceptualization of Illness
Bedside medicine	Patient	Practitioner	Private fees	Person	Prognosis and therapy	Total psycho-somatic disturbance
Hospital medicine	State; hospital	Clinician	Professional career structure	Case	Diagnosis and classification	Organic lesion
Laboratory medicine	State; academy	Scientist	Scientific career structure	Cell complex	Analysis and explanation	Biochemical process

Diagram 2: Medical Cosmologies, 1770–1870

	Bedside Medicine	Hospital Medicine	Laboratory Medicine
Subject matter of Nosology	Total symptom complex	Internal organic events	Cellular function
Focus of Pathology	Systemic—dyacrasis	Local lesion	Physico-chemical processes
Research Methods	Speculation and inference	Statistically oriented clinical observation	Laboratory experiment according to scientific method
Diagnostic Technique	Qualitative judgement	Physical examination before and after death	Microscopic examination and chemical tests
Therapy	Heroic and extensive	Sceptical (with the exception of surgery)	Nihilistic
Mind/Body Relation	Integrated: psyche and soma seen as part of same system of pathology	Differentiated: Psychiatry a specialized area of clinical studies	Differentiated: Psychology a separate scientific discipline

matched by the emergence of a new role for the sick-man, that of patient. As such he was designated a passive and uncritical role in the consultative relationship, his main function being to endure and to wait.

These social realignments were reflected within the cosmological system of Hospital Medicine. At the centre of the new medical problematic was the concept of disease. Interest in the unique qualities of the whole person evaporated to be replaced by studies of specific organic lesions and malfunctions. Diseases became a precise and objectively identifiable event occurring within the tissues, of which the patient might be unaware. The fundamental realities of pathological analysis shifted from the total body system to the specialized anatomical structures. The experiential[2] manifestations of disease, which had previously been the very stuff of illness, now were demoted to the role of secondary signs. The patient's interest in prognosis and therapy was eclipsed by the clinician's concern with diagnosis and pathology. The special qualities of the individual case were swallowed up in vast statistical surveys. In short the sick-man was no longer regarded as a singular synthesis of meaningful sensations. Instead the sick in general were perceived as a unitary medium[3] within which diseases were manifested. The consultative relationship took the form of a processing exercise in which the ambiguity and individuality of each case was systematically eliminated by the application of foreknown diagnostic procedures, the function of which was to allocate the patient to a category within the nosological system.[4] It was as a member of that category, i.e. as a suitable case for treatment, that he conducted the remainder of his relationship with his practitioner.

As medical investigators gained power over the conditions of their own recruitment, education and practise they became a much more homogeneous occupational group. A unified system of intellectual conduct could now be enforced throughout the system of production and distribution of medical knowledge by medical investigators themselves. Medical investigators obtained their posts through a system of selection which was under the direct control of senior members of the occupational group. Henceforth, therefore, the distribution of resources and rewards depended less upon the satisfaction of the patient than upon recognition among professional peers. The focal point of a career in medical innovation shifted away from the network of primary relationships with the sick toward a network of secondary relationships with other clinicians. In the era of Bedside Medicine discoveries were best kept as trade secrets to be exploited in the consultative relationship. Hospital Medicine, however, constrained medical investigators to make available their findings rapidly and openly to their occupational peers in the hope of attracting the attention of influential leaders of

---

[2] *experiential manifestations*: the symptoms experienced by the patient.

[3] *unitary medium*: an undivided or undifferentiated mass.

[4] *nosological system*: nosology was the categorisation of diseases according to their characteristic symptoms.

the profession. A battery of medical journals and societies established at the Parisian school in the second and third decades of the 19th century provided the institutional channels of this new type of career system.

[. . .]

A new phase in the emergence of an object orientated cosmology opened with the development of Laboratory Medicine . . . [W]hereas under Hospital Medicine the direction of the power differential between the sick and medical personnel had been reversed[5] under Laboratory Medicine the patient was removed from the medical investigator's field of saliency[6] altogether. This increase in the social distance between the sick and medical investigators was accompanied by a relocation of the fundamental realities of pathology in microscopical events beyond the tangible detection of patients and practitioners alike. . . . [Where] Hospital Medicine had celebrated the interests and perceptions of clinicians, Laboratory Medicine was founded upon the world-view of the scientific research worker. . . .

The introduction of Laboratory Medicine to German society may be illustrated by the example of Prussia. The role of patron was undertaken by a unifying and modernizing state. . . . In the early 19th century the Prussian state centralized the academic selection procedures and played a far greater role in evaluating candidates. . . . [U]niversity personnel likely to attain a continental reputation for their contributions to the advance of knowledge, rather than a local reputation for their pedagogic or therapeutic skills, were adopted as protégés by the Ministry of Education. In this manner a new breed of laboratory based medical investigators was created. Two distinct, and often mutually hostile, career systems emerged: that of research worker and that of medical practitioner. The former monopolized access to the laboratory facilities which rapidly became the essential means of production of the new medicine. Research workers grew into a self conscious and self confident elite, whose distinctive occupational ideology emphasized the value of scientific work for its own sake irrespective of its practical applications. . . .

---

[5] In bedside medicine, patients who had knowledge of their own symptoms and paid directly for practitioners' services held a position of power and were able to negotiate over both the diagnosis and treatment. In hospital medicine, where doctors made the diagnosis using instruments, and patients did not pay for their treatment, they had little say over the form of treatment prescribed.

[6] *saliency*: awareness, concern.

The conceptualization of sickness and health developed by the early 19th century French clinicians had been limited by the exigencies[7] of their occupational task, which restricted their gaze to morbid events occurring within gross anatomical structures. The imagination and curiosity of laboratory scientists were not bound within these restrictions, however. For them the study of illness became part of a much wider investigation into the organization and functions of organic matter. Morbid events were no longer regarded as a discrete area of enquiry but were studied in the context of a general analysis of both normal and abnormal physiological processes. . . .

The realignment of the boundaries of the medical investigator's quest were but one part of a general metamorphosis of work tasks characteristic of the shift from Hospital to Laboratory Medicine. The occupational activity of medical investigators henceforth took the form of the extension of certified knowledge rather than the servicing of clients.[8] The authority of the research worker was a function of his capacity to manipulate abstract symbols and concepts. . . . This development represented a significant gain in the social detachment of the medical investigator from the sick. It enabled him to conceptualize the sick-man as a material thing to be analysed, and disease as a physico-chemical process to be explained according to the blind inexorable laws of natural science. Thus whilst Hospital Medicine had dissolved the integrated vision of the whole man into a network of anatomical structures, Laboratory Medicine, by focusing attention on the fundamental particles of organic matter, went still further in eradicating the person of the patient from medical discourse.

This increase in social distance was accompanied by the erection of strong boundaries between the sick and medical investigators. Indeed the character of social relationships in the era of Laboratory Medicine gave the community of medical investigators the appearance of an insulated intellectual cocoon. Specifications for membership were exacting and exclusive. Significant communication about the causes and cures of illness was confined to the members of the group, legitimate publication outlets being reduced to a closely guarded few. The use of technical jargon and concepts served as a ritual mode of differentiation between the established and the outsiders.

---

[7] *exigencies*: necessities.

[8] Developing medical knowledge rather than providing information which would help in the diagnosis and treatment of patients.

1.2

Surgeons and the medicalisation of the hospital

Mary E. Fissell, *Patients, Power and the Poor in Eighteenth-Century Bristol* (Cambridge, Cambridge University Press, 1991), pp. 136–7, 140, 144, 146–7.

Mary Fissell's work has focused on 'medicine from below', exploring the work of ordinary practitioners, and the knowledge of lay men and women. This book is based on the premise that prior to the eighteenth century medical practice was shaped by patients as well as by practitioners. It is a study of the movement away from traditional, vernacular medicine as understood by all, to a medicalised system of diagnosis and treatment that devalued lay alternatives and thus disempowered the poor from an understanding of health and illness through a case study of Bristol. Fissell shows how this was accomplished within the creation of charitable institutions in the eighteenth century, where the patient was gradually denied a voice.

The Infirmary's new role in education had an unintended consequence: surgeons came to have a vested interest in the hospital. Neither the physicians nor the surgeons were paid for their Infirmary work; as aspirant members of the gentler classes, they donated their labor to the charity, in return for the gratitude of their patients and the attention – perhaps patronage – of the subscribers. The apothecary, on the other hand, was a salaried staff member, only a grade above the matron. The development of surgical education created a sort of hybrid role for the surgeon; technically unpaid, he in fact had a very strong interest in the Infirmary because it indirectly provided an important source of revenue in the form of pupils and lecture fees. Initially, pupils were assigned to all the surgeons, and the four guineas a year per surgeon was not princely. But it seems that this system rapidly fell apart, and individual surgeons began to sell their wares in the open educational market. Some surgeons, like Richard Smith, had at least two or three pupils per year, while others contented themselves with the occasional student. The profit to be made from pupils was not inconsiderable; over the period from 1744 to 1757, the surgeon James Ford earned over £700 from private pupils, not including lecture fees.

Professionally, then, the hospital became increasingly central to these surgeons' practices. For the Infirmary, this shift meant that, first, surgeons tried to gain control of the hospital, and, second, that they shaped the institution to serve their needs as surgeons and instructors. Conflicts between hospital subscribers and the surgeons in the latter part of the century serve as markers of this struggle for control.

Admissions constituted a perennial source of discontent. In theory, the subscribers controlled this process through their recommendations. But in practice, surgeons played a large role in deciding who would enter the Infirmary by the latter half of the eighteenth century. In theory, the non-casualty patient was admitted by the physician if a medical case, the surgeon if surgical, and the surgeons' admissions notes were countersigned by a physician. In practice, however, surgeons commandeered the admissions process. Richard Smith who as a surgeon does not offer an unbiased perspective, wrote 'The Physicians never from the first exercised any control or choice over the objects to be admitted but acted, in Signing the Notes under the direction of the Surgeons.' Long before Smith became an Infirmary surgeon in the 1790s, the house surgeons had been circumventing the physicians by admitting increased numbers of casualties. . . . These patients did not require a recommendation; they were admitted on the spot, usually by the surgeons. Virtually all of these patients were surgical.

Moving beyond casualty patients, the increase in the proportions of surgical to medical patients is suggestive of the surgeons' interests in maintaining an appropriate pool of teaching material. In the 1770s, only 28 percent of all inpatient admissions were surgical; this rose to 44 percent by the end of the century. Basically, surgeons packed the Infirmary with patients most likely to provide useful instruction for their pupils.

[. . .]

It was not just access to the bodies of living patients that surgeons longed to acquire. Cadavers became a very important teaching resource, and questions about the acquisition of such teaching material became a potent source of discord. When Godfrey Lowe gave his surgical lectures in the 1760s, he used bodies shipped down from London. But he was probably the last to do so. Regular body snatching was already a feature of an Infirmary education; anatomical training was a hallmark of the institution, and the dissections of patients' bodies commonplace. As Henry Alford, Infirmary pupil wrote:

> There were frequent operations at the Infirmary of almost every kind. As many acute and fatal cases were admitted, and there was an autopsy

7

in nearly every case of death, there were ample opportunities of getting a practical knowledge of the viscera, and also admitting of superficial dissections of many parts without any apparent injury or disfigurement of the body.[9]

In other words, both dissection and operative surgery were central to educational experience.

Surgeons emphasized anatomy, and anatomical training, because it was the subject that demarcated physic and surgery. Certainly physicians studied anatomy as well, but their focus was on what eighteenth-century doctors would have labeled the fluid constituents of the body, the humours and their precarious balance. Physicians regulated the body like a delicate and idiosyncratic machine, using evacuations to diagnose and rebalance the body. Surgeons cut. They needed both speed and accuracy for the few routinely performed operations – cutting for stone, reducing ruptures, doing amputations – if the patient were to survive blood loss, pain, and shock. As a contemporary description had it:

> The young surgeon must be an accurate Anatomist, not only a speculative but practical Anatomist; without which he must turn out a mere Bungler. It is not sufficient for him to attend Anatomical Lectures, and see two or three Subjects cursorily dissected; but he must put his hand to it himself, and be able to dissect every Part with the Same Accuracy that the Professor performs.[10]

Dissection meant the acquisition of anatomical knowledge, but it also provided lessons in manual dexterity and operative technique. As a London surgeon conflated dissection and surgery in the phrase, 'I was performing operations on a dead subject,' so too, the practice of anatomical dissection offered practitioners skills and techniques, as well as knowledge. This detailed anatomical experience came to define the surgeon.

For Bristol surgeons, this training seems to have meant a great deal of dissection, although evidence about such practices is difficult to evaluate. Richard Smith frequently alluded to dissections in his memoirs. He is a problematic witness, however, for he created and nourished much of the anatomical subculture in Bristol. His father had started an anatomical museum, furnished with the oddities of many years' worth of anatomical explorations, and Smith continued and expanded on his father's hobby. In his memoirs, Smith presented many body-snatching exploits with glee, eager to show how doctors triumphed over ignorance and superstition in their quest for knowledge. Although Smith may have

---

[9] Henry Alford, 'The Bristol Infirmary in my Student Days', *Bristol Medico-chirurgical Journal* 8 (1890), p. 167.

[10] R. Campbell, *The London Tradesman* (London, T. Gardner, 1747), p. 50.

overemphasized anatomy, other sources, such as newspapers and Infirmary records, show that dissection was often practiced and discussed. Indeed, Henry Alford recalled many years later that he had done far more dissection at the Infirmary than in his subsequent London training.

As far back as 1728, when an unfortunate shoemaker hanged himself and the body was buried at a crossroads, it did not rest for long before it was unearthed and dissected by surgeons. In this case, obviously, Infirmary surgeons were not the culprits, because the hospital did not yet exist. However, once the Infirmary was established, and in particular once it took on a teaching function, it was repeatedly linked with body snatching and dissection.

In 1761 the son of a collier had been brought to the Infirmary, a casualty with a head injury, who did not long survive. The boy's father stormed up to the home of the hospital surgeon, John Castelman, in the middle of the night. He had opened the coffin containing his son's body, and found the head was missing. The collier threatened to 'pull the Furmary down about thy ears!' if Castelman did not return the son's head immediately. Kingswood colliers were a notoriously riotous lot, and Castelman hurried to the hospital, returning with the head in a sack.

According to Richard Smith, such events were not rare. As a student, he had frequently stolen bodies or parts of bodies for anatomy lessons given by F.C. Bowles:

> use makes mastery, and we had reduced this to so regular a system that we practiced it two years without suspicion – we procured a key to the dead house and provided ourselves with screws – hammers – wrenching iron – nails, and everything likely to be wanted ... whilst the family were at dinner we stole into the Dead House – removed the Extremities, Head, or anything else we wanted, even the whole corps, and then made all fast, and in the same order as before.[11]

Because Bowles was not yet on the Infirmary staff, pupils smuggled him into the deadhouse, 'a mere coal-hole lit by a foot-square iron grating' where they 'spent hours in the ardent pursuit of anatomical knowledge.'

In 1806 ... the hospital treasurer received an anonymous letter saying:

> there is scarcely an unfortunate fellow creature who has died in the Infirmary for a considerable time past, whose remains have not been most Shockingly Mutilated by a Mr. Lawrence, Pupil to the Surgeons. Head, Arms, Legs in short all parts have been taken away from the Dead by him. Some of the nurses through bribery leaving the coffin unclosed.

[11] Bristol Biographical Memoirs, vol. 5, pp. 353–4, MS, Bristol Record Office.

This letter went on to detail how Lawrence had also stolen a body from the Infirmary burial ground and brought it to Richard Smith's coach house, where Smith had lectured and dissected.

[. . .]

Henry Alford, an Infirmary pupil in the 1820s, alleged that almost every patient who died in the hospital was anatomized. Even allowing for exaggeration, it seems that patients had become subjects for anatomic inquiry, what William Hunter called 'the passive submission of dead bodies.'

Hospital-based training not only reshaped surgical education; it created a new type of surgeon. . . . No longer men of the marketplace, the new surgeons saw themselves as professionals. On a practical level, these men also experienced rather different career paths than had their apprentice-trained forbears. The hospital was central to both self-image and working lives.

Young men trained in the hospital seem to have entered a rather crowded and competitive field. Very few of them would be able to emulate their teachers and take up lucrative city practices and affiliations with charitable institutions. These men, however, found their niches in other institutions: the army, navy, and militia, the Poor Law, the merchant marine.

[. . .]

It was not just the career structures that altered in relation to the hospital; surgeons' images of themselves changed as well. . . . [t]he rituals that made a surgeon were centered on the operating theater and the dissecting room, on a culture of anatomy and body snatching, rather than on visits to patients' homes and minding the shop. Their roles in the Infirmary helped to confirm their new status, both by emphasizing their charitable functions and by the authority conferred upon them by the city.

[. . .]

Thus, by the turn of the century, the hospital had become a medical workplace, run by and for the surgeons who had themselves undergone a transformation. Disputes continued well into the nineteenth century, suggesting that alignments of power within the Infirmary were by no means tidily or permanently arranged. Rather, I want to emphasize the transition from a charity, founded and run by philanthropically-minded laymen, to a medical institution that defined patients by their diagnosed diseases rather than their moral worthiness as objects of charity. This

10

transformation was achieved through the coincidence of two factors: the changing professional interests of the surgeons and the abdication of the governors.

1.3
The inpatient

Dora B. Weiner, *The Citizen-Patient in Revolutionary and Imperial Paris* (Baltimore and London, Johns Hopkins University Press, 1993), pp. 177–83.

The post-revolutionary Paris hospitals have long been seen as crucial in the development of the hospital as a centre for teaching medicine and surgery and research into pathological anatomy. Weiner's book surveys the politics of health in Revolutionary and Napoleonic Paris; she has a more positive approach than many late-twentieth-century historians who see physicians as abusing or at least misusing their power over patients in the new hospital. Weiner shows many practitioners to have been humane and concerned. She describes the creation of the citizen-patient in revolutionary Paris: in return for free health care, patients had a public duty to participate in research and teaching.

In the first eighteen months of the Hospital Council's existence, the admitting office at the Hôtel-Dieu hospitalized 21,888 women, men, and children, while an additional 16,143 persons gained direct entrance to Paris hospitals, pleading urgency. During the Consulate[12] and Empire,[13] the average total number of annual hospitalizations in Paris reached 32,500, of whom the admitting office processed two-thirds. The new inpatients and the administrators soon learned that physicians and surgeons now applied medical criteria, not only at the entrance door, but at every phase of the patients' hospital experience.

[. . .]

---

[12] In 1799 Napoleon became First Consul (and de facto ruler of the First Republic) to safeguard the moderate revolutionary state.

[13] Napoleon's republic became the First Empire in 1804 when he appointed himself Emperor. The First Empire ended with the abdication of Napoleon in 1814 and the return of the monarchy in 1815.

Under the new regulations, inpatients entering the hospital faced probing examination by the head physician or surgeon-in-chief, who 'alone confirmed their admission and assigned them to a ward.' If denied hospitalization, patients were sent away before morning rounds—that is, before 7 A.M. In practice, mercy often tempered these Draconian regulations. 'In case of doubt,' states the report of the Year XII, 'charity dictates that the patient be admitted.' Or, with regard to inmates of the Incurable Women's Hospital: 'The council felt it would be inhumane to reverse previous decisions or to demand the expulsion of persons admitted on flimsy evidence.'

The admitting interview was particularly thorough for assignment to teaching wards because the young doctor knew that he might have to present the new patient to his chief and colleagues: he needed plentiful information. The only official teaching services were located at the Hôtel-Dieu and the Charité; a third at the Hospice de perfectionement never opened for want of an appropriate locale. Therefore 'France never had a university clinic.' But unofficial or 'free' clinical teaching proliferated, at the Salpêtrière, St. Louis, Maternité, and Children's hospitals.

Bedside teaching made the inpatient the center of attention. Herman Boerhaave, the admired originator of modern clinical teaching, assigned twelve patients to such a service, Corvisart[14] forty, and Pinel[15] thirty. Students came daily to observe, to learn exactly what changes to look for, to watch and to listen as the professor used the patient to demonstrate the signs and symptoms and explain the natural history of each disease. Pinel suggested that some wards group only patients with the same illness so students could observe the gradations and complications of a single disease. How demoralizing it must have been for patients to learn from their neighbors how their illness might worsen and even prove fatal! But such considerations do not seem to have occurred to the Revolutionary doctors.

Leading clinicians all over Europe made special arrangements for the care of patients in teaching wards, assigning one or two advanced students to look after each patient and report to the professor on rounds. For clinical learning, there was no organization more important than the innovative and exclusive Society for Medical Instruction

---

[14] Jean Nicholas Corvisart (1755–1821) was one of the many distinguished teachers and researchers working in post-revolutionary Paris. Corvisart published on the diseases of the heart, correlating post-mortem findings with the sounds he could hear simply by pressing his ear to the patient's chest. This technique, called immediate auscultation, gave way to mediate auscultation using a stethoscope to clarify and amplify sounds.

[15] Philippe Pinel (1745–1826), a physician famous for his works on clinical medicine and for pioneering the humane treatment of the insane.

founded at the Charité on 29 May 1801 by Corvisart. Meant for fourth-year students and their elders, and directed by J.J. Leroux des Tillets (1749–1832) and Gaspard Laurent Bayle (1774–1816), the society provided rigorously structured clinical experience, heralding later nineteenth-century developments. Here the inpatient underwent the strictest admitting interview and continuing close scrutiny. For each patient, the young doctor in charge had to present the supervising professor with a brief, standardized admission record; initial observations (which the mentor would review and, if necessary, revise); daily records on a chart; and, lastly, a summary of the illness and autopsy. By 1818, over five thousand cases had been recorded. Nothing comparable had ever been attempted before. The admission of patients and their assignment to specific wards, long under the authority of a young assistant, developed into the position of chief of service. When autopsies became routine, the full-time positions of prosector and prosector's aide were added to the ranks. Among the earliest members of the Society for Medical Instruction were two outstanding clinical investigators of the early nineteenth century, François Magendie (1783–1855) and René Théophile Hyacinthe Laënnec.

It is thus clear that inpatients paid a price for the good medical care they now received and their new creature comforts. The intern in charge might come several times a day and explain to a group of students the signs and symptoms of a disease they were seeing for the first time: malaria, jaundice, scurvy; ulcers; a fracture or a malformation that required surgery; the manifestations of syphilis or sclerema neonatorum,[16] of depression, delusions, or hysteria. Then the physician-in-chief would come on 'grand' rounds and demonstrate the 'case,' expose the patient's body to general view, palpate, percuss, and auscultate;[17] point, demonstrate, and discuss. He might be gentle and sympathetic, or he might ignore the frightened, shivering person. These doctors used patients not only to teach their students, but for research as well. Even though the numerical method had been practiced for some years abroad (in Edinburgh and London, for instance), medical statistics could not have emerged without the hundreds of citizen-patients aligned on Parisian teaching wards. Sheer numbers amounted to a qualitative difference.

[16] *sclerema neonatorum*: a severe, sometimes fatal disease of the fatty tissues which occurs mainly in premature or debilitated infants.

[17] *palpate, percuss, auscultate*: Palpation, percussion and auscultation were among the first techniques of physical examination. Palpation involved feeling the body for any signs of internal disease. In percussion, the patient was shaken while the practitioner listened for sounds of accumulated fluid within the body. Auscultation involved listening for sounds, usually from the heart or lungs, either by pressing an ear to the patient's skin, or via a stethoscope.

Did these doctors experiment on their patients? Undoubtedly, as they always do, with regard to medication and diet, trying new drugs and dosages, varied foods or therapeutic strategies. The postgraduate hospital had the traditional mission of checking on new procedures and medications. Did doctors conduct dangerous experiments? That question is not easy to answer. . . .

A smallpox epidemic in the Year VI prompted the Paris Health School to conduct a public 'inoculation clinic'—that is, teach a public course, demonstrate the technique, and make inoculation[18] available to the working class. Medical students supervised the inoculated children and kept careful journals. . . .

The two doctors, Leroux and Pinel, used public wards from the St. Antoine orphanage and the Salpêtrière—young citizen-patients—for their experiment. And they reported their every move to the assembly of the medical school professors and proceeded only with the minister's permission. . . .

At the end of their report, the authors mention further experiments they wished to try, among them 'the inoculation of vaccine.' This was September 1799: the news of Edward Jenner's discovery had just reached Paris. The medical school launched experiments as soon as vaccine arrived from London. . . .

A 'ringworm clinic' with six beds was set up at the postgraduate hospital . . . and another at St. Louis in 1809–1813. There, 795 children were treated with Mahon's depilatory cream, which cured 527, while 196 had relapses. In the Year VII an experiment involving forty patients was tried at Cullerier's Venereal Diseases Hospital: ten patients were inoculated with syphilis, ten with 'sporic disease,' and twenty used as controls. And experimental therapy for mental patients was carried on at Charenton Hospice.

In all these cases, the decision to subject these citizen-patients to new or risky procedures for the advancement of knowledge and for the benefit of society was taken on their behalf by medical men convinced that the action was justified. They took it for granted that inpatients should serve to train young doctors. Trials of new medications and therapies occurred frequently and they involved risks. We have no evidence that physicians, around 1800, felt it necessary to ask for a citizen-patient's informed consent.

---

[18] Inoculation involved deliberately infecting children with smallpox, using material from a patient suffering from the disease, in order to provide future immunity. In vaccination, children were infected with cowpox – a much less dangerous disease – which also conferred immunity to smallpox.

The citizen hospitalized at public expense thus performed a hitherto rare public service. We have no documentation about the patients' feelings with regard to their new role: it would be as risky to conjecture resentment as it is to posit pride in a new usefulness. It was undoubtedly frightening to see doctors and students crowd around the bed and proceed to repeated and detailed examinations, and to be carried into an amphitheater for surgery, knowing that, whether one died on the operating table or in bed, one's body would be subject to autopsy. Without doubt the new 'hospital medicine' permanently altered the citizen-patient's role, and what had been exceptional gradually became the rule.

From the doctor's point of view, the patient also took on a different 'look,' as Michel Foucault has so brilliantly argued in *The Birth of the Clinic*. With his 'gardener's look,' the physician viewed individual patients as specimens that represented stages or aspects of one disease; then, with his 'chemist's look,' he analyzed and experimented *on* a 'case,' rather than *with* a sick person. After the patient died, there remained an instructive body.

'Paris had been the capital of the cadaver ever since the mid eighteenth century,' writes Pierre Huard.[19] Cadavers were needed at the Practical Dissection School, across the street from the new Health School: this establishment's enrollment rose from twenty-four students when it was founded in 1750, to 120 students in 1799, working in six new dissection pavilions. At the Hôtel-Dieu, the students' attention had, since Pierre Joseph Desault's day, been directed to postmortem examination, and at the Charité clinical school, after 1800, Corvisart autopsied every dead patient. Xavier Bichat performed this procedure on six hundred patients in twenty-one months: the results of his investigations form the basis of his five books; G.L. Bayle's research on pulmonary phthisis[20] was based on nine hundred cases; and Laënnec undertook twenty-two autopsies in September–October 1822 alone. By assembling a great many pathologic data, doctors gradually came to understand how a disease attacked the bodies of women, men, children, and babies and gained new ways of interpreting the signs and symptoms of living patients in the clinical setting.

[. . .]

The quest for legal 'subjects' has a long history. In 1760, the government empowered the Practical Dissection School to buy two bodies every ten

---

[19] Pierre Huard, a prolific French historian, has published on many aspects of medical history.

[20] *phthisis*: tuberculosis of the lungs.

days, for twenty-seven livres the pair. In 1768, the king ordered the Salpêtrière, which was under his jurisdiction, to provide a few cadavers to the Dissection School. But the Hôtel-Dieu, the main potential source of 'subjects,' steadfastly refused—a stance to be expected from nuns. To a believer, dissection and dispersal of a person's limbs created confusion on Resurrection Day. The nuns deemed dissection an outrage.

Under the Republic, the government did prevail and regulate the supply of cadavers. 'The Great Hospice of Humanity [Hôtel-Dieu] and the Hospice of Unity [Charité] are specially designated to supply [the medical school] and the other public establishments,' proclaimed a decree of 19 November 1798 (29 Brumaire, Year VII) drawn up by Dean Thouret. 'The school shall have first choice in all the other hospices, to obtain all the varieties of age, sex, constitution needed for the progress of its research'. Dean Leroux reported in 1813 that '1,320 cadavers were brought to the anatomy pavilions in the seven months when dissections were scheduled. They served the faculty's needs, in lectures, examinations, study sessions, and preparations. They were used in teaching 654 students how to dissect, and 96 students how to operate. If there had not been a shortage of subjects, a much larger number of students could have practiced anatomy and surgery.'

[. . .]

If we examine the registers of the Hôtel-Dieu in the years 1801–1815, we find over five thousand deaths a year. The regulations required that the bodies claimed by relatives be handed to them for burial. Prudence demanded quick disposal of the victims of contagious diseases. But there can be no doubt that thousands of cadavers dissected in the amphitheaters came from the Hôtel-Dieu. These were the bodies of citizen-patients who had served as object lessons when alive. They now served as objects when dead.

The inpatients' new role thus affected their hospital stay at every turn long before they paid the final price. They also helped impart new directions to medicine because their triage[21] into groups created new perceptions for the attending physicians.

---

[21] *triage*: the method of prioritising the care of injured soldiers in the battlefield (from the French verb 'trier' to sort). From the Napoleonic Wars, casualties were sorted by the severity of their wounds and their likelihood of survival. Here Weiner uses it to mean that patients were sorted according to their condition.

1.4

Mr Scott's case

Stephen Jacyna, 'Mr Scott's Case: A View of London Medicine
in 1825', in Roy Porter (ed.), *The Popularization of Medicine
1650–1850* (London and New York, Routledge, 1992),
pp. 254–65 [pp. 252–86].

Stephen Jacyna has researched into many aspects of the nineteenth-
century medical profession in Scotland and England. This article is
based on a collection of early nineteenth-century documents, held
in Glasgow University Library, concerning the case of James Scott,
an Edinburgh accountant, who travelled to the capital in 1825 to
seek further advice on the loss of strength he was experiencing in
his legs and back. The documents include accounts of consultations
between Scott and a number of London practitioners, and letters
from these doctors. They provide a rare insight into the clinical
encounter at this time.

It is unusual to have both the patient's and the practitioner's accounts of
a case in parallel; and much of the historiographic interest of Mr Scott's
case lies in the possibility it affords of comparing the two perspectives
on the same clinical event. A study of these documents permits an eval-
uation of many of our current presumptions about the nature of the
patient–doctor relationship in the early nineteenth century. It also
affords evidence of the forms of medical knowledge that mediated this
relationship. The date of these documents makes them especially valuable: 1825 can be considered either as standing at the . . . end of the
'long' eighteenth century or as at the outset of a new era in the history of
clinical medicine. Scrutiny of these documents confirms that there is
merit in both these views; Scott's case provides evidence both for the
survival of what is usually considered a typically eighteenth-century
absence of clear boundaries between lay and professional understandings of medicine and indications of the emergence of a more specialized
and segregated distribution of medical knowledge.

In an influential article N.D. Jewson has argued that a patronage model
is appropriate to an understanding of eighteenth-century clinical inter-
actions: 'By virtue of their economic and political predominance the
gentry and aristocracy held ultimate control over the consultative

17

relationship and the course of medical innovation'.[22] The physician was thus reduced to the role of a client whose professional success depended on his ability to satisfy the demands that the patient brought to the clinical encounter.

Patients were able to exert such control because they enjoyed epistemological parity with the practitioner. Medical knowledge did not constitute a discrete esoteric domain accessible only to the professional; it formed part of the common culture of gentlemen. In consequence it was possible for the polite patient to evaluate and criticize the diagnoses and prescriptions of his, or even her, medical adviser.

Although an accountant, James Scott was undoubtedly a gentleman; indeed, his lifestyle, as related in the documents describing his illness, approximates more closely to that of a country squire than to that of an urban professional. His clinical experiences should therefore supply some insights into how far the patron–client model of the élite patient–doctor relationship remained effective in the 1820s. . . .

. . . Scott's own account of his London experiences makes it clear that he approached each consultation with certain expectations and judged the practitioner by how far he attained these standards. In short, 'It was the patient who judged the competence of the physician and the suitability of the therapy'. Above all, Scott expected his medical adviser to be assiduous – to show in an obvious manner that he had applied his mind to the problems posed by the case. This application was manifested, in the first instance, by a careful scrutiny of the precirculated case history; this was to be supplemented by putting numerous searching questions to the patient. . . .

The practitioner's skill in interrogating the patient was a matter of special moment in shaping Scott's opinion of his accomplishment. Anthony Carlisle achieved particular approval by adding new details to Scott's clinical history that his other attendants had failed to elicit. 'One of his questions,' Scott remarked, 'brought out a circumstance that it had never occurred to me to mention, that while a boy I had frequently fainting fits, and that these were sometimes caused by swallowing anything very hot, or running myself out of breath. . . .' 'From the questions put and the earnestness of manner with which they were accompanied, I should,' Scott declared, 'conclude Sir A to be an extremely intelligent Physician.'

Scott's approval of [William] Maton and Carlisle's clinical method can in part be ascribed to the fact that they endorsed and reinforced deeply

---

[22] N.D. Jewson, 'Medical Knowledge and the Patronage System in Eighteenth Century England', *Sociology* 8 (1974) 382–3.

rooted perceptions of the causes of illness shared by patient and practitioner alike. Both practitioners took for granted that a long-term view of the patient's life history was necessary to an understanding of his present condition: indeed, Maton assumed that the health history of Scott's ancestors also had to be taken into account in making a diagnosis. Such concern with the 'deep' history of an individual is, as [Mary] Fissell has noted, typical of patients' narratives of illness in the eighteenth century.

The patient's narrative – the account he gave of his symptoms, biography, and family history – therefore remained central to the clinical encounter. . . .

However, Scott required more from his advisers than attention to his subjective experience of disease; he also expected them to subject him to a physical examination. According to Jewson, one consequence of the concentration upon subjective symptoms under bedside medicine was a neglect of physical signs. . . . The growing importance of physical examination in the nineteenth century was one aspect of the shift away from a 'subject' to an 'object' oriented medical cosmology: enquiry into the patient's subjective experiences mattered less in diagnosis than the identification of the objective causes of disease. . . .

Mr Scott's case provides a different perspective on the significance of physical examination in the patient–practitioner relationship. It is seen to coexist quite amicably with a continued preoccupation with the patient's narrative. Moreover, far from being resistant to medical intrusion upon his body or finding such investigation demeaning, Scott demanded such an examination from his advisers. When a practitioner failed to provide a physical examination, the patient regarded the doctor as remiss: thus Scott remarked with clear disappointment that William Lawrence 'did not put many questions, and did not examine my spine'. . . .

. . . A readiness to undertake a hands-on investigation of Scott's ailment was thus one criterion by which the practitioner's assiduity was judged. While the norms of polite behaviour were on the whole strictly observed, the clinical consultation was already emerging as a site where conventional restrictions on physical contact might with all propriety be systematically violated.

As well as evidence of technical competence and genuine application, Scott sought some token of a practitioner's personal concern with and involvement in his predicament. Thus he notes on several occasions that the doctor asked to be kept informed of the future progress of the case. . . .

A picture of the ideal physician begins to emerge: he is conscientious, skilful, courteous, and concerned. Most of the practitioners Scott saw in

London attempted to conform to this ideal; Maton and Carlisle perhaps came closest to satisfying their patient's expectations. William Lawrence was less successful. Scott's first consultation with him on 29 September seems to have been perfunctory and unsatisfactory. Lawrence managed, however, to emerge with more credit from a second meeting on 9 October. He showed his genuine application to the matter by insisting that he had 'again and again considered my case and that it was an extremely anomalous one'. He also showed his concern for the patient by asking to hear from Scott's Edinburgh advisers upon his return.

But there is a much more egregious exception to the conventional pattern of behaviour expected of the medical practitioner; the treatment Scott received from John Abernethy was *sui generis*.[23] Scott was accompanied on his visit to Abernethy by Goldsworthy Gurney, a surgeon whom he had previously consulted. Gurney,

> having made some observations in regard to the peculiarity of my way of walking, Dr [sic] Abernethy stopped him with a 'D-n you sir have I not read the statement, and read it with attention. I have not time to hear you speak, but wish to tell this gentleman what I think of his case.'
>
> Then addressing me he delivered a lecture of twenty minutes on disease in general, on his own case in particular as affected with rheumatism, and on some other cases which had come under his observation, but without any particular reference to the peculiarities of mine.

Leaving aside the gratuitous rudeness to a colleague in the presence of a patient, Abernethy's performance apparently violated the standards of behaviour Scott expected and on the whole received from his advisers. Abernethy had, it is true, read the case history 'with attention'; but he neglected to complement this with a careful interrogation of the patient. Instead of dealing with Scott's case in particular, he chose to deliver a monologue on disease in general; instead of making Scott the centre of attention, he presumed to speak about his own condition and about that of other patients; instead of stressing the individuality of Scott's condition, he sought to subsume it in a wider scheme

[. . .]

From other sources we know that Scott's treatment at the hands of Abernethy was by no means untypical. Indeed, he probably escaped relatively lightly: Abernethy seemed to have confined his customary rudeness during these consultations to the unfortunate Gurney; he was, however, quite capable of being offensive even to aristocratic patients.

---

[23] *sui generis*: of its type, unique.

Abernethy therefore seemingly violated the basic premises of the doctor–patient relationship – yet he prospered. Although some patients did flee his consulting-room in terror . . . Abernethy remained a fashionable practitioner; indeed . . . he 'had an amount of practice to which neither he nor any other man could do full justice.' This paradox can, in part, be explained in terms of the contrast Abernethy offered to the more conventional practitioner; in a normally sycophantic[24] society a reputation for bluntness could work in a practitioner's favour. This was the view taken by an obituarist who maintained that Abernethy's 'roughness of manner' was cultivated 'from inclination – habit – or perhaps DESIGN'.

[. . .]

There are, however, hints in Scott's account that Abernethy's departure from the conventions of patient–practitioner interaction was not as complete as might at first sight appear. . . . One is tempted to conclude that Abernethy played something of the role of a licensed jester in the court of élite medicine: he tacitly upheld the structures that he overtly subverted. Apparent lapses from the norms of accepted behaviour, such as Abernethy's digressions about his marvellous memory for past cases, might, for example, be viewed not as mere conceit but as an attempt to demonstrate his abiding long-term interest in his patients.

Mr Scott's case thus shows that the kind of power relations between patient and doctor that Jewson and others have seen as characteristic of eighteenth-century 'bedside' medicine were still evident in the 1820s. Just as a patron who commissioned a portrait would expect the painter to conform to certain conventions, so Scott required his medical advisers to observe certain patterns of behaviour. The medical men, for their part, by and large accepted this framework and sought to comply with their patron's demands. There is, however, an apparent difference in what was demanded by the patient: by the 1820s physical examination, far from being *infra dig.*, was *de rigueur*.[25]

The transition from a reliance on the patient's narrative in diagnosis to a preference for what can be derived by physical examination is usually considered as marking a fundamental shift in the epistemological basis of the clinical encounter. The initiative had passed from patient to doctor; the latter, moreover, now based his assessment of the case upon arcane knowledge accessible only to him using his special professional

[24] *sycophantic*: flattering.

[25] i.e. physical examination went from being inappropriate to being a required element of the diagnostic process.

skills. Obviously, on this reading, a major shift in power from layman to professional had also occurred. Scott's lay understanding of medicine, however, encompassed and endorsed physical diagnosis; and one way in which he manifested his continued strength in the clinical encounter was by requiring that his advisers employ these techniques.

There is evidence also that, early nineteenth-century developments in medical concepts and technique notwithstanding, the epistemological parity between doctor and patient remained intact. Scott felt competent to discuss his case on a basis of equality with his advisers, and they acquiesced. Thus the practitioners he saw accepted the need to explain and justify, rather than merely state and dictate, their diagnoses and treatments; Scott for his part felt free to question them and to make his own suggestions.

[. . .]

The fact that Abernethy advised Scott, as he did many of his private patients, to 'read his book' also indicates the extent to which medical knowledge remained the common property of all educated persons. The book in question – *Surgical Observations on the Constitutional Origins and Treatment of Local Diseases* – was not a 'popular' guide to medicine comparable to Buchan's *Domestic Medicine*.[26] It was a work written for the profession, but which also had a considerable lay readership. Its circulation among the educated classes 'served to give the *public* some notion of those principles which [Abernethy] was so beautifully unfolding to the younger portions of the profession in his lectures'. The 'public' in question was presumably the polite educated class of person who might consider consulting a practitioner like Abernethy in times of illness. Popularizing medical ideas could serve as a method of self-advertisement. . . .

This view of an equality between lay and professional knowledge needs, however, to be qualified. Even for the eighteenth century it is easy to exaggerate the degree to which doctors and patients shared a common discourse. William Cullen cast doubt on the extent to which even

> the acutest genius or the soundest judgment will avail in judging of a particular science in regard to which they have not been exercised. I have been obliged to please my patients with reasons, and I have found that any will pass even with able divines and acute lawyers; the same will pass with the husbands as with the wives. No person is qualified to judge of the

26 William Buchan's *Domestic Medicine* was one of the earliest and most popular handbooks of medical advice for laymen. First published in 1769, it was still being published in the middle of the nineteenth century.

soundness of a theory, unless he has been much exercised in reasoning upon the same subject.[27]

In other words, while educated laypeople might be able to comprehend medical doctrines, they were incapable of discriminating between them or of appreciating their application in a particular case. In order to gratify a patient's vanity or curiosity, the practitioner might discuss matters of medical theory with him; but this did not imply a concession of intellectual parity. There remained a 'higher' level of discourse in which only medical men could participate.

[. . .]

The operation of the two-tier system of discourse at which Cullen hinted is apparent in Mr Scott's case. Although Carlisle had discussed matters of diagnosis and therapy at length with Scott, he proposed to send a written opinion to his Edinburgh physician because 'he feels it necessary to explain himself technically . . . in place of putting into my hands a formal written opinion'. This implied that there were limits to what could be communicated about a case directly to the patient. The definition of this boundary gave the practitioner a useful tool in negotiating his relations with the patient.

[. . .]

Despite the obvious power enjoyed by the patient, the practitioners were not, therefore, entirely without resources. They could occasionally invoke a 'technical' discourse intelligible only to colleagues. Moreover, Abernethy's indiscretions notwithstanding, they could rely upon a certain professional *esprit de corps* which allowed them to structure their relations with members of the public. This solidarity, moreover, allowed doctors to exercise a degree of control over the patient's access to information about his case.

---

[27] Quoted in J. Thomson, *An Account of the Life, Lectures and Writings of William Cullen, M.D.* (Edinburgh, W. Blackwood & Sons 1859) vol. I, p. 503. William Cullen (1710–90) was a distinguished Scottish physician, successively holding chairs at the Glasgow and Edinburgh Medical Schools.

Part two
The changing role of the hospital

2.1
Rules for the admission and discharge
of patients

Rules and Regulations of the Huddersfield and Upper
Agbrigg Infirmary, 1834, pp. 16–20, Huddersfield Public
Library (Kirklees District Archives and Local Studies
Department) B.362.

The Huddersfield and Upper Agbrigg Infirmary, opened in 1831,
was a typical voluntary hospital. It was funded by charitable dona-
tions and staffed by doctors who gave their services free, out of a
sense of public duty. The patients had to be recommended by one
of the governors, and were expected to conform to a strict set of
rules concerning their behaviour. Here we see rules and regulations, not only for the patients, but also the doctors concerning
the type of patients who could be admitted and the times of
admittance and discharge.

Admission and discharge of patients

That in-patients be admitted and discharged every Friday, at the weekly
Board, between eleven and one o'clock.

That out-patients be admitted every day, Sundays excepted, provided
they bring their recommendations before ten o'clock in the morning;
the power of confirming or rejecting such admissions being vested in

the weekly Board. No recommendation to remain in force longer than two months.

That no patient be admitted without a recommendation, except in cases of accident or great emergency; and a certain number of beds shall be reserved for such cases as will not admit of delay. That Governors, recommending patients from distant places, be desired to send their cases drawn up by some Physician, Surgeon, or Apothecary, (post-paid,) to which an answer shall be returned, whether and when they may be admitted: but the Board shall be at liberty to reject such patients, if their cases appear to have been misrepresented, or their circumstances such as to enable them to provide for their own cure.

[. . .]

That where a certain number only of the cases duly recommended and qualified, can be admitted, those be first admitted whose cases will admit of the least delay; and in cases of equal exigency, the preference be given, first, to such as live at the greatest distance; secondly, to those recommended by such Governors as have not had an in-patient on the books within the year; and, thirdly, to those recommended by the largest contributors.

That such cases as cannot be admitted, be entered as out-patients, and be received into the house preferably to others, in equal necessity, upon the first vacancy, of which notice shall be given.

[. . .]

That no person be admitted either as in or out-patient, who is able to pay for medical aid. That no apprentices or domestic servants be admitted as in-patients, except for capital operations; in which cases, their master or mistress shall pay ten shillings and sixpence per week for their subsistence. That the medical officers be not required to visit apprentices or servants at the houses of their masters or mistresses.

That no soldier (except on furlough) be admitted as an in-patient, unless his officer, or some other responsible person, engage to pay one shilling per day for his subsistence during his continuance in the house.

That no woman advanced in pregnancy, no child under six years, (except in particular cases, as fractures, cutting for the stone, amputations, couching, or where some other surgical operations may be required,) or persons disordered in their senses, subject to epileptic fits, suspected to have the smallpox, measles, itch, or other infectious distemper, having habitual ulcers, syphilis, (except when requested by the faculty,) or those suspected to be in a consumption, or in an incurable or dying state, be admitted as in-patients; or, if admitted inadvertently, be allowed to remain, unless at the particular desire of the medical officers.

That all in-patients be discharged at the end of two months after their admission, unless their Physician or Surgeon certify to the weekly Board that there is great probability of cure, or considerable relief; in which case they shall be entered on the books as admitted a second time, on a renewal of their recommendation. And that whenever any patient is discharged, notice be sent to the recommender.

That it be recommended to all patients, when discharged, cured, or relieved, to return thanks in their respective places of worship, and to carry a letter of thanks to their recommending Governor, agreeably to printed forms to be delivered to them.

Rules for in-patients

That they strictly observe the directions of their Physicians and Surgeons; and also of the Apothecary, the Matron, and the Nurses.

That no patient go out of the Infirmary without leave from his Physician or Surgeon, or the Apothecary; or lie out of the house on any account whatever, on pain of expulsion.

That no men patients go into the womens' wards, nor women into the men's; nor be permitted to enter any ward but their own, without leave from the Apothecary or Matron.

That no patient sit up after eight o'clock in winter, or after nine in summer, unless by the Apothecary's permission; and every patient who is allowed to quit his bed, shall rise at seven in summer, and at eight in winter.

That there be no cursing, swearing, rude or indecent behaviour, on pain of expulsion after the first admonition.[1]

That there be no playing at cards or any other game within the limits of the Infirmary; nor any smoking, without leave from a Physician or Surgeon, first signified to the Apothecary: neither shall spirituous liquors, nor any provisions, be introduced by the patients or their friends.

That such patients as are able, be employed in nursing the other patients, washing and ironing the linen, cleaning the wards or any other work, but not without leave of the Physician or Surgeon.

That all patients provide themselves with proper changes of linen during their residence in the Infirmary, and with knives and forks.

---

[1] *admonition*: reprimand.

That such patients as are able, (each time obtaining leave of the Apothecary,) be permitted to go into the garden in suitable weather; but that they abstain from all improper conduct while there, and do not walk on the grass or borders.

That such patients as are able, shall attend divine service on Sundays, and whenever it shall be performed.

That the friends of patients may visit them on Tuesdays only, viz. between the hours of ten and twelve in the morning, and two and four in the afternoon; but that they shall not remain longer than one hour, nor enter any other ward.

That no patient who has been discharged for irregularity he admitted again, unless in an extraordinary case, not allowing delay.

That the rules for in-patients and for the nurses, be read every Friday evening, after the admission of new patients, by the Apothecary in the men's wards, and by the Matron in the women's wards; and that they be hung up in each ward.

Rules for out-patients

That all out-patients shall attend the Infirmary at such times as their Physician or Surgeon shall direct: if absent for three successive weeks, unless for some reason admitted as satisfactory by the Physician or Surgeon, they shall be dismissed.

That they provide their own phials[2] and gallipots,[3] and that no fresh medicines be given them unless they deliver their phials and gallipots clean, and return such medicines as are not used.

That no patient, in or out, loiter about the Infirmary or streets adjacent, or ask alms,[4] on pain of being discharged for irregularity.

[2] *phial*: small glass vessel, here used for holding medicines.
[3] *gallipot*: a small ceramic pot, probably used for ointments.
[4] *alms*: i.e. begging for money.

2.2
An appeal for funds

[W. Turnbull], *An Appeal on Behalf of the Intended Hospital at
Huddersfield* (Huddersfield, n.p. [c. 1825]), pp. 1–3, Kirklees
Central Library, Local History (Tomlinson Collection).

Dr William Turnbull graduated as MD in Edinburgh in 1814. He
practised as a medical officer in the Huddersfield Dispensary and
then in the Infirmary. The Dispensary had been opened in 1814 and
the Dispensary Committee proposed to set up new in-patient
facilities in the early 1820s. An appeal to raise funds for the
intended infirmary was set up in 1824. In April, 1825, a building accident in the town was responsible for 16 deaths and serious injuries.
This prompted the Dispensary's medical officers, including Dr
Turnbull, to write and circulate pamphlets in order to publicise
the infirmary appeal.

An appeal, in behalf of the intended hospital at Huddersfield

Feeling, like all well-wishers of humanity, the deepest interest in every
thing that has for its object the alleviation of human suffering, I hail,
with inexpressible pleasure, the efforts now making to establish a
public Hospital in Huddersfield.

Institutions, for the reception and relief of the diseased and
wounded, have long existed, under various names and regulations,
throughout Europe; and the benefit derived from them is so important,
the necessity for them so evident and urgent, that they seem to bear
almost a regular proportion to the increase, or, at least, the accumulation of society. Hence their number and magnitude in large cities, and
hence the interest taken in their welfare among all classes of the community, wherever free inquiry and the expression of public feeling
are allowed by the constitution of the state.——Benevolence, though
generally engaged in the formation and promotion of these establishments, is not the only agent to which they are to be ascribed; for
motives of a different kind, but perfectly compatible with it, and rendered imperative by the condition in which Providence has been
pleased to place our species, are equally obvious and powerful. Some of
these may be briefly noticed.

It is a duty of magistracy and police to prevent, as much as possible, the extension of contagious and pestilential disorders, though, unhappily, in the fulfilment of it, some of the dearest sympathies of life must be occasionally sacrificed to the common good. It is no less the duty than it is the interest of individuals, whose circumstances do not permit the adoption of the most efficacious measures for the cure of such disorders, and of any others of a formidable and threatening nature, to consent to a temporary separation from their families or friends, in the hope of successful treatment, and of a more speedy return to usefulness and comfort, than could have been effected while they remained in their own abodes.——All who have an opportunity of personally examining into the wants of the Poor, well know, that a large portion of their distress, in common times, arises from ill health. Many a decent family which has been long maintained in comfort by the exertions of the parents, has been brought to real misery by the sickness of the father or mother; or, as is frequently the case, the earnings of the parents are all consumed in the means of cure, or in alleviating the anguish of a child suffering under a long, painful, and necessarily expensive disease.—— In many of those instances, timely assistance would have rendered the cure short and easy; but unable to bear, and fearful to incur the expence of Medical Advice, they are often induced to delay their application, till the case is beyond the reach of remedial means. But supposing that a strong feeling of affection overcomes the consideration of their ability; and that application is made to the best Medical Assistance, every person must know, that the necessary expence of such Advice and Medicine, is far above the means of the labouring classes of society. Hence a poor family is driven, during sickness, to depend for the very necessaries of life upon their credit with the neighbouring Shopkeeper; and a system is thus introduced, which, more than any other, tends to degrade and demoralize the character. The feeling of compunction which at first arises at running into debts, which they have no prospect of discharging, wears off by degrees; and when the possibility of supporting themselves creditably is gone; when hope, the great stimulus to exertion, is no more, all further effort is palsied, a sort of moral despair succeeds, and they are contented to leave their debts unpaid, to forfeit all their independence of spirit, and idly to rely on a Parish for the future: thus they become useless, if not hurtful, members of the community. The expediency then, of aiding and accelerating the recovery of the health of the lower classes, especially those members on whose industry others are dependent for support, is quite unquestionable, though there were no higher reasons to enforce it than the policy of preventing or obviating the necessity of an augmentation of poor rates.[5]

Further, the instruction which such establishments afford those persons who are destined to practise the various branches of the healing art, besides being of a nature and degree unattainable, at least by many, in any other way, ultimately becomes advantageous to all ranks of society. Altogether, therefore, the policy of such establishments is as manifest, as the obligation to contribute to their support is clearly and imperatively deducible from the spirit and precepts of religion.

[. . .]

. . . [T]he great majority of the inhabitants, throughout the entire district, is employed in crowded and ill ventilated apartments,—nearly ten out of every twelve being engaged in trade and manufactures, or their subservient arts. Hence the constitutions of the people are generally weak and prone to disease;—and infectious disorders, when once introduced, spread with fearful rapidity; too often baffling the most skilful endeavours to arrest their devastating career.——It is, indeed, but too true, that where prosperity and population are on the increase, misery and misfortune keep a proportionate pace:—In proof of this, it is only necessary to look at the town of Huddersfield; the rapid extension of which, in wealth, population, and unwholesome industry, far from contradicting the observation, affords numerous and almost daily instances illustrative of its truth. The wail of the widow and the cry of the orphan still vibrate on the ear; and who can say—how soon we may be called upon to mourn over a similar catastrophe!

With regard to the practicability of founding and supporting an Hospital in Huddersfield, of a size sufficiently large to afford all the benefits these establishments are calculated to yield, a few remarks will suffice. Three months ago, it would have been a difficult task to have convinced the public that the design was at all practicable; and that there was sufficient either of opulence or liberality in the district for accomplishing so weighty an undertaking. The munificent and well-timed example, however, of a few philanthropic persons has set the question at rest, and has ensured the erection of a Building adequate to supply the wishes and wants of every indigent and lowly sufferer. Is then, the district capable of maintaining such an institution? On this head I have bestowed considerable pains to arrive at a sound conclusion; and, from authentic documents which have been shewn to me, I feel satisfied, that the annual expenditure of an establishment with twenty beds, and admitting as many out-patients as the present Dispensary, would not

---

[5] *poor rates*: a local tax collected on homes and businesses to pay for the support of local paupers.

30

exceed £900:—a sum which there ought to be little difficulty in raising in a community of 120,000 inhabitants. So far back as 1814, when the Dispensaries were established, the yearly subscriptions, congregational collections, and magistrates' fines, amounted to little short of £800. The town and neighbourhood surely, are not less opulent, or less populous, or less benevolent, than they were at that period. On the contrary, in all these they have wonderfully increased, and as no reflecting and generous mind can, for a moment, question the usefulness of such an institution, there is every reason to believe that the requisite amount will be obtained, with great facility.——The townships alone, if they follow, as it is hoped they will, the example of those around Leeds, and other places possessed of similar Charities, are almost sufficient to ensure its prosperity. Besides, it is not probable, that more than one-half of the contributions will be expended in the erection and fitting up of the edifice; the other half, therefore, would remain as a permanent fund, which, with occasional benefactions and legacies, would soon place the Charity in independent circumstances. If £200 a year were derived from this source, little more would be required than the Income which the General Dispensary easily obtained eleven years ago.

I think then, it may fairly be affirmed, that the district constituted of the Upper-Division of Agbrigg and the adjoining townships, is fully competent to the maintenance of such a Charity;—that the present period of peace and general prosperity is peculiarly favourable for its institution;—and that Huddersfield, from the easy access to it on all sides, from its large population, and from its central and healthy position, is well adapted for the site of such an Establishment.

In conclusion, I appeal to all who are friendly to the object in view; and urge them no longer to delay giving effect to their good wishes, but to hasten, by their patronage and support, the completion of an Institution, where the children of disease and poverty may reap those benefits, taste those blessings, and enjoy those privileges, which have descended upon other and more favoured districts in a much earlier period of their history.

2.3

The patient's experience

Martin Goldman, *Lister Ward* (Bristol and Boston, Adam
Hilger, 1987), pp. 36–7, 49–50, 58–9, 64–5, 67, 78–80, 84.

In 1877 Margaret Mathewson (1848–80) travelled from her home in
Shetland to Edinburgh to seek treatment for a diseased shoulder
joint. She was admitted to the city's Royal Infirmary, partly so her
case could be used for teaching. She was under the care of Joseph
Lister (1827–1912), then professor of Clinical Surgery and famous
for his development of antiseptic surgical technique. After eight
months, she was discharged, cured. She returned to Shetland but
died three years later, probably of tuberculosis. Margaret later
wrote about her experiences in hospital using a journal she kept at
the time – in one of the few accounts of surgery by a Victorian hospital patient. Her account is a reminder that although anaesthesia
and antisepsis made surgery less painful and much safer, it was
still an uncomfortable ordeal. When this extract begins, Margaret
has been examined by Lister and admitted to the hospital.

I went to the fire and sat down and took a look round. There were 9 beds
and 8 patients in bed. All the beds had nice white covers on, clean
pillow cases and clean sheets and the room so tidy and neat; also a big
fire on . . . Under the beds was wood flooring. Down the centre was flag-
stone. On this stood a long table, on one end of which were lots of lotion
bottles and dressing stuffs. . . . All the patients seemed to be quite at
home and not to be suffering very much but no one spoke to me but all
looking as if wondering if I was to be one of their number.

[. . .]

Then the dinner bell rung, and the nurse came in with 9 basins of soup
and bread on a tray. Then she came back with potatoes and meat. At
4.30 p.m. the tea bell rung and nurse McConnachy again came with tea,
bread, and butter.

   At 5 p.m. visitors came and stayed till 6.30 p.m. when a bell rung for
them to leave. At 7.30 supper came, bread and milk. At 8 p.m. all had to
go to bed that were walking about. 8.30 a change of nurses – the day
nurses went off duty and the night nurses came on. I lay awake about
1½ hours then went asleep.

Next morning I was awoke by the night nurse . . . at 5.30 a.m. 'Get up and make yourself generally useful.'

[. . .]

For breakfast we first for a basin of porridge and milk, then coffee and bread. About 9 a.m. there was a change of nurses again also the morning post called with letters for the ward. At 9.30 a.m. Miss Logan came on duty.[6] At 10 she came with an armful of gauze 40 yds to the patients to tear into lengths of 20 yds each, some about 3 inches wide and others less for bandages. These were smoothed, then rolled on a little hand machine for the purpose, then put into a little basket and set on the table with other dressings stuffs.

10.30 people began to call to see Prof. Lister. 11 and 11.30 there was a great commotion. Doctors driving in to the door, students by scores walking down from the college arm in arm. Then the two surgical Professors came each in his own open carriage, viz. Prof. Spence and Prof. Lister. At 11.40 a.m. all was very quiet. 12.45, Prof. Lister, Dr. Cheyne and about 40 students came downstairs, and into our ward, examined some of the patients, then came to me and the Prof. said 'Undress please.' . . . The Prof. then asked me almost the same questions as on the previous day,[7] then said to the students 'Gentlemen, this is a case of consumption of the lungs[8] but is providentially turned from the lungs to the shoulder joint. There it has formed a circumficial abscess. Also here is another glandular abscess on the collar bone which makes this a very interesting case for us all. Dr. you will dress it antiseptically this afternoon.'

They all went out. The Doctor came and dressed it with carbolic lotion and it felt much easier.

[. . .]

Next day I was called upstairs to be lectured on, and was put into a dark room where I found by their voices there were others before me. . . . I sat about 2 hours and then Dr. Cheyne[9] came and told me I was not wanted today as there were so many others.

[. . .]

[Next day] I sat two hours in the dark hole again. Then Dr. Cheyne came and told me I was not wanted today yet as there were so many to be

---

[6] The nurse in charge of the ward.

[7] i.e. on her initial examination.

[8] *consumption*: tuberculosis.

[9] Dr Cheyne was Lister's assistant.

done. I was truly glad as I was shaking with fear and cold as well. When I came downstairs I found I had lost my dinner. . . . Next day I was called again, and was also called into the big theatre and lectured on before about 40 gentlemen and all the lecture was in English so I had the benefit of it too. Prof. asked me almost the same questions . . . as he had done previously; then again explained the case as before.

[. . .]

I was very much excited by this time, so much so that I felt the cold perspiration running down my forehead which the Prof. observed then patting me on the arm said: 'Now turn your back on these gentlemen.'

I was thankful to hear this but on turning round my feelings were more aroused by looking on the blackboard and seeing the diagram of my arm chalked in its then swelled state, also the natural state, then special marks where it had to be operated on. Seeing this I almost fainted as until then, I had a hope it would not be so serious an operation. . . .

[. . .]

[A]bout 10.30 a.m. Nurse Kilpatrick came and told me to undress as usual and be quick as I would soon be called, but it was 1 p.m. ere Dr. Cheyne came and called me. . . . The big theatre door was open and we went in. Prof. bowed and smiled. I returned the bow. He then told me to step up on the chair (set at the side of the table on which was a blanket and 2 pillows) then lie down on the table. I did so and saw that my turn had come at last and now was the time to be cool and as collected as possible. . . .

There were a lot sitting in the gallery and four gentlemen sitting around the table. Dr. Cheyne came and laid a towel saturated with chloroform over my face and said 'Now breathe away.' . . .

I felt myself growing weaker and weaker and every nerve and joint relaxing and breaking up as it were, a very solemn moment thus staring death in the face and I believed I never should awaken to look on the things of time any more but was indeed entering eternity. . . .

[. . .]

I was conscious of no more until I awoke in bed in a strange ward, viz. No. 2. My first thought was 'My arm is it off or not?' I at once sat up to feel for it. I could not find it at all, but I was all bandaged up from the waist to the neck. It must be away.

I then found it bandaged to my waist and breathed a sigh of thankfulness to God for this renewed instance of His goodness to me. . . .

[. . .]

. . . I felt very sick and kept on vomiting. The nurse brought a jug of ice and gave me always a teaspoonful as soon as I stopped vomiting. . . .

I got more feverish and sick, and felt the vomiting more – straining on the stomack, and always grew weaker. Dr. Cheyne came and took my pulse, marked it down on the card. . . .

I vomited all the evening now and again. I went asleep but soon awoke and felt more feverish, also a bad headache, a strange pain about the joint and smarting all around as if it were cut. As the night wore on the pain increased, and at times I was on the eve of shouting, the pain was so severe. I then thought 'I shall not shout as long as I can avoid it.' I thus hid my mouth in the sheet. . . .

[. . .]

About 12.45 Professor came and a train of students with him. . . .

[. . .]

Prof. then dressed it with the spray, then put on chloride of zinc and moved the arm to and fro. The pain was indescribable. I never felt such excruciating pain before. I also felt the arm quite loose from my body. The pain caused me almost to faint.

Prof. said to the students: 'Gentlemen, I have a great fear of putre-faction setting in and you all know its outcome. Thus I will look anxiously for the second day or third day between hope and fear. I hope the chloride of zinc will preserve it but it is only an experiment. However we will see if spared.'

[. . .]

I thought over the last of Professor's speech seriously. Evidently he has very poor hopes of my recovery indeed. I thus better now look over my hopes of eternity, where probably I will soon be in reality and see if my hope will stand the test of 'The Judgement Day'.

[. . .]

About 11.45 Prof. came to dress me and a great many students. When Prof. had taken off the bandages, he said, 'Gentlemen to my glad sur-prise you see there's neither colour nor smell here and it is preserved entirely by the chloride of zinc.' . . .

Prof. then moved it (which caused excruciating pain and ever after I dreaded the moving). Prof. then bandaged it up, then said, 'Gentlemen, I had great fears of the patient standing the operation . . . She took a very small quantity of chloroform at first only about ½ an ounce, but that was not near enough to keep her quiet, the time I required for the operation. Thus I had to repeat the dose often until I feared to give more for getting her back. And after all it required an hour and ten minutes to restore her, and it's [sic] effects must have been heavy and will be felt for some time yet to come, but I trust it will now be a successful case.'

2.4
Designing the ideal hospital

Florence Nightingale, *Notes on Hospitals*, 3rd edn (London, Longman, Green, Longman, Roberts and Green, 1863), pp. 32–6, 43–4.

Florence Nightingale's image as the 'Lady with the Lamp' and the heroine of nursing reform has been questioned by many recent historians who have shown that she was more concerned with questions of hospital design and administration than with nursing. Nightingale's ideas on health and disease encompassed nine-teenth-century notions that connected the physical, the moral and the psychological. She explicitly rejected the germ theory of disease, and held to a belief that disease was attributable to poisons in the air. Nightingale also held that responsible and moral behaviour were equally important in the avoidance of disease. *Notes on Hospitals* was originally published in 1859; along with her *Notes on Lying-in Institutions* (a study of 1871) her works became the authority on hospital design and administration.

Construction of Hospitals on such a Plan as to prevent Free Circulation of External Air.—To build a hospital with one closed court[10] with high walls, or what is worse, with two closed courts, is to stagnate the air even before it reaches the wards.

This defect is one of the most serious that can be committed in hospital architecture; and it exists, nevertheless, in some form or other in nearly all the older hospitals, and in many even of recent construction.

The air outside the hospital cannot be maintained in a state sufficiently pure to be used for internal ventilation, unless there be entire freedom of movement. Anything which interferes with this is injurious. Neighbouring high walls, smoking chimneys, trees, high ground, are

---

[10] i.e. courtyard.

all more or less hurtful; but worse than all is bad construction of the hospital itself.

[. . .]

Even in the true separate pavilion structure,[11] unless the distance between the pavilions be double the height of the walls, the ventilation and light are seriously interfered with.

For this, among other reasons, two stories are better than three; and one is preferable to two. . . .

To build a hospital in the midst of a crowded neighbourhood of narrow streets and high houses, is to ensure a stagnation of the air without, which no ventilation within, no cubic space, however ample, will be able to remedy.

[. . .]

Defects in Ward Construction injurious to Ventilation.—One of the most common causes of unhealthiness in hospitals is defective construction and arrangement of the ward-space of such a nature as to lead to difficulty of ventilation, or want of light. The expression, 'a good ward,' comprehends something quite different from mere appearance. No ward is in any sense a good ward in which the sick are not at all times supplied with pure air, light, and a due temperature. These are the results to be obtained from hospital architecture, and not external design or appearance. . . .

Defective Height of Wards.—It is not possible to ventilate sufficiently a large ward of ten or twelve feet high. . . . A ward of thirty beds can be well ventilated with a height of about fifteen or sixteen feet, provided the windows reach to within one foot of the ceiling. Otherwise, the top of the ward becomes a reservoir for foul air. . . .

Too Great Width of Wards between the Opposite Windows.—It does not appear as if the air could be thoroughly changed, if a distance of more than thirty feet intervenes between the opposite windows: if, in other words, the ward is more than thirty feet wide. . . .

[. . .]

Defects in Drainage, Water Closets, Sinks, &c.—Hospital Sewers may become cesspools of the most dangerous description, if improperly made and placed. In one hospital I knew, if the wind changed so as to blow up the open mouths of the sewers, such change was frequently marked by outbreaks of fever among the patients, and by relapses

---

[11] Hospitals designed with separate wings (or 'pavilions') which housed the wards.

among the convalescents from fever. Where there are no means for externally ventilating the sewers, no traps, no sufficient water supply, no means for cleansing or flushing them, and where the bottoms are rough and uneven, such occurrences cannot fail to take place. The emanations from the deposits in the sewers are in such cases blown back through the pipe-drains into the water-closets and sinks, and thence into the wards. Where sewers pass close to or under occupied rooms, the walls or covers being defective, exhalations will infallibly escape into those rooms. There are hospitals where such things exist at the present time.

There can be no safety for the sick if any but water-closets of the best construction are used, as also if they are not built *externally* to the main building, and cut off by a lobby, separately lighted and ventilated by cross windows, from the ward. The same thing may be said of sinks. I have known outbreaks of fever even among the healthy from an ill-constructed and ill-placed sink in this country.

2.5

Gateways to death?

John Woodward, *To Do the Sick no Harm. A Study of the British Hospital System to 1875* (London and Boston, Routledge Kegan Paul, 1974), pp. 123–36, 139–40, 142.

In this book John Woodward, an economic historian, tried to go beyond the usual, laudatory histories of individual hospitals, which focused on their administration and the careers of eminent members of staff. Instead, he analysed the work and development of British voluntary hospitals, exploring all aspects of their function. In this extract he questions whether nineteenth-century hospitals deserved their reputation for high mortality.

Medical historians have tended to view the hospitals in the eighteenth and nineteenth centuries as being horrific institutions in which most of the patients died. This dismissal of the work of the voluntary hospitals has been stated in the strongest of terms:

> Indeed, the chief indictment of hospital work at this period is not that it did no good, but that it positively did harm ... The common cause of death was infectious disease; any patient admitted to hospital faced the risk of contracting a mortal infection ... it was not until much later [than the

eighteenth century] that hospital patients could be reasonably certain of dying from the disease with which they were admitted.[12]

However, the evidence upon which this damning conclusion is based needs to be examined . . . The practice of St Bartholomew's Hospital of admitting cholera patients to the general wards in 1854 is used to support the view that hospitals did not appreciate the necessity of sep-arating infectious and non-infectious cases. This is highly misleading, for the hospitals varied in their attitudes towards infectious disease and policies changed according to experience. 'Contemporary accounts of the unsatisfactory conditions in eighteenth century hospitals . . . in the writings of Percival, Howard, etc.' are given as further evidence without any form of criticism. Although John Howard[13] found that conditions in the London hospitals were not above reproach, his reports on the provincial hospitals he visited disclose a mixed picture of good and bad conditions . . . On the mortality after surgery, evidence is taken from a book, published in 1874, by the senior surgeon at University College Hospital, John Erichsen.

> He showed that mortality following all form of amputation was between 35% and 50%, and following certain [unspecified] forms it was as high as 90%. Results of other types of operation were equally bad; Erichsen's observations were based upon the third quarter of the nineteenth century; there is no reason to suppose that earlier results were better.[14]

The notion that these high rates of surgical mortality were preceded by even higher rates in the eighteenth century is highly misleading. Mortality after surgery in the early years of hospital practice was not high, and even the figures presented by John Erichsen were not representative of the voluntary hospitals in the third quarter of the nineteenth century.

Florence Nightingale, in a perfect example of the abuse of statistics, attempted to show that mortality in hospitals was disgracefully high and that improvements would have to be made. A reviewer of her book wrote that 'It is sad to see a work of so much value – full of such useful information – disfigured by a few serious and elementary mistakes'. . . . [T]he reviewer noted that the statistics were based on the *Report of the Registrar-General for 1861* and 'therefore, perhaps Miss Nightingale can hardly be held responsible for it'. He continued:

---

[12] T. McKeown and R.G. Brown, 'Medical Evidence Related to English Population Changes in the Eighteenth Century', *Population Studies*, 9 (1955–56), p. 125.

[13] John Howard (1726–96) is more famous for his campaign for prison reform, but he also reported on conditions in hospitals.

[14] McKeown and Brown, 'English Population Changes', p. 120.

In 1861, returns were made from 106 Hospitals, giving the number of inmates in each on April 8. The number of deaths registered in each Hospital during the year 1861 is also given. Our readers will hardly believe that on these two bases a percentage of mortality is struck. The inmates of a single day are balanced with the deaths of a whole year, and no wonder the results are 'striking enough'. . . . There is something audacious in the last column of this table, where twenty-four London Hospitals are accredited with a mortality per cent on inmates of 90.84. No doubt it will be said this is the quotient of the figures employed; but we entirely deny their validity and the accuracy of the impression thus conveyed.[15]

This damning criticism was refuted by William Farr, the Registrar-General, who thought that the method used admitted 'of no ambiguity'. . . .

[. . .]

Thus, the evidence used to support the pessimistic case, though of formidable repute, received a severe criticism at the time of its publication and the statistics presented in it are open to great doubt. . . .

[. . .]

A review of the figures issued by the voluntary hospitals during the eighteenth and nineteenth centuries shows a consistent picture of relatively low mortality among patients – the impression of the hospitals killing more than they cured created by William Farr and Florence Nightingale being completely erroneous. . . .

The Salisbury General Infirmary treated 66,455 in-patients and 132,185 out-patients from its opening on 2 May 1767 to the end of the hospital-year 1875–6. Of the in-patients 26,811 were claimed to be cured and 3,428 relieved, while 2,014 patients had died under its care, a death-rate of approximately 3 per cent. . . .

From 1747 to 1846 the Salop Infirmary discharged 29,161 in-patients as cured and 21,096 as relieved. The deaths totalled 2,481 out of 56,819 completing their stay in the hospital, a death-rate of about 2.5 per cent. . . . From 1827 to 1836 out of an annual average of 855 patients admitted 30 died.

These figures are representative of the smaller provincial hospitals in the eighteenth and nineteenth centuries, and it is noticeable that even in the larger provincial and metropolitan hospitals the claimed mortality-rates were only a little higher.

. . . [A]t Manchester Infirmary in the year 1769–70 12 patients died and 16 were found to be incurable, but 286 were cured or relieved and

[15] *Medical Times and Gazette*, 1864, p. 129.

193 were made out-patients. By the year 1874–5 a grand total of 1,522,504 patients had been treated, of which 959,346 were claimed to have been cured, 126,770 relieved and 49,744 had died. The Bristol Infirmary generally exhibited mortality-rates of between 8 and 10 per cent annually; for example, figures of 8.4 per cent and 9.4 per cent were recorded in 1811 and 1828 respectively . . .

Improvements were made in hygiene and cleanliness at St Thomas's Hospital in 1783, and a comparison was made between the mortality in the ten preceding and ten subsequent years by its famous physician Sir Gilbert Blane.

I found the former to be in the proportion of one to fourteen, the latter of 1 to 15.6. The average rate of mortality for the next ten years was 1 to 14.2; but in the last ten years, that is from 1803 till the present year, 1813, it has been 1 in 16.2.[16]

[. . .]

The impression that mortality was lower in the smaller voluntary hospitals in the provinces than in those in the larger provincial towns is maintained by a survey made by a committee established by the Birmingham General Hospital in 1844. For the hospital-year 1841–2 three hospitals, the Bedford General Infirmary, the Suffolk General Infirmary (Bury St Edmunds), and the Gloucester Infirmary recorded death-rates of under 2 per cent. The Birmingham General Hospital itself and the Manchester Royal Infirmary recorded figures of 8.65 per cent and 8.12 per cent respectively.

An interesting survey of the experiences of hospitals was published soon after the revelations of Miss Nightingale and William Farr. Though this study by Fleetwood Buckle completely refuted the statistics produced by the two illustrious figures of Miss Nightingale and Mr Farr, it has not received its due share of publicity, even at the time of its first appearance. In 117 hospitals in England and Wales, which completed a questionnaire, 95,661 in-patients were treated in 1863, of which 7,361 died, a death-rate of 7.607 per cent. When this figure is broken down to its constituent parts, it is found that the eighteen metropolitan hospitals treated 53,031 in-patients and recorded a death-rate of 9.19 per cent; the 92 English provincial hospitals treated 59,681 in-patients and recorded a 7.672 per cent mortality-rate; and the 7 Welsh hospitals treated 12,524 in-patients and recorded the low death-rate of only 3.58 per cent. . . .

Some explanation is needed of the disparities in the death-rates between the voluntary hospitals and over time. . . .

[16] Gilbert Blane, 'On the Comparative Prevalence and Mortality of Different Diseases in London', *Medico-chirurgical Transactions* 1 (1813), p. 142.

The hospitals in London and in the large provincial centres of population were more likely to receive a greater proportion of accidents which were potentially more fatal than hospitals in rural areas. Even within London the experience of hospitals was different. Thus, the London Hospital in Whitechapel Road 'which is placed in the centre of one of the densest and poorest districts, and in close proximity to the Docks, and a large number of serious accidents than any other hospital in London', recorded high death-rates. . . . [B]y 1863 the total of accident cases treated at the London Hospital had reached 12,488. . . . In contrast, at Guy's Hospital in the same year only 4,704 accident cases were treated.

The hospitals situated in the manufacturing towns had a similar problem. At the Sheffield Royal Infirmary it was stated for the year 1844–5 that '196 In-Patients, with sudden Accidents, &c., have been admitted during the past year without any recommendation; some of them with fractured limbs, and others with dislocations, wounds, contusions, burns and scalds'. . . .

[. . .]

The second influence on mortality in the voluntary hospital system . . . is . . . bed occupancy. The voluntary hospitals in London and . . . the the large provincial towns had the greatest turnover of patients as the demand for beds always appeared to exceed the supply available. . . . As an example in an important provincial town, Leeds, the General Infirmary reported in 1786 that 'During the two last Years, the average Number of In-Patients on the Books, waiting their turn for Admission into the House, has not been less than Twenty-five at a Time'. This, undoubtedly, would have had effects on the time that a patient was allowed to convalesce after treatment in a hospital; though the cases likely to be admitted to hospitals in metropolitan or large provincial hospitals were usually of a more serious and acute character than those entering the smaller rural hospitals. . . .

The mortality attendant on surgical cases was less than that on medical cases and this was reflected in the overall mortality of a hospital by the proportion of each type of case, i.e. surgical or medical, admitted. . . .

[I]n 1862 at Guy's Hospital in London and at the Sheffield Royal Infirmary overall mortality was virtually identical at 9.61 per cent and 9.5 per cent respectively. The mortality in each hospital, in both the medical and the surgical cases, was again very similar; at Guy's the mortality was 14.49 per cent for medical cases and 6.16 per cent for surgical cases, while at the Sheffield Royal Infirmary the respective mortality figures were 14.6 per cent and 6.3 per cent. . . .

Again, the admission or exclusion of cases of infectious diseases forms a very important item in regulating the mortality of a hospital; and this is not merely because infectious diseases, such as typhus and small-pox, present normally a far larger percentage mortality than most other cases admitted into hospitals, but because practically, the admission or non-admission of this class of affections regulates in no small degree the admission of other acute medical diseases. . . . So that the hospital which declines to receive fever cases into its wards, ceases in large proportion to receive cases of acute internal inflammation which really form the great bulk of the urgent cases which physicians are called upon to treat.[17]

Mortality from fever was subject to great fluctuation as at the London Fever Hospital from 1805 to 1876 when the death-rate varied from 9.0 per cent to 25.5 per cent

[. . .]

It was usually the practice of the voluntary hospitals to refuse admission to persons suffering from incurable diseases – 'Now such diseases include organic affections of the heart in their later stages, advanced Bright's disease,[18] cancerous affections, and especially confirmed phthisis. It is notorious that the affections here enumerated . . . constitute the chief causes of death in those who have passed beyond the age of puberty.'[19] If consumption is considered at the Glasgow Royal Infirmary, the death-rate from this disease was 34.8 per cent from 1829 to 1832, which constituted 7.8 per cent of total deaths; 43.1 per cent from 1844 to 1849, constituting 14.0 per cent of total deaths; and 30.1 per cent from 1871 to 1876, constituting 16.6 per cent of total deaths.

[. . .]

If a hospital admits a large proportion of such ailments as venereal diseases, eye diseases and skin diseases where the prospects of a fatal termination are remote, the mortality-rate of such a hospital will be less than that of a hospital which does not admit such cases. Thus, at Guy's Hospital in 1862, 395 eye cases were admitted, none of which proved fatal. . . . Some of the voluntary hospitals developed a speciality in one form of disease and as a result admitted a large number of cases of that particular type. The Devon and Exeter Hospital found that a large percentage of cases admitted were for skin diseases as the physicians of that hospital had acquired a reputation for treating skin affections.

[17] a disease of the kidneys.
[18] J.S. Bristowe and T. Holmes, *The Hospitals of the United Kingdom*, p. 518.
[19] *consumption*: tuberculosis.

[. . .]

Although mortality in voluntary hospitals was not unduly high, consideration must be given to the method used in the compilation of the figures and to the possibility of 'adjustment'. The voluntary hospitals were dependent on financial support from private individuals and success had to be seen if subscriptions were to be maintained and new ones encouraged. The figures used to calculate the death-rate prevailing in a hospital could be adjusted in a number of ways. Bristowe and Holmes wrote

> in the majority of hospitals, it is we believe, the custom to reckon among their deaths those who have been brought dead to the institution; but there are many hospitals where such cases are not reckoned, and there are some indeed where even those who die within 24 hours are, on the ground that they were moribund at the time of admission, excluded from computation.[20]

In the annual reports of the voluntary hospitals such cases were listed under a separate category and allowance has been made for these cases in the calculations used. A large percentage of the deaths in the larger metropolitan and provincial hospitals was provided by this category, and if these cases were excluded from the compilation of the returns a considerable improvement in the death-rate recorded could be engineered.

[. . .]

Thus, the conclusions to be reached about the experience of the voluntary hospitals during the eighteenth and nineteenth centuries . . . are favourable towards their contribution to the health of the community. The hospitals did achieve what appears to be a remarkable degree of success in treating their patients and the mortality remained at a low level throughout the period, generally being under 10 per cent of the patients admitted.

[20] Bristowe and Holmes, *Hospitals of the United Kingdom*, p. 527.

Part three

The emergency of modern surgery

3.1
Surgery and medicine

Christopher Lawrence, 'Democratic, Divine and Heroic: The History and Historiography of Surgery', in his *Medical Theory, Surgical Practice: Studies in the History of Surgery* (London, Routledge, 1992), pp. 20–3 [pp. 1–47].

Christopher Lawrence has researched and published on many topics within the history of medicine. This edited collection of papers explores the history of surgery from the seventeenth to the twentieth century. Lawrence's essay charts how the history of surgery has been constructed and reconstructed by successive generations of historians. In this section he shows how historians have refined Owsei Temkin's argument that the development of surgery in the late eighteenth century was closely linked to changes in medical thinking.

Temkin's . . . much cited paper, 'The role of surgery in the rise of medical thought'[1] . . . begins to tackle the general issue of the surgeon's success by way of the local French context. In it, Temkin claimed an important role for what he called 'the surgical point of view', an anatomical and local pathological approach to disease, in the rise of modern medicine. Temkin claimed that this view had been gaining ground during the eighteenth century, especially in France. Temkin also made a subtle linkage between medical knowledge and medical

---

[1] Owsei Temkin, 'The Role of Surgery in the Rise of Modern Medical Thought', *Bulletin of the History of Medicine*, 25 (1951), pp. 248–59.

power. He argued that when, at the end of the eighteenth century, French surgeons gained power and prestige they, and the aspiring physicians they taught, employed the ancient concept of *anatomical* reasoning, coupled with their familiar nosography of external diseases ... to explore and give shape to the internal disorders of the body. ... Temkin's approach suggests that the historian might consider how 'the surgical point of view' was not a timeless, or value-free way of describing the body and disease but a partial or interested perception, which shaped bodily knowledge in a particular way. Temkin argued, however, that there was more to the intellectual invasion of the body by surgeons than the use of local pathology. In Temkin's opinion the surgical point of view was not the only intellectual 'determining factor in the reorientation of medicine'. Chemistry and physiology were important and above all 'localized pathology was in need of general pathology'.

Temkin's observation pointedly raises the issue of the significance of attempts to localise disease in the eighteenth century both through post-mortems and at the bedside. This approach, ... was not simply confined to surgeons; Morgagni[2] often attempted to identify the physical limits of disorders in the living. It remains debatable, however, whether eighteenth-century localism can be equated with that of the nineteenth century. Eighteenth-century practitioners recognised diseases such as arterial ossification and aneurysm, with their seats in the parts. Yet most diseases, by nature of their history or by good or bad management, could change their bodily site. This rather obvious point has been eloquently laboured by [Michel] Foucault, who insists that the local pathology of the Paris clinic is epistemically[3] distinct from that of Enlightenment medicine.[4] It is the gulf that separates Morgagni from Bichat,[5] not their proximity, that is striking. For Morgagni, according to Foucault, 'Morbid kinship rested on a principle of organic proximity.' Thus 'asthma, pleuropneumonia, and haemoptysis[6] formed related species in that they were all three localized in the chest'. For Bichat, famously, 'Since every organized tissue has everywhere a general

[2] Giovanni Battista Morgagni (1682–1771), professor of Anatomy at Padua, Italy, was one of the first practitioners to systematically investigate the effects on the body's organs and tissues of diseases. His *De sedibus et causis morborum* [On the seats and causes of disease] (1761) was based on around 700 post-mortem examinations.

[3] *Epistemically* (epistemic): relating to knowledge.

[4] Michel Foucault, *Birth of the Clinic* (London, Tavistock, 1973).

[5] Marie François Xavier Bichat (1771–1802) devised the doctrine of tissues, distinctive types of structures – cellular tissue, skeletal tissue, cartilage – some of which were dispersed throughout the body. Bichat discovered that diseases attacked particular tissues rather than specific organs, one of the founding principles of modern pathology.

[6] Inflammation of the lungs and spitting of blood (a symptom of advanced tuberculosis).

arrangement, and, whatever its situation may be, retains the same structure and properties, &c, its disease must unquestionably be every where the same. The difference between this and the pathological model employed thirty years earlier by Alexander Monro *secundus*[7] is striking:

> our several organs are supported from, and in a great measure composed of branches of the same hydraulic system, so that a disease primarily influencing a single organ may in various degrees be communicated to others or to the whole.

Historians, while absorbing Foucault, have been relatively loath to address themselves directly to the epistemic issues he raises. None the less, Foucault's claims coincide with Temkin's assertion that a new general pathology was required to make localism of the eighteenth-century sort the basis of a new medicine. More recently Russell Maulitz's work can be read as elaboration of this position.[8] Maulitz has argued that the establishment of Bichat's membrane or tissue pathology was based on its value as intellectual cement to the medical and surgical communities in France, thrown together by the Revolution. Maulitz argues that the membrane pathology employed by early nineteenth-century French physicians and surgeons is not to be construed, as histories of pathology and surgery have often done, as simply a refinement of the organ pathology of the eighteenth century. Echoing Foucault, Maulitz calls this earlier surgical pathology 'natural historical'. Maulitz thus cuts the thread, spun in the nineteenth century and employed by historians of ideas ever since, that provides intellectual continuity between Morgagni and Bichat and between Bichat and Virchow.[9] For different reasons, however, John Pickstone had earlier cut the same thread in a different place, arguing that the epistemological assumptions of Bichat's tissue pathology were fundamentally different from those of Virchow's cell theory.[10] Pickstone seated Bichat firmly back in the Enlightenment where, presumably, he shared his assumptions with Morgagni. . . .

Resolution of these difficulties must certainly take account of a significant element in the general pathology of the nineteenth century: the view

---

[7] Alexander Monro *secundus* (1733–1817) was the most distinguished of three professors of anatomy of that name at Edinburgh University (father, son and grandson). Monro lectured on anatomy and surgery, and was interested in localised pathological change.

[8] Russell C. Maulitz, *Morbid Appearances: the Anatomy of Pathology in the Nineteenth Century* (Cambridge, Cambridge University Press, 1987).

[9] Rudolf Virchow (1821–1902) developed the theory that all cells arose from other cells. Pathology resulted from abnormal changes within cells.

[10] John Pickstone, 'Bureaucracy, Liberalism and the Body in post-Revolutionary France: Bichat's physiology and the Paris School of Medicine', *History of Science* 19 (1981), pp. 115–42.

that each and every part of the body, whether tissue or cell, was living. Only when physicians and surgeons used this concept was pathology made synonymous both with altered functioning and, crucially, with the changed appearance of the ultimate units of life itself. A further question now arises: how far were developments elsewhere identical to those in France? In particular, were the intellectual refashionings taking place in London and Edinburgh only superficially similar to those occurring in Paris? At first sight there seem to be great similarities. In both British cities there was a limited coalescence of medicine and surgery. Physicians were proclaiming the value of local pathology and surgeons were showing interest in reshaping theories of general disease. Yet recent work on London suggests that the Channel separated rather different orientations. Maulitz has argued that 'John Hunter[11] folded enough physiological theory into his surgical system to make clear to all professional comers the elevated, esoteric status of surgical science.' Hunter and his work were invoked by his illustrious successors anxious to establish their status as scientific practitioners. Yet that 'did not *necessarily* translate . . . into the further step, taken in France . . . by which surgical theory might methodically be integrated into medical theory. . . . In Maulitz's account John Hunter, Matthew Baillie and their circle were eighteenth-century taxonomists and natural historians. Only in the 1830s with the work of, for example, Bright, Hodgkin and Carswell,[12] did French pathology enter English medicine. In Edinburgh, where the tight hold of the grandees of the medical school and the College of Physicians collapsed during the Revolutionary years, French pathology seems to have had an earlier reception. Outsiders, such as John Thomson,[13] who were seeking to create a new general pathology seem to have used French ideas in part to attack the Tory establishment.

---

[11] John Hunter (1728–93), the leading surgeon-physiologist of the late eighteenth century. Hunter researched into the physiology of blood, the teeth, wound healing and venereal disease.

[12] Richard Bright (1789–1858), Thomas Hodgkin (1798–1866), Robert Carswell (1793–1857) all researched into pathological anatomy in London in the early nineteenth century.

[13] John Thomson (1765–1846), Professor of Military Surgery at Edinburgh University. Thomson researched into pathology and wrote an influential book on the processes of inflammation.

3.2

Surgery and experimental medicine

Claude Bernard, *An Introduction to the Study of Experimental Medicine*, trans. H.C. Greene (New York, Dover Publications, 1957; first edn 1865), pp. 168–9.

The Frenchman Claude Bernard (1813–78) has a reputation as an eminent pioneer of experimental physiology and an important spokesman for the role of the laboratory in medical research. Trained in Paris, he held many distinguished posts, including a chair at the Sorbonne University. Bernard developed new techniques of animal experimentation to investigate the physiology of the blood, the localised action of drugs, the breakdown and storage of sugars in the body, and the ability of the body to regulate its own physiology. In this essay he presented his experimental method as the new scientific basis of medicine. The booklet is still regarded today as one of the fundamental texts of modern biomedicine.

About the year 1852, my studies led me to make experiments on the influence of the nervous system on the phenomena of nutrition and temperature regulation. It had been observed in many cases that complex paralyses with their seat in the mixed nerves are followed, now by a rise and again by a fall of temperature in the paralyzed parts. Now this is how I reasoned, in order to explain this fact, basing myself first on known observations and then on prevailing theories of the phenomena of nutrition and temperature regulation. Paralysis of the nerves, said I, should lead to cooling of the parts by slowing down the phenomena of combustion in the blood, since these phenomena are considered as the cause of animal heat. . . . If my hypothesis is true, I went on, it can be verified by severing only the sympathetic, vascular nerves[14] leading to a special part, and sparing the others. I should then find the part cooled by paralysis of the vascular nerves, without loss of either motion or sensation, since the ordinary motor and sensory nerves would still be intact. To carry out my experiment, I therefore sought a suitable experimental method that would allow me to sever only the vascular nerves and to spare the others. . . .

---

[14] The sympathetic nervous system supplies the involuntary muscles and glands.

Accordingly, I severed the cervical sympathetic nerve[15] in the neck of a rabbit, to control my hypothesis and see what would happen in the way of change of temperature on the side of the head where this nerve branches out. On the basis of a prevailing theory and of earlier observation, I had been led, as we have just seen, to make the hypothesis that the temperature should be reduced. Now what happened was exactly the reverse. After severing the cervical sympathetic nerve about the middle of the neck, I immediately saw in the whole of the corresponding side of the rabbit's head a striking hyperactivity in the circulation, accompanied by increase of warmth. The result was therefore precisely the reverse of what my hypothesis, deduced from theory, had led me to expect; thereupon I did as I always do, that is to say, I at once abandoned theories and hypothesis, to observe and study the fact itself, so as to define the experimental conditions as precisely as possible. To-day my experiments on the vascular and thermo-regulatory nerves have opened a new path for investigation and are the subject of numerous studies which, I hope, may some day yield really important results in physiology and pathology. . . .

3.3
The impact of anaesthesia

Martin S. Pernick, *A Calculus of Suffering. Pain, Professionalism and Anesthesia in Nineteenth-Century America* (New York: Columbia University Press, 1985), pp. 208–21.

Martin S. Pernick, an American historian of medicine, has written about the links between medicine and mass culture, including the dissemination of public health information in film. His work is also concerned with the role of values and ethics in medicine. His book, *A Calculus of Suffering*, does not share earlier historians' assumptions that the arrival of anaesthesia brought immediate benefit to all. Using patient records from American hospitals, Pernick reveals the complex factors shaping the use of anaesthetics in the mid-nineteenth century. For example, he demonstrates that not all patients were equally likely to receive anaesthetics. Pernick's

---

[15] The cervical sympathetic nerves originate from the cervical region of the spinal cord.

work is based on American records but all the evidence suggests that the introduction of anaesthesia to Europe followed a similar pattern.

From the nineteenth-century cartoonist who portrayed 'Furor Operativus'[16] to the latest histories of nineteenth-century American medicine, most observers have suspected that anesthetics created an enormous boom in surgery. Nineteenth-century surgeons generally shared in this assessment. The *Annual Report* of the Massachusetts General Hospital in January 1848 declared that the discovery of ether 'greatly increased the actual number of operations,' a judgment seconded by John Collins Warren. Fear that ether had provoked an irresponsible spree of unnecessary procedures was a major concern of those who felt there was already too much art and not enough nature in surgery. Critics of the supposed epidemic of surgery brought on by anesthesia included natural healers like the hydropaths,[17] as well as influential conservative surgeons like Henry J. Bigelow. Bigelow feared that 'the annihilation of pain' would upset the careful conservative balance between benefits and risks. . . . As early as March 1847, British surgeon Tyler Smith observed a 'general rush towards the operating room' he attributed to ether.

But there is a major conceptual problem in interpreting these charges that anesthesia led to a proliferation of surgery. Do such claims accurately reflect a real increase in surgery, or do they simply reflect the growing hostility of midcentury observers toward an unchanged number of operations? How much did surgery really increase after 1846, and to what extent was anesthesia responsible for this increase? The few attempts to document the actual yield of this surgical harvest have been very inadequate. In one recent effort, William G. Rothstein calculated that, before anesthesia, the Massachusetts General Hospital performed 6.2 amputations annually, while after anesthesia, the figure rose to 20.7. This 'much more frequent' resort to the knife, he implied, was due largely to ether.

Such evidence is very inconclusive. First, there is no reason to assume that changes in the tiny number of amputations really reflected changes in the treatment of the overwhelming majority of surgical patients for whom removal of a limb was never contemplated. Second, even in the limited realm of amputations these data are almost

---

[16] A cartoon showing doctors operating on patients with a pile of coffins – illustrating the widely-held view that surgeons were 'experimenting', with the loss of patients' lives.

[17] *hydropaths*: a sect of unorthodox healers who believed that cold water, applied by baths, showers and wrapping the body in wet sheets, would restore a natural balance of heat in the body and thus cure disease. The practice flourished in the late nineteenth century.

worthless because they use 1850 rather than 1846 as the dividing line between the pre-anesthetic and postanesthetic eras and because they are based on the entire timespan from the founding of the hospital in 1821 until the Civil War. Use of such a long time period is highly suspect because any number of other events besides Morton's discovery[18] that occurred in those years might have altered the number of operations performed. Among the changes that might explain a rise in amputations, the most obvious are the rapid growth of Boston's population, especially following the Irish famine migration of 1848; the enormous increase in serious injuries due to the growth of railroads and industry; and the expansion of the hospital with the opening of its new wing in 1847 . . .

On the other hand, developments such as the growing acceptance of conservative professional standards during the 1830s and thereafter may well have helped hold down the total number of amputations performed and thus made Rothstein's estimate of the impact of anesthesia too low.

Nineteenth-century attempts to measure the influence of anesthesia on the rate of surgery suffered from this same inability to control for the effects of other changes. . . .

It is possible, however, to distinguish the effects of anesthetics from the effects of other events that might have influenced the number of operations performed at the Massachusetts General Hospital. . . . By controlling for the total number of patients and by examining only the year before and the year after Morton's discovery, the influence of extraneous variables on the rate of surgery can be minimized. The results show that there was indeed a sharp and sudden increase in surgery at Massachusetts General immediately following the introduction of anesthesia, independent of the simultaneous large increase in the overall number of patients. Before October 16, 1846, less than 16 percent of patients on the surgical wards received any operative treatment. After that date, almost 40 percent of those admitted went under the knife. Thus, the rate of surgery per admission considerably more than doubled. By contrast, at the Pennsylvania Hospital, where anesthesia came into use much more gradually and on a much more limited scale than in Boston, there was no such increase in the operation rate, at least among fracture cases. New York Hospital, which fell between its Boston and Philadelphia counterparts in its adoption of anesthesia, experienced an intermediate upsurge in operations. From June 1845

[18] William Morton (1819–68), a Boston dentist, is one of a number of individuals credited with discovering the anaesthetic properties of ether.

to May 1846, 18 percent of patients admitted underwent surgery; for 1847–48, the figure increased to almost 22 percent.

Of particular interest, the rate of increase in surgery differed greatly for different types of patients. With one minor exception, the boom in surgery at Massachusetts General was most marked among those patients most likely to receive anesthetics: the aged, women, native-born Americans, nonlaborers, and amputees. For example, the increase in major limb amputations following the discovery of ether far exceeded the increase in any other type of surgery. Just before the use of anesthetics, only 1.3 percent of Massachusetts General patients were subjected to the loss of a limb—and the rate of amputation per admission had been *declining* relatively steadily since the 1830s. In the year following the introduction of ether, nearly 7 percent of all patients received amputations, an unprecedented jump of almost five times the previous rate. Put another way, the proportion of amputees among all patients receiving surgery nearly doubled following the introduction of anesthesia. The increase in the frequency of amputations was dramatically larger than that calculated by Rothstein, largely because of his failure to take into account the declining amputation rate and growing conservatism of surgeons between the 1830s and 1846.

Women patients, another group that received anesthetics proportionally more often than other patients, likewise experienced a greater proportional increase in surgery rates following the introduction of ether. Before anesthesia, about 16 percent of all patients got operations, with no noticeable difference between the sexes. After ether, one-third of the men but more than one-half of the women were subjected to surgery. Thus, while the rate of surgery for men doubled following the discovery of anesthesia, the rate for women more than tripled. In other words, women received a much larger share of the total number of operations after anesthesia than before (controlling for admissions).

Less dramatic, but still marked, was the proportional rise in the rate of surgery on native-born Americans. Before anesthesia, Massachusetts General surgeons operated on American- and foreign-born patients at roughly the same rate. But following Morton's innovation, surgery became 1.5 times as common on natives as on immigrants. While the rate of surgery for immigrants doubled, the rate for natives almost tripled. Nonlaborers too received slightly more than their share of the increase in surgery.

Thus the rate of surgery did increase enormously following the introduction of anesthesia, and the increase was most marked for those types of patients most likely to receive anesthetics.

[. . .]

Nineteenth-century critics and modern historians not only claimed that surgery increased following anesthesia but also that this increase was unjustifiable and unnecessary. Many observers feared that anesthesia had unleashed a horde of knife-happy experimenters, eager for fame and experience, who performed needless and incompetent surgery on their helpless victims. The rise in operations on women in particular seemed to confirm the worst fears of medical nihilists, surgical conservatives, feminists, and moralists, all of whom saw anesthesia as giving vent to the profession's 'lust for operating.'

Such charges actually contained a number of separate elements; it is best to examine them one at a time. First, to what extent did the use of anesthesia contribute to a rise in experimental or unproven types of operations? In the case of gynecology there is evidence that anesthesia did indeed lead to more new and untested operations. The rise in ovariotomies is perhaps the most dramatic case in point. In this operation, a woman's sex organs were removed, either as the result of a specific physical lesion or for the cure of general systemic and emotional problems. Before 1846, ovariotomy had been done only as an heroic last resort, limited to cases of life-threatening tumors. Perhaps 100 had been performed in the entire history of medicine. With the discovery of anesthesia, the practice of ovariotomy expanded enormously. Between 1849 and 1878, Dr. Washington L. Atlee alone removed the ovaries of 385 women. Many of these were frankly experimental operations, and while most were the result of painful or life-threatening tumors, a few were ventures in 'normal ovariotomy.' Not surprisingly, Atlee was among the first gynecologists to use surgical anesthetics. His colleague Augustus K. Gardner of New York, an even more outspoken advocate of experimental gynecological surgery, was also a pioneer of anesthesia, who claimed to have been the first New York physician to use chloroform in obstretrics. 'I have no doubt that the use of anaesthesia will strip [ovariotomy] of most of its dangers, and render it simple and safe . . .,' Atlee wrote in 1849. Anesthesia itself had been an experiment; thus it is not too surprising that many of its earliest users conducted other experiments as well.

Without anesthesia, the number and scope of surgical experiments undertaken by Atlee, Gardner, and others would have been conceivable only in an extermination camp. One British text of 1859 went so far as to claim that 'our large and tedious plastic operations[19] in the female, are all the result directly of the discovery of anaesthetics.'

[19] *plastic operations*: i.e. reconstructive operations.

But even with anesthesia, these experiments remained controversial among conservative surgeons, and were infrequently performed by most, before the introduction of antiseptic techniques. At the Massachusetts General Hospital, of the two women diagnosed as having ovarian disease in the year following the discovery of ether, one was dismissed without treatment, even though she demanded an operation. The other was treated by the nonexperimental, noncastrating method of 'tapping.' After two such treatments, she too requested an ovariotomy; upon its 'not being considered prudent' by the surgeons, she was sent home.

In cases of less controversial research, anesthesia also led to a rise in experimentation, even at Massachusetts General. Before 1846, the hospital surgeons had begun to experiment with new techniques in palate, lip, and vaginal fistula repair. Following Morton's discovery, the rate of such experimental surgery increased 1.5 fold. George Hayward attributed the increase in his own vesico-vaginal fistula experiments to the availability of ether.

However, the rate of increased experimentation ran considerably behind the overall increase in surgery. While experiments grew 1.5 fold, the overall rate of surgery more than doubled. Thus, ether did increase the number of experiments, but not by as much as it increased the frequency of surgery in general. Consequently, minor experimental surgery constituted a smaller share of the total number of operations performed after anesthesia than before (controlling for admissions). The major reason anesthesia did not increase the proportion of such minor experimental surgery may well have been the fact that anesthesia was usually contraindicated for minor surgery in general and for mouth operations in particular.

Thus, while the discovery of anesthesia did lead to a rise in untested operations by some surgeons, the increase in hospital experimentation was less than the increase in routine surgery. Experimental operations remained an insignificant segment of the overall postanesthetic upsurge in hospital surgery.

A second and more subtle criticism of the postanesthetic surgical boom was that painlessness prompted operations on patients who would have recovered equally well without such interference. For example, nineteenth-century critics and some recent historians have pictured a postanesthetic world in which every bruise or fracture was likely to prompt amputation. But before judging whether the increase in surgery after 1846 was 'necessary,' it is important to remember that the midcentury profession was bitterly divided over the standards by which to judge the legitimacy, value, and 'necessity' of surgery. Opponents of surgery, including the more dogmatic hydropaths, homeopaths, and therapeutic nihilists, regarded almost all operations as unnatural and unnecessary. At the opposite pole, heroic surgeons saw the scalpel as a saber with which to lead the charge against the ramparts of disease. Thus, nineteenth-century criticisms must be seen in context; the very same operation that one doctor called legitimate and necessary, might be denounced by another as excessive and irresponsible. Furthermore, by making operations less distasteful and easier to perform, anesthesia probably further muddled the definition of surgical necessity.

This nineteenth-century debate over the standards of surgical legitimacy makes any assessment of the postanesthetic surgical boom more interesting and more difficult for the historian. The task is compounded by the fact that our own standards of what constitutes 'necessary' surgery are very controversial; witness our current concern over 'second opinions' for elective surgery and over what types of operations ought to be covered by medical insurance.

In one sense, of course, the question is unanswerable—no one can say for sure what would have happened if an operation that was in fact performed had not taken place. But by looking at the experiences of large enough groups of patients with similar medical conditions, it is possible to make some likely inferences. A variety of such evidence indicates that, at the Massachusetts General Hospital, the introduction of ether was followed by a dramatic increase in the proportion of surgery that was performed on those patients who were least likely to recover on their own. In that sense, it may be said that these operations were not unnecessary.

One good indication of this trend is the treatment of emergency and acute injury cases. Through almost all of the nineteenth century, such victims were universally regarded as the single class of patients most likely to die. They generally had the poorest prognosis for recovery regardless of treatment, because they were the most susceptible to infection and to shock. For example, at the Massachusetts General Hospital in the year before Morton's discovery, acute and emergency cases accounted for almost two-thirds of all deaths, though they comprised less than one-third of the patients admitted.

Before the introduction of anesthesia these emergency patients were generally seen as too seriously ill to warrant any surgical treatment. During 1845–46, the Massachusetts General Hospital operated on only 4 of the 66 emergency and acute surgical admissions. Once anesthesia became available, the operation rate on this group of patients jumped to almost 1 in 4. The rate of surgery for emergency cases virtually quadrupled, while the rate for others increased only 2.4 times. In other words, emergency cases made up a much larger share of the surgery done after anesthesia (controlling for admissions) than before. Thus, the sharpest increase in the rate of surgery took place on the class of patients generally recognized to be the least likely to recover on their own. And, following ether, these 'sickest' patients accounted for a greatly increased proportion of the total number of operations performed.

An unnecessary operation may also be defined as one more extensive in scope than 'necessary.' In this sense, many nineteenth-century surgeons insisted that ether actually decreased the amount of unnecessary surgery. Anesthesia made more practical the prolonged and intricate conservative procedures required to preserve limbs a preanesthetic surgeon would have simply cut off. Many practitioners claimed anesthesia enabled them to substitute bone excisions and resections for amputations,[20] Caesarian section for craniotomy,[21] and so on. But while the conquest of pain made such operations feasible, the available records suggest that they became only slightly more common in practice.

In summary, the development of anesthesia probably increased the proportion of operations done on the sickest patients—those least likely to recover without surgery. In that sense, charges that the increase in surgery was unnecessary are not justified.

But this conclusion is not the same as saying that the increased number of operations did anything to *help* those on whom they were performed. Perhaps, for example, surgeons began to operate more frequently on the sickest patients merely because they regarded such hopeless cases as expendable material for teaching and for practicing their technique. There are two logically separate and distinct issues. Having shown that anesthesia led to a disproportionate increase in operations on people likely to die without aid, we must next judge whether these operations prevented or speeded the deaths of their recipients. Even if postanesthetic surgeons operated only on the sickest patients, their operations may still have been 'unjustified' in the sense of worsening rather than improving the recipients' already slim chances for recovery. . . .

The third, and most serious criticism leveled against the additional surgery that followed the introduction of anesthesia was that it increased the surgical death rate. Many mid-nineteenth-century professional and lay periodicals agreed that death resulted from the immediate

---

[20] *excisions and resections*: conservative operations involving the removal of small amounts of bone in order to preserve limb function.

[21] *craniotomy*: the operation to remove a foetus from the birth canal by breaking the bones of the skull, in order to save the life of the mother. It was used only as a last resort.

effects of inhaling chloroform in 1 of every 2,500 to 10,000 cases; ether deaths were variously given in the range of 1 in every 10,000 to 30,000. However, some surgeons suspected the long-term effects of anesthesia might be far more serious. Virtually all the published mid-nineteenth-century American hospital statistics indicated that, following the introduction of anesthesia, more patients died from surgery than ever before. Summarizing printed data on operations performed between 1821 and 1850 at hospitals in Boston, New York, and Philadelphia, Dr. FitzWilliam Sargent placed the death rate at 27.6 percent for nonanesthetized amputations and 32.3 percent for amputees who received an anesthetic—an additional 5 deaths in every 100 operations, due to anesthesia.

Recent historians have accepted such statistics at face value. William Rothstein repeated an 1864 report that claimed to show that the Massachusetts General Hospital amputation mortality rose from 19 percent before ether to 23 percent afterward—that is, an additional 4 deaths in every 100 operations due to the anesthetic. On the basis of similar sources, John Duffy concluded that the increase in surgery following anesthesia 'was not immediately beneficial to patients.'

Nineteenth-century explanations of why anesthesia should have increased surgical mortality varied and have changed further since then. Most observers then and now agreed that the additional deaths were from infection and/or shock, but there the agreement ends. Many antebellum surgeons tended to blame the anesthetic itself for lowering the patients' 'vitality.' Other midcentury observers, however, claimed that anesthesia had made doctors overeager, careless, and sloppy.

With the gradual acceptance of antiseptic techniques and the germ theory of disease in the late nineteenth century, the explanation for these deaths changed. The modern interpretation, first stated by John Collins Warren's grandson, stresses the fact that antebellum surgeons lacked understanding of the causes of infection. Mid-nineteenth-century surgeons would operate on several patients in a row, using the same instruments, often without even pausing to wash. The more operations done, the less likely it was that even rudimentary sanitary precautions would be taken; thus the opportunity for the spread of germs was greater. By boosting the amount of surgery performed, the development of anesthesia supposedly led to a higher surgical infection rate.

But despite the seeming impressiveness of this explanation, the evidence on which it rests is very thin. None of the figures purporting to show an increase in deaths after anesthesia is statistically significant. Careful reexamination of the data leads to the conclusion that the introduction of anesthesia had little or no effect on the death rate from surgery, and that it actually lowered the overall death rate from serious injuries by making it possible to perform life-saving operations on patients who would otherwise have died untreated.

As already pointed out, nineteenth-century printed statistics on anesthetic use contain two enormous flaws. First, they cover the entire period from 1821 to the 1850s or 1860s. Second, they make little or no attempt to assess the role of other important changes taking place in those years, inside and outside the hospital. Anesthesia certainly was not the only new development of the 1840s that could have contributed to a higher surgical death rate. The most important of these other considerations was undoubtedly industrialization.

Nineteenth-century surgeons were uniformly horrified by the grisly body count of the industrial revolution. 'Everyone who has had frequent occasion to amputate for railroad accidents,' knew that 'a wheel of a locomotive engine or railway car. . . . in most instances produces a compound and comminuted fracture of the worst kind,' according to George Hayward of Massachusetts General. George W. Norris of the Pennsylvania Hospital agreed that 'the most desperate kind' of surgery was that 'resulting from railroad accidents, machinery, &c.' Norris did not know any bacteriology, but he recognized that the extreme tissue damage caused by industrial accidents made infection far more likely in such injuries than in any other type of surgery. Midcentury hospital reports often listed 'R. R. accident' and 'machinery' as separate categories of disease, distinguished from all other types of accidents and other causes of surgery.

Railroads, factories, and anesthetics appeared at virtually the same time in American urban history. Noting this coincidence, a few medical observers suspected that ether might be getting the blame for deaths actually the result of industrial accidents. Samuel D. Gross absolved anesthesia and attributed the rise in surgical death rates to the 'fearful increase in railway and other terrible accidents, many of which are necessarily fatal, no matter to what treatment they may be subjected.' The records of the Massachusetts General Hospital lend strong support to Gross' explanation. If the accident cases are separated from the others, it becomes clear that the introduction of anesthesia made almost no difference in the surgical death rate; indeed there seems to have been a very slight downturn in operative mortality.

Both before and after anesthesia, between 1821 and 1850, accident victims died at nearly four times the rate of any other amputees. But, between 1821 and 1846, accidents had caused only one-third of all amputations; after 1846 they accounted for fully half of the limbs lost. Between 1849 and 1854, the percentage of hospital admissions due to accidents more than doubled. Over the entire antebellum era, the proportion of accident victims among patients increased steadily each year.

In the most sophisticated nineteenth-century analysis of postanesthetic death rates, Dr. Samuel Fenwick of Newcastle, England, also found that accidents, not anesthesia, explained the rise in surgical mortality. He examined the records of Newcastle Infirmary for 1823 to 1856 and reported that anesthesia lowered the disease-amputation death rate, from 19 to 13 percent and the trauma-amputation death rate from 32 to 31 percent. Fenwick's results were largely unknown in the United States. But his data seem to confirm that it was the growing seriousness of the injuries, and not the use of ether or the growing number of operations per se, that most likely accounts for the rise in surgical mortality. *Punch* was more accurate than he could possibly have realized when he joked, in January 1847, 'The establishment of the fact that surgical operations may be performed without pain has been properly described as "Good News for Travelers by Railway." '

[Data from the Massachusetts General Hospital] and Dr. Fenwick's study still probably under-estimate the life-saving value of postanesthetic surgery. These data cover only deaths following surgery—patients who died after an operation are counted, but those allowed to die without surgery are omitted. As we have seen, however, after the introduction of ether, doctors began to operate more often on people whom they previously had considered too seriously injured for surgery. This new willingness to operate on such high-risk cases probably led to more deaths following *surgery* but fewer deaths overall. Unfortunately, the available evidence is too slim either to confirm this explanation or to rule it out. Among the very worst injuries—compound fractures— the overall death rate for all patients admitted did drop from 40 percent to 32 percent at the Massachusetts General following the introduction of anesthesia, but the number of cases was far too small for statistical significance.

In summary, the evidence examined so far suggests that, following the discovery of anesthesia, operations previously done largely on the strongest and most insensitive patients could now be done on those formerly regarded as too delicate, such as women, old people, and badly injured accident victims. The result was an overall increase in surgery, including some additional experimental operations and some undoubtedly unnecessary interventions. But these latter cases were proportionally rarer after anesthesia than before.

The growing frequency of operations did not cause the rise in the surgical death rate; the more frequent resort to surgery in fact may have saved a number of lives that would otherwise have been lost. It was the industrial revolution, and the growing ability of surgeons to operate on previously hopeless cases, not increased careless or unnecessary surgery, that accounted for the rise in surgical deaths following 1846.

Yet, if anesthesia did improve the ability of surgeons to save lives, the numbers could not have been very great. And while statistics can measure the quantity of life saved, they tell us nothing about the quality of that life. Did the increase in surgery following 1846 enable more people to return to useful happy lives, or did it produce agonized invalids? On this question the records are silent. And while anesthesia may have saved some lives, its major influence was not in the area of life and death but in the removal of pain, an advantage that is not directly measurable.

Despite our conclusions to the contrary, the historical fact remains that many mid-nineteenth-century American physicians thought anesthetic surgery did kill about 5 percent more patients than nonanesthetic operations did. Whereas present-day detective work reveals their conclusions to have been wrong, these original statistical reports are still vital to an understanding of nineteenth-century attitudes toward anesthetics and the importance of pain. Even though their figures may have been erroneous, the early reports provide an invaluable measure of the risk nineteenth-century physicians *thought* they were running by using anesthetics. While a few anti-utilitarians like Meigs considered even 1 death in 10,000 too many to justify anesthesia, Sargent's data indicate that most practitioners considered even a 5 percent increase in the risk of death an acceptable price to pay for avoiding the pain of amputation. Thus, nineteenth-century mortality reports, while inaccurate from our viewpoint, provide an excellent indirect measure of the relative value midcentury surgeons placed on the prevention of pain when weighed against risk to life; they provide a numerical solution to the calculus of suffering.

3.4

Surgery and research

Emil Theodor Kocher, 'Concerning Pathological
Manifestations in Low-Grade Thyroid Diseases', Nobel
Lecture, 11 December 1909, in *Nobel Lectures, Including
Presentation Speeches and Laureates' Biographies.
Physiology or Medicine, 1901–1921* (Amsterdam, London
and New York, Elsevier Publishing Company, 1967),
pp. 330–1.

Emil Kocher (1841–1917) was Professor of Surgery and head of
the University Clinic in Berne, Switzerland. He was famous for his
pioneering operation to remove the thyroid gland, and had a particular interest in surgical infections. He was an enthusiastic fol-
lower of the aseptic principles proposed by Joseph Lister. Kocher
published papers on experimental and clinical work in many surgical fields and in orthopaedics. He received the Nobel Prize for
Medicine in 1909 for his work on the physiology, pathology and
surgery of the thyroid gland. The extract is from his Nobel lecture,
given in December 1909.

Pasteur's investigations . . . [22] into the cause of the fermentation of wine,
and his findings in connection with this concerning the processes of
decomposition in general, have prepared the ground for the greatest,
and certainly the most beneficent, advance in Medicine. From Lister's[23]
spirit of inquiry originated the idea of applying to human pathology, in
a way that was as simple as it was ingenious, Pasteur's concepts about
the importance of the smallest organisms in the decomposition of
liquids: he studied the decomposition of urine under the influence of the
dust particles in atmospheric air and established, using measures that
have now been long abandoned, that the fluids in human wounds, the
so-called wound exudate, was also preserved from decomposition by
keeping dust away; and, as a result of this, healing of wounds took place
with a hitherto unknown speed and reliability.

The results of Pasteur's and Lister's investigations, which sprang from
practical requirements and purely clinical observations, have shown

[22] Louis Pasteur (1822–96) was one of the great pioneers of bacteriology.
[23] Joseph Lister (1827–1912) developed antiseptic techniques to prevent wound infection,
especially after surgery.

themselves to be more fruitful than one would have ever dreamed possible, thanks to the energetic cooperation of numerous investigators (among whom R. Koch on the theoretical side and R. Volkmann on the practical side are outstanding).

The first powerful advance was, it is true, a practical one. Surgical treatment underwent a vast expansion, as not only could the dangers be eliminated within the province of treatment for accidental wounds, which had been under the care of the surgeons till then, but also a surgical method of treatment, which was crowned by the most brilliant cures, was made possible in the great majority of the so-called internal diseases. It has become possible within less than half a century to expose all the organs of the body, brain and heart not excepted, without danger, and carry out the necessary surgical measures on them.

But it was just this ability to make all the organs accessible to direct observation, and to alter the conditions in which they exercise their functions, that broadened our knowledge of the *physiology* of the body extraordinarily. The physiologists have even learned from the surgeons to set up their animal experiments under the influence of narcosis[24] and asepsis[25] in such a way that unnecessary pain during, and disturbances after the operation do not occur, and the physiological activities of the organs can be brought to light without any distortion at all. It is only necessary to recall the amazing results concerning the function of the organs of digestion obtained by Pavlov,[26] whose merits have also been duly acknowledged in this place.

It was also due to strict asepsis that one of the most serious, and, before Lister, most dangerous operations could be undertaken without substantial risk, that is the removal of a goitrous thyroid,[27] which so often proves urgently necessary on account of severe respiratory disturbances. We ourselves have communicated a continuous series of 300 and more goitre operations without a fatality. Important though this result has been for suffering humanity, yet it has been far exceeded by the understanding which has grown, anew on practical and clinical soil, concerning the vital *physiological* function of the thyroid. It is true that Schiff, the physiologist, had already initiated experiments into the acute ill effects of thyroid withdrawal in dogs, but they have been disregarded. They were in fact communicated merely incidently in an

[24] *narcosis*: a loss of sensation or consciousness due to the application of a narcotic.

[25] *asepsis*: a set of techniques used in modern surgery based on the idea of preventing any contact between the body and bacteria.

[26] Ivan Pavlov (1849–1936), Russian physiologist, famous for his experiments on conditional or learned reflexes, which showed the physiological response to various stimuli.

[27] *goitrous thyroid*: a condition in which the thyroid gland becomes greatly enlarged.

essay on sugar formation in the liver (1859). With the passage of time it has become clear that these effects were essentially related to the parathyroid glands, and proved that the lack of these is not compatible with life. Schiff himself only really understood the significance of his experiments and extended them further with more exhaustive investigations, after our communications had appeared. Early in 1883, at the Congress of the Deutsche Gesellschaft für Chirurgie we announced that some 30 of our first 100 patients operated on for goitre, whom we were able to follow up and reinvestigate, presented a syndrome which can be precisely characterized, and which we designated simply with the name *cachexia strumipriva*. This appeared in a well-marked form only in those patients from whom we had removed the whole thyroid, and on the other hand only with temporary manifestations in those in whom the whole goitrous structure was supposed to have been removed, but where in fact a portion had remained, which continued to grow.

Part four

The role of the laboratory

4.1
The power of the laboratory

Claude Bernard, *An Introduction to the Study of
Experimental Medicine* (trans. H.C. Greene)
(New York, Dover publications, 1957; first edn 1865),
pp. 142–3, 145–9.

Claude Bernard (1813–78) was an eminent pioneer of experimental physiology, who developed new techniques of animal experimentation to investigate problems including the physiology of the blood and the localised action of drugs. This essay was an extended argument for the importance of laboratory research as scientific basis of medicine.

[S]cience, which stands for what man has learned, is essentially mobile in expression; it varies and perfects itself in proportion to the increase of acquired knowledge. Present day science is therefore necessarily higher than the science of the past; and there is no sort of reason for going in search of any addition to modern science through knowledge of the ancients. Their theories, necessarily false because they do not include facts discovered since then, can be of no real advantage to contemporary science. No experimental science, then, can make progress except by advancing and pursuing its work in the future. . . .

[W]e need not ourselves be poets or artists to judge literary or artistic work, but this is not true of experimental science. We cannot judge of a memoir on chemistry without being chemists nor of a memoir on physiology if we are not physiologists. In deciding between two different scientific opinions . . . we must above all be deeply versed in technical science; we must even be masters of the special science and ourselves be able to experiment and do better than the men whose opinions we discuss. Some time ago I discussed an anatomical question concerning the anastomoses[1] of the pneumogastric and spinal nerves. Willis, Scarpa and Bischoff had expressed different and even opposite opinions on this subject. A mere scholar could only have quoted these various opinions and more or less correctly compared the texts; that would not have answered the scientific question. It was therefore necessary to dissect . . . and to compare each anatomist's description with nature. This is what I did, and I found that the difference between the authors in question came from their not having assigned the same limits to the nerves. So anatomy, carried further, explained their anatomical dissension. . . . To be really useful, criticism in every science must be done by men of science themselves, and by the most eminent masters.

[. . .]

The experimental point of view is a coronation of perfected science; for we must not deceive ourselves; true science exists only when man succeeds in accurately foreseeing the phenomena of nature and mastering them. Noting and classifying natural bodies and phenomena is not at all the equivalent of complete science. True science acts and explains its action or its power: that is its character, that is its aim. . . .

The spirit of man follows a necessary and logical course in the search for scientific truth. It observes facts, compares them, deduces appropriate results which it controls by experiment, to rise to more and more general propositions and truths. In this advancing labor, a man of science must, of course, know and deal with his predecessors' work. But he must be thoroughly convinced that this work is merely a support from which to go farther, and that new scientific truths are not to be found in study of the past, but rather in studies made anew on nature, i.e., in the laboratory. Useful scientific literature, then, is preëminently the scientific literature of modern work which enables us to keep up with scientific progress; and even this must not be carried too far, lest it dry up the mind and stifle invention and scientific originality. But what use can we find in exhuming worm-eaten theories or observations made without proper means of investigation? That may, of course, be helpful in learning the mistakes through which the human mind has passed in its evolution, but it is time wasted for science, properly speaking. I deem

---

[1] *anastomoses*: joining together.

it highly important to guide the minds of students early toward active experimental science, by making them understand that it develops in laboratories, instead of leaving them to believe that it awaits them in books or in the interpretation of ancient writings. . . .

A physiological laboratory, therefore, should now be the culminating goal of any scientific physician's studies . . . Hospitals, or rather hospital wards, are not physicians' laboratories, as is often believed: as we said before, these are only his fields for observation; there must be held what we call clinics, i.e., studies of disease as complete as possible. Medicine necessarily begins with clinics, since they determine and define the object of medicine, i.e., the medical problem; but while they are the physician's first study, clinics are not the foundation of scientific medicine; physiology is the foundation of scientific medicine because it must yield the explanation of morbid phenomena by showing their relations to the normal state. We shall never have a science of medicine as long as we separate the explanation of pathological from the explanation of normal, vital phenomena.

Here then lies the real medical problem; this is the foundation on which modern scientific medicine will be built. As we see, experimental medicine does not exclude clinical medicine; on the contrary, it comes only after it. But it is a higher science, and one necessarily more vast and general. We easily imagine how an observational or empirical physician, never leaving his hospital, may think medicine completely shut in there, as a science distinct from physiology, of which it feels no need. But for a man of science there is no separate science of medicine or physiology, there is only a science of life. There are only phenomena of life to be explained in the pathological as well as in the physiological state. By putting this fundamental idea and this general conception of medicine into the minds of young people at the outset of their medical studies, we shall show them that the physico-chemical sciences which they have learned are tools to help them analyze the phenomena of life in its normal and pathological states. In frequenting hospitals, amphitheatres and laboratories, they will easily grasp the general connection uniting all the medical sciences, instead of learning them like fragments of detached knowledge with no relation between them.

In a word, I consider hospitals only as the entrance to scientific medicine; they are the first field of observation which a physician enters; but the true sanctuary of medical science is a laboratory; only there can he seek explanations of life in the normal and pathological states by means of experimental analysis. . . . In my opinion, medicine does not end in hospitals, as is often believed, but merely begins there. In leaving the hospital, a physician, jealous of the title in its scientific sense, must go into his laboratory; and there, by experiments on animals, he will seek to account for what he has observed in his patients, whether about the action of drugs or about the origin of morbid lesions in organs or tissues. There, in a word, he will achieve true medical science. Every scientific physician should, therefore, have a physiological laboratory; and this work is especially intended to give physicians rules and principles of experimentation to guide their study of experimental medicine, that is, their analytic and experimental study of disease. The principles of experimental medicine, then, will be simply the principles of experimental analysis applied to the phenomena of life in its healthy and its morbid states.

[. . .]

[L]et me end by saying that one truth is well established in modern science, namely, that scientific courses can only serve to introduce and to create a taste for the sciences. By pointing out, from a professional chair, the results as well as the methods of a science, a teacher may form the minds of his hearers and make them apt in learning and choosing their own direction; but he can never make them men of science. The laboratory is the real nursery of true experimental scientists, i.e., those who create the science that others afterward popularize. . . . [I]t is to-day everywhere recognized that pure science germinates and develops in laboratories, to spread out later and cover the world with useful applications. We must, therefore, first of all attend to the scientific source, since applied science necessarily proceeds from pure science. . . .

Only laboratories can teach the difficulties of science to those who frequent them; they show that pure science has always been the source of all the riches acquired by man and of all his real conquests over the phenomena of nature. This is also excellent education for the young, because it makes them understand that the present, very brilliant applications of science are merely the blossoming of earlier labors, and that those who reap the benefits to-day owe a tribute of gratitude to their predecessors who painfully cultivated the tree of science, but never saw its fruits.

4.2

Laboratory knowledge

Andrew Cunningham, 'Transforming Plague. The Laboratory
and the Identity of Infectious Disease', in Andrew
Cunningham and Perry Williams (eds), *The Laboratory
Revolution in Medicine* (Cambridge and New York,
Cambridge University Press, 1992), pp. 224–30 [pp. 209–44].

In the 1980s Bruno Latour, a sociologist of science, showed that
the knowledge generated in the laboratory was not 'self-evident' –
scientists had to persuade the public that their findings – produced
in the highly artificial environment of the laboratory – were
relevant to practical problems in hospitals and agriculture. In this
article, Cunningham explores the circumstances surrounding the
generation of one piece of knowledge – the identification of
the bacteria causing plague.

How was plague transformed from a disease whose identity was symp-
tom-based into one whose identity was cause-based? The transformation of the identity of plague took place in the laboratory, and from that
moment on plague would only be identifiable in the laboratory. It is
common to see this event as a simple 'unmasking' or a 'drawing back
the veil' on what had been known all along to be there but which had
hitherto simply evaded the light of science, and that is the language that
was also used by many contemporaries about the event just after it had
happened, and which has been regularly used since. But it was not a
simple 'unmasking'. Instead, the new view of the disease, its new identity, was a *construction* since it involved, and depended totally on, a
new way of thinking and seeing, the laboratory way of thinking and
seeing. . . . The laboratory was the instrument used to attribute responsibility to micro-organisms. Yet the laboratory is never a mere instrument: it is also a *practice* which defines, limits and governs ways of
thinking and seeing. Plague acquired its new identity from this new
activity, this new practice. Therefore the laboratory had to precede,
both in time and conceptually, the 'causative micro-organism' identity
of the disease. It was necessary to take the laboratory to the disease,
and then to take the disease through the laboratory.

The transformation of the identity of plague happened in Hong Kong
in the summer of 1894. Plague broke out in early May, being immedi-

ately identified by the native population, who at once took to flight. The outbreak was of especial interest to those colonial powers with major interests in the region: Britain (the 'lessee' of Hong Kong), France and Japan.

[. . .]

The two investigators who (to use the customary phrase) 'discovered' the plague bacillus in Hong Kong in 1894 were Shibasaburo Kitasato and Alexandre Yersin. The rivalry between [Robert] Koch and [Louis] Pasteur in Europe, on nationalist and scientific grounds, was continued here in Hong Kong by their volunteer champions: the German school of Koch was represented by Kitasato, a Japanese, and the French school of Pasteur by Yersin, a Swiss who had become a naturalised Frenchman. . . .

As Kitasato was a bacteriologist and Yersin was a microbiologist (these were the preferred terms used in their respective German and French schools), on the very first day that they could, they each *looked for* a micro-organism. As Yersin wrote, 'It was obvious that the first thing to do was to see whether there was a microbe in the blood of the patients and in the pulp of the buboes. And in order for them to search for a causative micro-organism it was necessary for each of them to have available to them a *laboratory*: that is, a dedicated space (a room) with special equipment in it. Kitasato, arriving first, made friends with Dr Lowson of the Colonial Medical Service, who 'put everything needful at our disposal in the most friendly spirit. A room in the Kennedy Town Hospital (one of the plague establishments) was given to us, and there we began our work on June 14th.' Yersin, however, was denied space in the Kennedy Town Hospital. . . . But he made friends with a long-established Catholic priest, and was thus able to build a laboratory of his own. As he wrote to his mother on 24 June, 'After having stayed at the hotel for some days, I have built myself a straw hut near the hospital for the plague victims and there I have set up my living quarters and my laboratory. . . .

The equipment to transform inner space into a laboratory each investigator had brought with him. The most important item in a bacteriologist's arsenal was his microscope; it was virtually his emblem of office: indeed when Yersin got off the boat he was carrying his microscope in one hand and his autoclave[2] in the other.

---

[2] *autoclave*: a device for sterilising equipment. This is crucial in bacteriological research, to ensure samples are not contaminated by other bacteria from the environment.

Thus they both arrived, transformed certain areas into laboratories and established themselves inside them, and they both started looking for a causative micro-organism. On the very first day, at the very first autopsy, each of them found one. Kitasato reported:

> On that day we were able to see a post-mortem examination performed by Professor Aoyama [one of the Japanese team]. I found numerous bacilli in the bubo (in this case a swelling of the inguinal[3] glands), in the blood of the heart, in the lungs, liver, spleen, &c.

When Yersin eventually got started with his investigations he too immediately found a candidate micro-organism . . . It was never a problem for Yersin to see the bacillus: 'I always find it; for me there is no doubt.'

Looking down his microscope each man could see a micro-organism of a particular known form (rod-like, i.e. a bacillus) but with its own unusual and distinctive properties. It could be uniquely characterised in the laboratory according to its motility,[4] staining reactions and behaviour when cultivated, and these characteristics gave it its unique identity, making it distinguishable from all other micro-organisms. This unique identity was described by each investigator. Kitasato's micro-organisms

> are rods with rounded ends, which are readily stained by the ordinary analine dyes, the poles being stained darker than the middle part, especially in blood preparations, and presenting a capsule sometimes well marked, sometimes indistinct . . . I am at present unable to say whether or not 'Gram's double-staining method' can be employed . . . The bacilli show very little movement, and those grown in the incubator, in beef-tea, make the medium somewhat cloudy.

Yersin's micro-organisms were

> short, stubby bacilli which are rather easy to stain with analine dyes and are not stained by the method of Gram. The ends of the bacilli are colored more strongly than the center. Sometimes the bacilli seem to be surrounded by a capsule . . . In broth, the bacillus has a very characteristic appearance resembling that of the erysipelas[5] culture: clear liquid with lumps depositing on the walls and bottom of the tube.

Both investigators thought that the bacillus they had found was the causative agent of plague that they had come to Hong Kong to find. But before their rod-shaped micro-organisms, their bacilli, could be deter-

---

[3] *inguinal*: the groin. Buboes or swellings of the lymph glands in the armpit and groin were one of the characteristic symptoms of plague.

[4] *motility*: ability to move spontaneously.

[5] *erisypelas*: a serious streptococcal infection, causing bright red patches on the skin.

mined to be the causative agent of plague, they had to be put to and pass certain other tests, which both investigators employed. These were the tests to fulfil 'Koch's postulates'[6] Kitasato wrote, 'I still had doubts about the true significance of what I found; I therefore made a cultivation . . .' This was the first test he applied: could his bacillus be cultivated artificially, would it grow in a pure form outside the human body? Kitasato found that it would:

> The growth of the bacilli is strongest on blood serum at the normal temperature of the human body (37 °C): under these conditions they develop luxuriantly and are moist in consistence and of a yellowish grey colour; they do not liquefy the serum. On agar-agar jelly (the best is good glycerine agar) they also grow freely. The different colonies are of a whitish-grey colour and by a reflected light have a bluish appearance; under the microscope they appear moist and in rounded patches with uneven edges . . . If a cover-glass preparation is made from a cultivation on agar-agar, and, after having been stained, is observed under the microscope long threads of bacilli are seen.

Yersin too had success in making his bacillus grow in pure cultures outside the body:

> The pulp of buboes, seeded on agar, gives rise to transparent, white colonies, with margins that are iridescent when examined with reflected light. Growth is even better if glycerol is incorporated into the agar. The bacillus also grows on coagulated serum . . . Microscopical examination of the cultures reveals true chains of short bacilli interspersed with larger spherical bodies.

Once each bacillus had been successfully cultivated there was a second test to be made, the test on live animals. Kitasato mainly used the experimental animal which Koch had made indispensable, the white mouse:

> The mice, which were inoculated on the first day with a piece of spleen and some blood from the finger-tips [of the first corpse post-mortemed by Professor Aoyama], died in two days' time, and at the post-mortem examination upon them I found oedema[7] round the place of inoculation, and the same bacilli in the blood, in the internal organs, and in the oedematous part around the place of inoculation. All animals which had been inoculated with the cultivations (pigeons excepted) died after periods extending from one to four days, according to the size of the animal. The same

---

[6] A series of rules, devised by Robert Koch, to prove that an organism was the cause of disease.

[7] *oedema*: a swelling due to the collection of fluid under the skin.

state of the organs after death and the same bacteriological observations always obtained as in the case of the mice.

Yersin too turned to animals to test whether his bacillus was the true causative micro-organism of plague. He found it was.

> If one inoculates mice, rats or guinea pigs with the pulp from buboes, they die, and at autopsy one can note the characteristic lesions as well as numerous bacilli in the lymph nodes, spleen and blood. Guinea pigs die in 2 to 5 days, mice in 1 to 3 days.

So when the bacillus was inoculated into healthy animals it produced 'the characteristic lesions'; it killed the animals in a few days; it produced 'the same state of organs after death', and 'the same bacilli' were found in the blood and in the internal organs of the dead animals.

The third test each bacillus had to pass was whether it was present in all cases of the disease. Kitasato found that his bacillus was indeed always present (well, almost always):

> Every day I took blood from many plague patients and examined it, and almost every time I found the bacilli as above described, sometimes in great numbers, sometimes only few in number . . . On the other hand, these same bacilli were to be found at every post-mortem examination (of which we had upwards of fifteen) in great quantity in the bubonic swellings, in the spleen, the lungs, the liver, in the blood contained in the heart, in the brain, intestines – in fact, in all internal organs without exception – and every cultivation from any particle of these parts invariably produced the same bacilli.

Yersin too found his bacillus everywhere present in the body of humans or animals suffering from the plague: 'The pulp of the buboes always contains masses of short, stubby, bacilli . . . One can find them in large numbers in the buboes and the lymph nodes of the diseased persons', and in inoculated animals 'at autopsy, one recovers the bacillus from the blood, the liver, the spleen and the lymph nodes'.

Yersin, as a true Pasteurian, subjected his bacillus to one further question: did it exist naturally in, or could it be cultivated into, forms with lesser virulence, and which could thus be used to give animals and humans immunity against the plague? Kitasato, as a true Kochian, asked and answered a different final question: 'What means are to be employed against the plague? – preventive measures, general hygiene, good drainage, perfect water-supply, cleanliness in dwelling-houses, and cleanliness in the streets.'

The bacillus that Kitasato found and the bacillus that Yersin found passed all the tests of Koch. 'From this evidence', wrote Kitasato, 'we must come to the conclusion that this bacillus is the cause of the disease known as the bubonic plague; therefore the bubonic plague is an infectious disease produced by a specific bacillus'. Yersin concluded similarly that 'Plague is thus a contagious and transmissible disease', whose cause is the bacillus he had found.

As soon as they were each certain that they had discovered the causal micro-organism of plague, each of them got into print as quickly as possible. Yersin, typically for a Pasteurian, placed his report in the *Annales de l'Institut Pasteur*. Kitasato, however, had been befriended by the British Dr Lowson, who encouraged him to let him translate his original German text into English and to send it to London to be published in *The Lancet*. Yersin and Kitasato sent not just descriptions of their successful hunt for 'the causative micro-organism' of plague but, most importantly, pictures. What was portrayed in these pictures was not the *symptoms* – the patients suffering the disease – but the *microbe*, a thing which could only be seen down the microscope. And the message of these pictures is this: 'here is the micro-organism = here is the disease (plague)'. They had taken into their laboratories a disease whose identity was constituted by symptoms; they had emerged with a disease whose identity was constituted by its causal agent.

After Kitasato and Yersin had each found their plague bacillus, the tiny micro-organism was given its new scientific name. That name was in Latin. Hitherto what had been named in Latin or Greek was the disease (*pestis*); henceforth it was the micro-organism. The name given to the micro-organism directly expresses its causal relation to the disease. Its first name was *Bacterium pestis*, the bacterium of the plague. In 1900 it was renamed *Bacillus pestis* the bacillus of the plague. From 1923 it was called *Pasteurella pestis*, which is short for 'the Pasteur-genus causative micro-organism of the plague'. A new genus, *Yersinia*, was proposed in 1954, and today the bacillus is increasingly referred to as *Yersinia pestis*, the 'Yersin-genus causative micro-organism of plague'. (Evidently the Pasteurians won the naming contest over the Kochians.)

4.3

The rationale for the laboratory

Richard L. Kremer, 'Building Institutes for Physiology in
Prussia, 1836–1846. Contexts, Interests and Rhetoric',
in Andrew Cunningham and Perry Williams (eds),
The Laboratory Revolution in Medicine (Cambridge and
New York, Cambridge University Press, 1992), pp. 89–100
[pp. 72–109].

Richard Kremer has worked on the history of the biomedical
sciences in France and Germany. In this study, he shows that
researchers could not assume that German states – often portrayed
as generous patrons of laboratory science – would pay for new
facilities and chairs. Instead, researchers had to make a good case
for laboratories. This article explores three proposals for new physiological institutions submitted by three researchers. They show
the range of functions claimed for the laboratory. Jan Purkyně
(1787–1869), then working in Breslau, became famous for his
research into the microscopic anatomy of the brain. Karl Heinrich
Schultz (1798–1871) was a botanist and physiologist in the faculty
at Berlin when he submitted his proposals. Julius Budge (1811–88)
was an assistant professor at Bonn.

Among the three proposals to create physiological institutes, Purkyně's
rhetorical strategy of 1836, richly developed in a lengthy twenty-seven-
page memorandum . . . is undoubtedly the most complex. Purkyně's
1836 manifesto reflects a strategy of caution, as if he did not want to
appear too radical in seeking to establish a new institution for physiological teaching and research.

Physiology needed such an institute, Purkyně began, because the
subject (*Fach*) had undergone massive change. In some earlier unspec-
ified time, physiologists had engaged primarily in 'idle speculations' and
'literary-philosophical' disputation. The subject had been 'discursive', a
'lecture doctrine [*Kathederdoktrin*] which dealt only with disputable
concepts', an 'axiomatic teaching method'. It had floated between the
extremes of 'intellectual [*geistige*] commentary on anatomy' and
the 'otherworldly independence of *Naturphilosophie*'. But recently,
continued Purkyně, citing no specific examples, physiology had left
those heights for an 'earthly and material but living and organic home'.

It had become a 'demonstrative *Fach*', an 'experimental science', a 'science of experience'. Like the other experimental sciences – Purkyně listed variously anatomy, therapeutics, physics, chemistry, botany, mineralogy 'and others' . . . – physiology now based its practice on experiment and observation. In this new status as an 'Erfahrungs-wissenschaft', physiology thus 'must demand [from the state], with the same right as other natural sciences, a complete set of experimental and demonstration apparatus, and a suitable locale for experiments and demonstrations and for storing instruments, models and preparations'. . . . With such rhetoric, Purkyně asked not for radical innovation; he would have the Cultural Ministry believe that he simply wanted what had long become standard for other sciences, in both the medical and philosophical faculties. He merely wanted to claim his 'rights'.

Realising that physiology at nearly every university except Breslau was combined with the anatomical chair, Purkyně carefully described the independent status of physiology as the new *Erfahrungs-wissenschaft* and its relation to the other disciplines. A 'partly historical, partly statistical overview' of Europe's scientific institutions revealed four separate patterns for anatomy and physiology, ranging from total separation and isolation to one person simultaneously filling both roles. According to Purkyně, the former, the most common arrangement, leads to one-sidedness with anatomy alone treating the material elements and physiology becoming completely abstract and literary. The latter, although it might reduce costs since apparatus can be shared, usually requires too much of one person. Much better, he implied, is the arrangement in which both physiology and anatomy have their own institutional support, and relate as 'sister sciences', united in love rather than regulations. Throughout this analysis, Purkyně referred to anatomy and physiology as clearly distinguished subjects (*Fächer*) intellectually; the problem was to provide adequately for their institutional separation. Always cautious, Purkyně nowhere referred to specific universities or professors; nowhere did he discuss systematically how the particular subject matters of anatomy and physiology might be distinguished (even though his students were mostly writing dissertations in what might have been called microscopic anatomy). Apparently he wanted to justify the institutional separation of anatomy and physiology as modestly as possible. Interestingly, he did not exploit the already existing separation of the *Ordinarien* at Breslau by arguing that since physiology had its own chair it also needed its own institute.

Just as physiology could not be reduced to anatomy, so too could it not be reduced to the physical sciences. In some detail, Purkyně outlined the complex tasks of physiology. 'General physiology' deals with broad concepts of life; 'special physiology' includes physiological morphology, physiological physics, physiological chemistry, physiological dynamics, physiological psychology and physiological anthropology. The last of these deals with 'complete humanity as a total organism'; psychology treats the soul, consciousness and the free will, dynamics considers not only physical agents such as light, heat, electricity, but also 'vital forces' and 'specific energies', drawing analogies with physical forces where possible. Embryology (morphology) requires the 'doctrine of teleology of organic forms'. Clearly, physiology has its own subject matter, expansively ranging from embryology to anthropology, and its own explanatory tools. As such, it has a 'real existence', is an 'autonomous' *Fach* (wrote Purkyně as early as 1831), and thus requires its own institute.

For his final rhetorical justification for an institute, Purkyně turned to status, in both a local and larger sense. On pragmatic grounds, he wrote, it is impossible to expect the physiologist to meet his 'scientific needs' in the already established institutes of anatomy, botany, physics or chemistry. Directors of these institutes are already too busy to accommodate a physiologist, they lack space, costly instruments are difficult to share, etc. But more importantly, it is 'unworthy', even 'barbaric', to expect representatives of 'so important a branch of natural science as physiology' to work in other institutes. Any respectable, independent science deserves its own state-supported institutes at the university. Furthermore, in this 'progressive generation', in the present 'upturn of scientific life in Europe', such institutes have become the 'spirit of true science [*Wissenschaftlichkeit*]'. 'It would be doubly important', Purkyně concluded, 'if through Your Excellency's decision the beginning of such a worthy position for physiology could occur in our Prussian state, partly on account of science and its teachers, partly on account of the good example, which like so many others, would spread from here to all sides all the more effectively.

Significantly, Purkyně in this memorandum did not try to justify a physiological institute on the grounds of its utility for medicine, the state or pedagogy. In his opening sentence, he did note that physiological demonstrations and experiments are important for the education (*Bildung*) of medical students. And he did briefly mention the clientele for the institute: not only the director, but also medical students (how they would be selected was not specified), other faculty and 'amateurs of science' would have hands-on access to the apparatus. Conspicuous by its absence, however, is any mention of the service of physiology to the medical enterprise. . . . Chemistry, physics, botany – these were the sciences Purkyně emphasised as the model for the new physiology: the more physiology became like them, the less connected it seemed to medicine. Furthermore, Purkyně specifically urged the state not to support physiology on grounds of utility. He suggested that the state, only recently having moved to support natural science, had acted primarily from two motives. It had first begun to underwrite those 'doctrines' which had 'obvious utility' – medicine, surgery, obstetrics, anatomy, physics, mineralogy and later chemistry. Or it had supported sciences like zoology simply because of the pleasures they offered. Physiology, however, fitted neither of these categories and thus had received minimal state aid. But a 'higher progress' occurred, Purkyně argued, when 'pure science for itself [*reinen Wissenschaft um ihrer selbst willen*]' is supported. . . . In his rhetoric, then, Purkyně called on Prussia to support the new physiology simply for its own sake.

Finally, given Purkyně's well-known interest in Pestalozzian educational reforms . . . it seems surprising that he did not explicitly discuss pedagogy or the pragmatic Pestalozzian theme of learning through active engagement with the surrounding world. According to Pestalozzi, the keystone of the epistemological process is *Anschauung*, a term used broadly by the reformer to mean both mental operations relevant to forming ideas (sense impression, observation, perception, intuition) and a more active, higher mental process which makes perceptions conscious. In the 1836 document, Purkyně does occasionally refer to the new physiology as based on 'sensory *Anschauungen*', and to the importance of enhancing lectures with models or demonstrations (*Veranschaulichung*) to aid in the formation of an '*Anschauung* and concept [*Begriff*] of life'. The new physiology did progress by seeing rather than by abstract philosophising, and it should be taught by seeing. But Purkyně's rhetoric here does not make this a primary *raison d'être* for an institute.

[. . .]

The rhetorical strategy employed by Schultz differs sharply from Purkyně's, as did, undoubtedly, their interests. Rather than welcoming the new status of physiology among the natural sciences, Schultz deplored recent trends in his field. Explicitly concerned with pedagogy, Schultz frequently wrote of *Anschauung*. He envisioned a new type of *Bildung* based on organic principles rather than the dead, reductionist philosophy of the Greeks, a philosophy which, he later wrote, leads only to 'communism, aetheism and Judaism'. Indeed, Schultz dreamed of the medical faculty replacing the philosophical faculty as the site in which all students, not just those studying medicine, could acquire the integrated, moral *Bildung* necessary for the survival of life, society and Christianity.

78

[. . .]

Unlike Purkyně's, Schultz's rhetorical strategy was based squarely on his view of medical education. He attempted to justify his *Observatorium* by appealing to the needs of medicine, not those of physiology. Medicine, Schultz began, urgently requires two types of unities – of teaching and research, and of theory and empiricism. The 'true purpose of [medical] study is the application of science in life'. Since medical science is not a 'closed, finished building' but a 'continuously growing tree', so too must medical instruction change. This can only occur if the professor is also a scientific researcher. The research imperative, Schultz was claiming, belongs in the medical as well as in the philosophical faculty. The professor also must reject a purely empirical medicine and not shy away from medical theory. Every 'reasonable' physician is driven to theory simply by the need to seek reasons for his actions in natural laws. It is essential, therefore, that the medical student receive 'theoretical *Bildung*', based not on the opposition of theory and empiricism, but on their unity.

To unite teaching and research and theory and praxis, Schultz continued, medical faculties must offer 'organic studies of nature', taught with proper pedagogical methods. The only way to teach theoretical medicine is through '*Naturanschauungen* and studies of nature', not through 'mere tradition and books'. This has been realized in anatomical, chemical and clinical instruction, but not in physiology, pathology or pharmacology (the three subjects for Schultz's *Observatorium*). Learning via experiment and experience will provide *Anschauungen* or 'living pictures' that are 'just as indelible and complete' as bookish descriptions are 'blurred and incomplete'. Learning by *Anschauungen* is easier, faster, and longer lasting than is memorising from books. *Naturanschauungen* of physiological actions are essential for all of medicine. Medical praxis is based on knowledge of the normal 'inner course of organic actions'; anatomical structures cannot be understood without a view of the development of organs (embryology); to understand deviations in illness, knowledge of the 'inner machinery of physiological processes' such as muscle and nerve action, or movement of the blood, is essential. And most importantly, unsubstantiated prejudice can most easily be combated by sensory *Anschauungen*. 'The path of research is thereby shown to students, and their desire for their own testing will be stimulated. This lays the foundation for further scientific training (*Fortbildung*), through which sensory *Anschauung* itself finally dissolves into rational theory'. Here, then, is a rhetoric filled with Pestalozzian principles.

Such visualising experimentation also indicates for Schultz that reductionist physiology must be rejected. Chemical experiments treat neutral, dead matter which never exhibits the 'fire of organic activity'. Experiments on living bodies, however, always reveal a 'self-activity through the interaction of elements of form', forms which never appear in dead matter (*Stoff*). The exterior matter merely acts as a stimulus to awaken the 'energy of life'. Schultz's rhetoric here becomes animated, as he castigates those who claim life itself is merely a chemical, physical or mechanical process. Rather, these physical sciences deal only with the conditions of life and the material residue of life after death. They cannot explain the 'life principle' or the 'excitation of life [*Lebenserregung*]'. The relations between chemistry and physiology, Schultz concluded, are like those between a carrier of supplies and a field marshal in a war – an analogy guaranteed to catch the attention of a Cultural Minister. . . .

For Schultz, then, a new institution for theoretical medicine would serve far greater purposes than simply meeting the needs of physiology. By making physiology *anschaulich*, the *Observatorium* would become the centre of medical education. And by teaching the 'true organising principles' for society, it would also become the centre of *Bildung* in the university. Schultz's rhetorical strategy was much more expansive and aggressive than the cautious tack taken several years earlier by Purkyně.

Budge presented the most moderate rhetoric and the shortest (only ten pages) of the three proposals. . . . His justification for taking the step in 1846, however, was narrowly focused and almost exclusively pedagogical – teaching medical students the 'art of observation'. The most difficult task for young students, argued Budge, is learning to observe at the sick-bed. There the cases shown to students are isolated, and physiological processes are highly disturbed by illness. Likewise, at smaller universities like Bonn, students in the anatomical institutes rarely have time to use microscopes or learn the 'most commonplace' chemical analyses. Budge's criticism of current teaching practices within Bonn's anatomical institute could not have been more direct; it might have been overly harsh.

To emphasise further the importance of skills in microscopy and chemical analysis, Budge noted how medical praxis and instruction had changed. Clinical professors, he wrote, now spend days studying pathological tissue, and employ assistants in their institutes or clinics to conduct chemical or microscopic investigations. This has greatly benefited medical science, argued Budge, citing Schönlein's clinic at the Charité (in 1842, the latter had brought the recently qualified (habilitated) chemist, Johann Franz Simon, into his clinic) and the upswing of pathological anatomy at the Austrian universities. Students must enter these practical clinics already possessing the basic skills of chemistry and microscopy, and only a physiological institute in an 'intermediate station' can offer such training at the correct point in the process of medical education. Like Purkyně and in contrast to Schultz, Budge sought to support recent changes in the practice of physiology as a medical science with the creation of a new institute.

4.4

The role of the laboratory in the hospital

L.S. Jacyna, 'The Laboratory and the Clinic: The Impact of Pathology on Surgical Diagnosis in the Glasgow Western Infirmary, 1875–1910', *Bulletin of the History of Medicine* 62 (1988), pp. 389–94 [pp. 384–406].

It is often assumed that the laboratory fitted quickly and easily into diagnostics. This case study of the role of the pathologist in a Glasgow hospital shows that, at the end of the nineteenth century, clinicians used the laboratory only in a limited way and for specific tasks.

Coats [the pathologist to the infirmary], performed all the other functions expected of a hospital pathologist. Most of his time was occupied by autopsies: in 1876, the first full year of the Pathology Department's operation, 130 of these were performed. Coats noted that in addition to these cadavers, he received in that year 43 'morbid products' to examine. . . .

The bulk of the specimens sent to the pathologist . . . were the by-products or detritus of surgery. Amputated limbs, evacuated fluids, and excised joints figure prominently. The largest category was composed of the various tumors excised on the wards. Of the 23 specimens for 1876 for which descriptions survive, 22 were of this kind. A surgeon who dispatched a tumor expected the pathologist to examine it and provide an account of its macroscopic and (in some instances) microscopic appearances. . . .

In some cases of a dubious nature the pathologist was clearly expected to identify a growth; for example, a multiple ovarian cystoma

81

'was sent to the pathological department, so that its nature could be ascertained.' The motive, often, was simple curiosity. George Buchanan, Professor of Clinical Surgery at Glasgow, in October 1890 sent Coats 'a small fungiform tumour from the dorsum[8] of the tongue.' 'It does not seem to present any evidence of malignancy but it is not a simple wart,' Buchanan wrote. 'Can you define exactly what it is[?]' On other occasions, the pathologist was asked to establish whether a tumor was malignant. . . . Thus, Dr. Walter Sandeman of the village of Bridge of Weir in April 1895 sent the pathologist a mass of hemorrhoids passed *per rectum* with the specific request that he 'let [Sandeman] know if there [was] anything of a malignant nature about the specimen.' This is a common plea in the letters that accompanied the specimens regularly sent from the Peterborough Infirmary to Glasgow for pathological examination during the 1890s.

More often, however, the clinician was satisfied as to the character of what he had excised. The pathologist in these cases was expected to elaborate upon this diagnosis by specifying the gross and histological[9] features of the tumor. In such instances the pathologist also served as a check upon the clinical diagnosis, usually confirming it, but sometimes correcting the surgeon's view.

When the pathological did differ from the clinical diagnosis, the authority of the former was put to the test. Some surgeons were ready to defer to the pathologist. Hector Cameron[10] in two similar cases in 1888 altered the diagnosis recorded in the ward journal in the light of a contradictory pathological report. . . .

In cases where clinicians could not agree on a diagnosis, the pathologist was occasionally requested to act as arbiter. . . . In February 1896, Horace Abel wrote from Peterborough to ask Lewis Sutherland, one of the department's pathologists, his opinion on the

enclosed specimen removed this afternoon from the Vagina. . . . [The patient] was examined under Ether and a hard growth found on upper part of Vagina which was clinically pronounced malignant disease. . . . The case has been seen by a specialist in Town and pronounced non-malignant. A microscopic examination has been made elsewhere and confirmed Dr. Walker's original diagnosis. . . .

[8] *dorsum*: upper surface.

[9] *gross and histological*: features that can be seen by the naked eye, and at the cell or tissue level, observable only through a microscope.

[10] Hector Cameron was surgeon in charge of one of the female surgical wards at the Western Infirmary.

Sutherland's reply to this appeal was cautious. The portion of tissue sent to him had 'mainly the characters of an inflammatory tissue,' he wrote. 'There is at places a considerable amount of epithelial[11] tissue regarded by Dr. Coats as probably cancerous.' This seemed to satisfy Dr. Abel.

[. . .]

Thus, the pathologist was important, yet he remained incidental to the clinical process. His opinion was sought only after the crucial decisions had been made on purely clinical criteria. The surgeons to a great extent still regarded the pathologist as the Keeper of the Dead. The tumors they sent to him were, in effect, little cadavers. The continuity between these excision 'biopsies' and the long-established practice of autopsy is underlined by the fact that until the turn of the twentieth century no special stationery was provided to accompany such specimens: the same request form that accompanied cadavers, slightly modified, was employed. The pathologist's contribution was to identify the specimens' nature with more sophistication than the surgeon could muster; to corroborate or correct the clinical diagnosis; and to add to the stock of medical knowledge. The pathologist's judgment could lead to a revision of the clinical diagnosis or settle a difference between clinicians, but, so far as the patient was concerned, such post facto adjudication mattered little. At most, the pathologist might contribute to the prognosis of a case that had already received surgical treatment.

Cases did occur, however, that deviated more radically from the traditional view of the relation of the pathologist to the clinician. On these occasions, pathology contributed to the formulation of the surgeon's diagnosis and thus to the making of therapeutic decisions. A trickle of specimens sent for diagnostic purposes began to arrive at the pathology laboratory during the mid-1890s. Sometimes they were accompanied by frank confessions of bewilderment on the part of the surgeon. In a case of an extensive tumor of the thigh. Hector Cameron admitted that he 'was unable to decide whether he had to deal with a periostitis: an osteomyelitis or possibly a diffuse sarcoma.'[12] . . . A note of urgency enters into some of these requests, reflecting the new importance being attached to the pathologist's response. His judgment upon a specimen was no longer merely part of a retrospective exercise of no immediate

---

[11] *epithelial*: cells covering the internal and external surfaces of the body.

[12] Periostitis is an infection of the connective tissues surrounding the bones. Osteomyelitis is an inflammation of the bone itself. A sarcoma is a cancer in the supportive tissues of the body, such as bone, muscle and fat.

moment: the course of future treatment depended upon it. As G.H. Edington remarked when asking for an opinion on a growth he had removed, 'Tubercle, Gumma,[13] or Sarcoma – as if the last, something more radical may need to be done.'

Cases can be found where the surgeon did heed the voice of the pathologist in the course of treatment adopted. . . . A particularly clear illustration of this is found in a case on Alexander Patterson's ward in October 1900. In the course of an operation on a swollen knee joint on 24 October, 'a mass of soft granulations were extracted and in the depth of the wound thus made necrosed[14] bone was found. The probability of sarcoma was discussed and it was decided to get the specimen examined.' On 31 October the following notation was made: 'The pathologist's report of sarcoma to hand. It was considered advisable to amputate at the hip today.'

On the basis of such examples it is easy to conclude that by the end of the nineteenth century 'laboratory' medicine had triumphed over the scepticism and opposition of 'clinical' purists. This, however, would be a gross oversimplification. The cases cited above where the pathologist was consulted and where his opinion played a crucial part in the clinical process need to be contrasted with others where clinical judgment remained stubbornly autonomous.

One of the most obvious applications of histopathology lay in the field of differential diagnosis. Syphilis and tuberculosis were both endemic at the end of the nineteenth century; these diseases were sometimes difficult to distinguish by clinical criteria alone. Thus, in 1895, Dr. A.B. Kelly confessed himself to be 'in difficulties' in the case of a man who presented an evidently syphilitic ulcer of the tongue, but who claimed that he was free of the disease (the social stigma attached to syphilis made clinicians more than usually sceptical about their patients' testimony in such instances). Kelly sent a scraping from the tongue and a piece of epiglottis[15] to the pathologist to find out whether the lesion was tubercular. The pathologist reported: '[The] fragment of tissue from the epiglottis shews an exceedingly typical tubercular structure. A few tubercle bacilli are found among the epithelial cells of the tubercles.' Pathologists were also called upon to differentiate among various forms of chronic inflammation (whether specific or otherwise) and malignant formations.

---

[13] Tubercle is a chronic local inflammation caused by the tuberculosis bacterium. Gumma is a soft tumour, usually caused by syphilitic infection.

[14] *necrosed*: dead.

[15] *epiglottis*: the flap of tissue which protects the voice box.

In other areas, however, clinicians showed what seems an almost willful blindness to the possibility of establishing the nature of a complaint by reference to the pathologist. In the case of M.N., a past history of syphilis was enough to occasion a course of anti-syphilitic treatment for an ulcer of the scrotum. This continued for fifteen months before the ulcer was removed and sent to the pathologist, who pronounced it epitheliomatous. . . .[16]

The impression obtained from these examples is that when clinicians were reasonably confident of the nature of the lesion, they saw no reason to consult the pathologist before making a diagnosis. It was only in doubtful cases, when they found themselves 'in difficulties,' that clinicians deemed such extraneous assistance necessary. If the clinical diagnosis in what had seemed a patent case was subsequently called into question, then a belated recourse might be had to pathology.

4.5
The impact of vaccine therapy

Michael Worboys, 'Vaccine Therapy and Laboratory Medicine in Edwardian Britain', in John Pickstone (ed.), *Medical Innovations in Historical Perspective* (Basingstoke, Macmillan, 1992), pp. 96–102 [pp. 84–103].

It is now generally accepted that in the early decades of the twentieth century many practitioners saw little or no role for the biomedical sciences in medical practice, arguing that clinical skills produced a more accurate diagnosis. In this article, Michael Worboys explores the debate over vaccine therapy – a new technique which involved injecting patients with vaccines made from killed bacteria in order to stimulate an immune response.

The evidence . . . suggests that vaccine therapy, if judged by the extent of its practice and duration of popularity, was a significant, though minor, medical innovation. However, the treatment was promoted as more than a single innovation, it was a new kind of medicine. . . . In 1907, R.W. Allen . . . claim[ed]

---

[16] *epitheliomatous*: tumour in the epithelial tissues.

The medicine of the future is the medicine of vaccines and of sera. The empiricism of the past will give way to methods based upon scientific knowledge and the public will no longer look upon medicine with a sceptical eye and dose themselves with ineffective nostrums.

[. . .] Wright,[17] his followers and his supporters saw vaccine therapy as nothing less than the vanguard for the reconstitution of medicine, leading it to be more scientific and research-based, with the laboratory its central agency and symbol.

Studies of the late Victorian and Edwardian marriage of medicine and science now recognise that this union was not without its problems. It is now argued that the reaction of many clinicians to science, the laboratory and technology was ambivalent, even hostile. It is certainly possible to find evidence of differences of opinion over the relative merits of clinical signs and symptoms, as against laboratory tests. However, it seems that this issue was more in the nature of an underlying tension than a conflict. This was because the two 'sides' – bedside and bench – were not that distinct, nor were they evenly matched. Most medical bacteriologists were clinically trained and held only part-time appointments. A significant number of physicians, surgeons, general practitioners and state medical officers dabbled in bacteriological technique and speculated on aetiologies.[18] An indication of the extent to which laboratories were used is that in the early 1900s over 4000 doctors, approximately one in five, subscribed to use the diagnostic laboratories of the CRA.[19] In most settings, including the hospital and in public health, bacteriological diagnosis was normally described as an adjunct to clinical methods. Besides, clinicians were far too powerful to be challenged by the lower-status and usually more junior staff in the laboratory. In some universities, bacteriological laboratories were run by senior and often distinguished scientists: however, these facilities were often isolated institutionally and had few links with, let alone influence on, clinical teaching or practice. With regard to laboratory diagnosis, it was clinicians who requested tests in the first place and who interpreted and selectively absorbed the findings. . . .

---

[17] Almroth Wright (1861–1947), British director of the Institute of Pathology at St Mary's Hospital, London. Wright developed a series of vaccines to treat a wide variety of conditions, including a widely-used anti-typhoid vaccine.

[18] *aetiologies*: causes.

[19] (CRA) Clinical Research Association, a commercial laboratory providing pathological and laboratory services to general practitioners and local authorities.

Several features distinguished vaccine therapy from other bacteriological and laboratory activities. The position and character of Wright
was undoubtedly important. Wright was an international scientific
celebrity; it was said that his laboratory and clinic was 'a place of
scientific pilgrimage'. Through contacts with Ehrlich[20] St Mary's
enjoyed a near-monopoly of the earliest supplies of Salvarsan in Britain,
even though Wright himself had no time for this latest German chemical remedy. Arguably, it was Wright's promotion of tuberculin treatment, which came to be seen as a special case of vaccine therapy, that
led to the inclusion of medical research in the 1911 National Insurance
legislation. . . . However, the main difference between vaccine therapy
and other clinical laboratory work was that it was 'therapy', and as such
directly encroached on the domain of the clinician.

Many of the issues surrounding the treatment, and its implications
for medicine in general, were aired at two sessions at the Royal Society
of Medicine (RSM) in 1910 and 1913. At both meetings vaccine therapy
was said to have been 'on trial'. Wright began the first meeting with an
address attacking clinicians' ignorance of bacteriology and of medical
science in general. He pointed out that the most celebrated achievement of modern medical science, antiseptic surgery, had been adopted
as a mere technique and that most clinicians still failed to understand
the underlying bacteriology. . . . [W]ith vaccine therapy the laboratory
had overtaken the clinic. . . . [T]he new vaccinist-bacteriologist could
offer exact diagnosis, even of incipient[21] disease, and the precise tar-
geting and monitoring of treatment.

[. . .]

Apart from Wright's opening address, the discussion at the RSM in 1910
was not on relations between bench and bedside, but on clinical concerns – the mechanics of the treatment, and did it work? . . . To the
charge that the treatment worked only for a few chronic and relatively
trivial diseases, the St Mary's workers replied with a long list of conditions said to benefit: pneumonia, typhoid fever, rheumatism, endo-
carditis, tubercular infections, dermatitis, tooth abscesses, hay fever,
urinary calculi, food poisoning, epilepsy and the complications of
cancer, gonorrhea, influenza, whooping cough, catarrh and glycosuria.
Most supporters gave detailed and optimistic case reports, whilst the

---

[20] Paul Ehrlich (1845–1915), a German researcher who established many of the fundamental concepts of chemotherapy. He also developed many ground-breaking new drugs, including
salvarsan, the first effective treatment for syphilis.

[21] *incipient*: just beginning or at a very early stage.

relatively few critics present commented on the dearth of published papers, the absence of animal experiments and the ambiguities in those studies that had been published.

[. . .]

The debate at the RSM had revealed other tensions within the medical community. There were suggestions that the treatment was seen by some as offering physicians the means to claim back from surgeons certain diseases which the latter had taken over in recent decades. Vaccine therapy implied that infections had to be combatted by systemic treatments and Wright argued that neither the knife nor anti-septics could ever remove all infective material. However, leading surgeons, like Arbuthnot Lane (Guy's) and C.B. Lockwood (St Bartholomew's) were enthusiasts and thought anti-streptococcal and anti-staphylococcal vaccines might strengthen the battle against wound infection by providing internal asepsis. . . . It was clear, too, that vaccines could be seen as challenging public health campaigns, like that against tuberculosis. . . .

Another tension highlighted was generational, between younger doctors trained in the new laboratory techniques and their older, more clinically-oriented, colleagues. Bacteriology as a laboratory subject had been introduced as a formal part of the medical curriculum only in the late 1890s, so it was only from the early years of the century that Britain had graduates conversant with bacteriological techniques. . . .

The RSM met to discuss vaccine therapy again in 1913. This time a different verdict was delivered,

> Failures . . . are more common than successes, and though there is no doubt about the efficacy at times of vaccine treatment, still in the mass the results are disappointing. This seems to be damning with faint praise: but we may put it less harshly, and say that the early enthusiasm and hopes excited have been tempered by experience.

What had brought about this revision? There had been no sudden increase in critical reports of vaccine therapy. These had always existed – what had changed is that more notice was now taken of them. In part, it was because there were different speakers and a different audience. A complaint in 1910 was that the opponents of vaccine therapy had not turned out, three years later they did. . . . Opponents may have gained confidence from the fact that the uses of therapeutic vaccines had become more circumscribed and that medicine had not been reshaped. A more modest estimation was being reflected in the literature, and it has been shown earlier that there had already been a levelling off and decline in the sales of vaccines after 1910. Certainly, the indeterminate effects of vaccines contrasted with the obvious effects, intended and unintended, of the new chemotherapeutic agents, like Atoxyl and Salvarsan. These shifts reversed the roles at the RSM by 1913, vaccine therapists were now on the defensive; significantly, though, the critics spoke out against the style of vaccine therapy as much as its results.

Part five

The emergence of a modern profession

5.1

Occupational closure and the 1858 Medical Act

Ivan Waddington, *The Medical Profession in the Industrial Revolution* (Dublin, Gill and Macmillan, Humanities Press, 1984), pp. 138–43, 147–52.

Ivan Waddington, with his colleagues at Leicester University, S.W.F. Holloway and N.D. Jewson, has helped to bring a sociological approach to the study of the history of medicine. Waddington has written on the development of hospitals, the profession and medical ethics in the nineteenth century. In this extract, he challenges the old assumption that the registration of practitioners was introduced to benefit the public.

In recent years . . . a number of social scientists have begun to develop a more sceptical analysis of the significance of registration. Thus, in their work on the medical profession in Britain, Noel and José Parry have suggested that registration may best be viewed as part of 'an occupational strategy which is chiefly directed towards the achievement of upward collective social mobility and, once achieved, it is concerned with the maintenance of superior remuneration and status'. The importance of registration, they suggest, lies in the fact that it enables practitioners to achieve 'a degree of monopoly with respect to the provision of particular types of services in the market'.[1] . . .

[1] Noel Parry and Jose Parry, *The Rise of the Medical Profession* (London, Croom Helm, 1976), p. 79.

... On the basis of this examination, it will be suggested that the campaign for medical registration did indeed have strong monopolistic elements, and that a major thrust of medical politics in the first half of the nineteenth century was concerned with the perceived need to restrict entry into what was seen as an overcrowded profession. Thus it will be argued that medical practitioners were concerned both to control the number of qualified practitioners entering the profession and to reduce the competition from practitioners who were not qualified. It will further be argued that most practitioners were clearly aware of the effect which this process of occupational closure would be likely to have in terms of raising both the status and the incomes of medical men, and that the establishment of a medical register under the control of the General Medical Council proved to be a very effective way of restricting entry to the profession. In order to understand this point more fully, it will be useful to examine briefly what many medical men saw as the problem of overcrowding within the profession, especially from the 1830s.

In the early 1830s, the *Lancet* argued that 'the members of the medical profession are not a body of wealthy individuals, and, as we have seen, there is indeed considerable evidence to indicate that whilst the incomes of consultants were often very high, many general practitioners were forced to live on extremely modest incomes. The two most frequently identified causes of what medical practitioners saw as the depressed level of medical incomes were an oversupply of qualified practitioners and what was seen as unfair competition from those who were not qualified. ... The evils of excessive competition, arising from an oversupply of qualified practitioners, were ... pointed out by the author of an article published anonymously in the *Quarterly Review* in 1840. The author – believed to have been Sir Benjamin Brodie – argued that 'the supply of medical practitioners is in fact not only very much beyond the demand, but very much beyond what is necessary to ensure a just and useful degree of competition ... and to this cause may mainly be attributed the present restless and uneasy state of the profession. In this, as in all other pursuits, a certain degree of competition is required for the security of the public; but in the medical profession it is easy to conceive that the competition may be not only beyond what is really wanted, but so great as to be actually mischievous. ...

[T]here may have been some substance in these complaints, for in the 1820s and early 1830s there was a very rapid increase in the number of persons who took out a licence to practise medicine. Thus the Royal College of Surgeons estimated that in 1824 some 5000 persons held the diploma of the College; by 1833 this number had increased to 8125, an increase of more than 62 per cent in a ten year period. A similar story emerges if we examine the number of medical men who took out a licence from the Society of Apothecaries. . . .

[. . .]

. . . By the 1840s there was a general consensus amongst medical men on the need to restrict entry to the profession, and the issue was discussed frequently and openly in the medical journals. Thus the *Lancet* held that 'It is admitted on all hands that many of the evils under which the medical profession now labours, are owing to the teeming multitude of practitioners. This necessarily involves an impoverished state of the profession, and has, doubtless, contributed largely to that depression of intellect and morals among its members. . . . The means of restraining this superfluity of doctors, and rendering the number of the profession more proportionate to the population, become, therefore, very important objects of medical legislation.' The *Lancet* then went on to review a number of schemes for restricting entry to the profession . . . the *Lancet* argued that the best way to restrict entry was by 'making the standard of qualification high, as well in medicine as in letters and science'. If this scheme were adopted, 'the numbers of the profession would be effectually limited without any injurious exclusions; the character of the profession would be greatly elevated, and the public welfare would be promoted'. This was, of course, a relatively sophisticated statement of what was essentially an economic argument for restricting entry to the profession. . . .

A second aspect of the campaign for registration which involved a clear element of monopolisation was the attempt to prevent unqualified practice, and here, once again, economic considerations were of major importance. Thus in 1843, the *Lancet* argued: 'That "the profession is overstocked" we daily hear exclaimed, and the assertion is true. The "profession" is overstocked, and with a superabundance of unqualified men, mere speculators in drugs and chemicals.' The result was that 'educated practitioners are deprived of their legitimate means of obtaining a subsistence'. Medical men, continued the *Lancet*, 'who scorn to make their liberal profession a trade, complain of this usurpation of their rightful field of profit, and of this degradation of medicine, in vain'. . . . The view that medical education was an investment, and that unqualified practitioners were denying qualified practitioners a legitimate return on that investment was, in fact, a recurrent theme. This idea was, for example, very precisely expressed by one contributor to the *Lancet*, who held that 'no person should risk the expenditure of time, labour, and money necessary to the attainment of his qualification or licence to practise, unless he felt himself to be effectually

guarded by the laws against the competition of unlicensed and ignorant, though impudent and plausible empirics'.

[. . .]

Although many general practitioners were dissatisfied with the fact that
the 1858 Act[2] did not make unqualified practice illegal, the exclusion of
unqualified practitioners from all government medical services was, in
the long term, to assume greatly increased importance with the continual expansion of the public sector of health care in the late nineteenth
and twentieth centuries . . . [T]he Act conferred an advantage on registered practitioners 'by providing them with apparent state approval;
that is, the prestige of the state was thrown behind members of the
organised medical profession.

In conferring these advantages on those who were registered, the Act
followed closely the principle laid down by Sir James Graham[3] in 1844,
when he argued that the law should not be used to prohibit unqualified
practice, but it should be used to 'discourage it by securing exclusive
advantages to the regular practitioner'. Thus the effect of the 1858 Act
was not only to exclude unregistered practitioners from the steadily
expanding public sector of medical care but also, in the private sector,
to give registered practitioners 'a competitive advantage in the open
market'. . . .

[T]he impact of the 1858 Act on the level of recruitment to the profession appears to have been one which took effect almost immediately.
Thus, in the twenty years or so following the passage of the Act, the
growth in the number of medical practitioners in England and Wales
was quite minimal, and was far outstripped by the growth of the total
population. In 1861, there were 14,415 medical practitioners in England
and Wales. In the decade from 1861–71, this number increased by just
269, or 1.8 per cent, and in the period from 1871–81, there was a further
increase of 407, or 2.7 per cent. Thus, over the twenty year period from
1861–81, the number of medical practitioners in England and Wales
increased by under 5 per cent, compared with a 24 per cent increase in
the employed male population, and an increase in the total population
of no less than 29 per cent over the same period.

[. . .]

There is some evidence to suggest that . . . this restriction of entry to the
profession was associated with a significant improvement in both the

[2] The 1858 Medical Act established the medical register and the General Medical Council.

[3] Sir James Graham (1796–1861) was Home Secretary in Sir Robert Peel's Conservative government. He was closely involved in the debate over medical reform in the 1840s and 1850s.

earnings and the status of medical practitioners. Thus St. Thomas's Hospital, in the evidence which it submitted to a Government Committee in 1878, pointed to the 'steady and progressive decrease of the number of medical practitioners in the United Kingdom, proportionately to the population', and went on to note that 'It is certain that within the same period the remuneration of medical men occupied in civil practice has greatly increased. . . . The social status and influence of civil medical practitioners has undoubtedly increased with their increased earnings.

[. . .]

In conclusion, therefore, we may suggest that those writers who have argued that the 1858 Act was passed for the benefit of the public have offered at best a grossly oversimplified account of the significance of registration, for they have ignored not only the fact that the profession derived significant monopolistic advantages from registration but equally importantly the fact that these monopolistic advantages were clearly recognised within the profession from the very beginning of the campaign for registration.

5.2

The Medical Act of 1858

Irvine Loudon, *Medical Care and the General Practitioner 1750–1850* (Oxford, Clarendon Press, 1986), pp. 298–301.

Irvine Loudon worked as a general practitioner, but has produced many works exploring the lives and careers of general practitioners in the eighteenth and nineteenth century. His research fits into the genre of works on 'medicine from below' and explores the experiences of ordinary provincial doctors.

Until quite recently the Medical Act has been applauded as one of the great landmarks in the advance of medicine whereby the medical education and ethical behaviour of medical practitioners came under firm control for the benefit of the public. It was an Act by which the profession put its house in order. Now, it is more usual to describe the Medical Act as a prime example of professional consolidation and monopolization based on motives of self-interest; which, of course, it was. But the two views are not incompatible, especially when considered within the mid-nineteenth-century climate of opinion. Then it was commonly agreed that a professional man's self-interest was the best guarantee of good public service. The efficient would prosper and the bad go to the wall. It was not the purpose of the state to interfere more than possible in social transactions between customer, client, or patient, and the provider of services. In medicine it was necessary only to ensure a minimum standard of competence—a belief which became enshrined in the concept of 'the safe general practitioner'. Such arguments concerning the state and the provisions of health care are still familiar today. Was the Act, therefore, of benefit to the public and the profession?

In the long term the answer must be in the affirmative, even if it is an affirmative with reservations. The disciplinary powers of the General Medical Council have a powerful deterrent effect on professional misbehaviour, even if the decisions of the disciplinary committee have sometimes appeared to be capricious. The primary purpose of the Act, the regulation of medical education, is clearly important although (except as a last resort) the Council only has power to advise, not to compel. Until recently the method of appointing members of the Council was not representative, and the part played by the medical corporations was excessive. But the public is much better served and protected than it would have been if medicine had been totally free from the control of a Medical Council. Did the Act, however, confer immediate advantage on the profession?

Those who support the thesis that the Act was the triumphant product of a movement based purely on medical self-interest are forced to the logical conclusion that it was welcomed by the profession for the benefits it bestowed on them. They emphasise that, as a result of registration, outdated legal restrictions on medical practice were removed, and practitioners could sue for fees and apply for public service; but these were not important issues. It is also said, and is hard to deny, that registration conferred a certain psychological advantage on the registered practitioner, and it is certain that the medical corporations[4] gained greatly by the passing of the Act; the Act virtually guaranteed their continued existence and rubber-stamped their authority. The suggestion that the Medical Act was responsible for introducing modern medical education is so wide of the mark that it needs only to be mentioned to be dismissed. Finally, it is sometimes suggested that, for all its failings, at least the Medical Act was responsible for unifying the profession; but this is nonsense, confusing causes with results. The

---

[4] *corporations*: the Colleges of Physicians and Surgeons and Society of Apothecaries.

Medical Act of 1858, like the Apothecaries Act of 1815, was the product, not the cause of changes in the profession. In any occupational group, unification is promoted by a common pathway of entry and an ethos which provides a sense of corporate identity, purpose, and pride. At best the Medical Act contributed to a very minor degree to these components of professional unity. But it would be hard to justify an assertion that, in the short term, the Act conferred material advantage on practitioners in terms of better education, more patients, higher fees, reduced competition from irregulars, greater respect from the public, or even greater ability to control the development of the profession. Certainly, neither the practice nor the position of physicians and surgeons was affected materially by the Act; nor, contrary to received opinion, did the general practitioners gain anything. Indeed, they lost the opportunity for social and professional mobility which, in the 1820s and 1830s was their source of optimism and vitality. The authentication of the corporations and medical qualifications had the effect of fossilizing the prospects of the general practitioner and ensuring that he remained as a subordinate grade. To this extent the general practitioners were disappointed people who had challenged the medical corporations and lost. Their views of the Act were forcibly expressed by a London practitioner, Edwin Lee, who wrote in 1863 that the Medical Act had added no advantages to medical men, had not altered medical education, and provided only a means of levying an extra tax. Lee provided an impressive body of evidence from the press, lay and medical, deriding the Act as 'a very considerable failure'. 'Depend upon it,' wrote one practitioner, 'the Medical Council will make it their duty to serve only the interests of the medical corporations they represent.' Another complained, 'The Medical Council . . . are supposed to be our representatives. What have they hitherto represented? The monopoly and exclusiveness of effete corporations.' A writer to the Dublin medical press complained that the Council was 'not accountable to those who compose the medical body politic' and the *Medical Circular* asserted that the Act, far from promoting unity, had 'increased the evil of multifarious qualifications . . . [and] . . . helped to exasperate the lamentable divisions that have made our profession the reproach of society'. 'We have got our protection,' wrote a Dr Wilks, 'We have obtained our registration at last; but as for advantage it may be of to the profession. I, for one, value it at a straw.'

5.3
An operation by Bransby Cooper

Editorial, *The Lancet*, 1827–28, vol. II, pp. 20–2.

In 1828 Bransby Cooper, surgeon at Guy's hospital, performed an operation to remove a bladder stone from Stephen Pollard, a farm labourer. The operation took almost an hour and the patient subsequently died. Thomas Wakley, editor of the *Lancet*, seized on the incident to criticise the elite staff of London's hospitals. The operation was held up as proof that Cooper owed his position more to the patronage of his uncle, Sir Astley Cooper, one of the hospitals senior surgeons, than his surgical skills. Astley Cooper sued Wakley for libel damages of £2,000 but was awarded just £100.

'Our report of the operation of lithotomy[5] at Guy's Hospital, in which Mr. Bransby Cooper, after employing a variety of instruments, extracted the stone at the end of fifty-five minutes, – the average *maximum* time in which this operation is performed by skilful surgeons being about six minutes; has . . . excited no ordinary sensation in the minds of the public, as well as among the operator's professional brethren. An attempt has been made to call into question the accuracy of our report, in a letter signed by a number of the dressers[6] and pupils of the [hospital] . . . Some of the young gentlemen who have affixed their signatures to this letter, were present at the operation; others, who were *not* present at the operation, have nevertheless, with a generosity more characteristic of their age than of their discretion, added the weight of their testimony to that of the eye-witnesses. . . . The letter in question may be regarded as a testimonial of the estimation in which a good-natured lecturer is held by the young gentlemen who attend his class. But the question is not whether Mr. Bransby Cooper is popular among his pupils, but whether he performed the late operation with that degree of skill, which the public has a right to expect from a surgeon of Guy's Hospital; whether, in short, the case presented such difficulties as no degree of skill could have surmounted in less time, or with less disastrous consequences; or whether the unfortunate patient lost his life, not because his case was one of extraordinary difficulty, but because it was

---

[5] *lithotomy*: the operation to remove stones from the bladder.
[6] *dressers*: junior doctors and senior pupils.

the turn of a surgeon to operate, who is indebted for his elevation to the influence of a corrupt system, and who ... would never have been placed in a situation of such deep responsibility as that which he now occupies, had he not been the nephew of Sir Astley Cooper. This is the question, the only question, in which the public is interested; and if Mr. Bransby Cooper is desirous of bringing this question to an issue in a Court of Justice, it will be for Mr. Benjamin Harrison, the treasurer of Guy's Hospital to enlighten the minds of the jury as to the circumstances under which the nephew of Sir Astley Cooper was elevated to his present situation ... We contend, as we have repeatedly contended on former occasions, that the inevitable tendency of making the patronage of hospital surgeoncies an affair of family influence, jobbing, and intrigue, is to occasion a cruel and wanton augmentation of human suffering, and to render frequent such heart-rending spectacles as that which was lately exhibited at Guy's Hospital.

[...]

Suppose it had been stated that, instead of employing fifty-five minutes in extracting the stone Mr. Bransby Cooper had performed the operation in the usual time. ... Suppose it had been stated that, instead of manifesting great perplexity and embarrassment, Mr. Bransby Cooper had exhibited the utmost coolness and self-possession; that the patient appeared to suffer very slightly during the operation, and was removed from the theatre with every prospect of a favourable issue to the case. Let us suppose these and similar *false* representations, to have been made in this Journal, and we will ask whether any of these young gentlemen, friendly as their feelings are towards a teacher, whose good nature is a matter of greater notoriety than his science, and interested as they are in obtaining his good will, and his certificates to enable them to pass their examinations at the College before his 'uncle', who is the president of that benighted body; – we will ask whether any of these young gentlemen ... would have come forward to contradict a favourable, though false, report.

5.4
Medical ethics

W. Fraser, 'Queries in medical ethics', *London Medical Gazette*, 1849, II, pp. 181–3, 186–7, 227–8.

Many historians have claimed that in the early nineteenth century, books on medical ethics were really about the etiquette of working with other practitioners at a time when the relative status of different practitioners within the profession was in flux. This, one of the many works on medical ethics which appeared at this time, shows that writers were concerned with the responsibilities of practitioners towards their patients – as well as the rules of professional decorum.

Query 1. – If a patient wishes you to call into consultation a medical man, of whose qualifications in the circumstances of the case you may have an unfavourable opinion, is it proper and honourable to decline doing so, or to endeavour to alter the opinion of your patient?

Ans – If your patient expresses a very decided wish to have a particular person called in, you ought to acquiesce, provided there be no professional stain on his character sufficient to warrant you to decline doing so. His being junior to yourself, either in age or professional capacity, is certainly no sufficient reason.

[. . .]

Query 4. – When a medical man is called into consultation by another, and supposing they entertain a difference of opinion as to the nature of the case . . . is either of them justified in giving an unfavourable impression of the practice of the other to the patient, or his friends, or to any other person?

Ans – No.

[. . .]

Query 8. – When a medical man called, during the progress of a case, into consultation with another practitioner, persists . . . in continuing his services after the danger is over, and when the person first in attendance thinks his further assistance both unnecessary and inconvenient — what is the proper resource for the latter?

Ans – The most effectual hint would be paying him his fee; but if he declare the case still to be in need of his attendance, you can have no resource without coming to a rupture with him.

Query 9. – When a medical man is called to a case on an emergency, during the absence of the practitioner in attendance – what is the proper etiquette to be observed by the two?

Ans – The person called in should do what is *necessary* in the urgency of the case, and nothing more, nor should he repeat his visit. . . . The ordinary attendant . . . should not neglect to thank the other . . . for his assistance; and moreover, if this has been of great consequence, and the patient's circumstances are such as to justify it, he should advise the latter to send him a suitable fee.

[. . .]

Query 11. – When a patient labouring under a complaint tending, if the proper means are not used, to a fatal termination, calmly and deliber-ately tells you that he does not wish his life protracted – what duty remains for you?

Ans – To endeavour, in the first place, to bring him to a more hopeful and healthy frame of mind; and, whether you succeed in this or not, to tell him that so long as you continue in attendance, you must and will use the proper means for his recovery. The friends, at the same time, should . . . be made aware of the state of affairs.

[. . .]

Query 21. – If it should come to the knowledge of a medical man that a case under the management of some other person is evidently misun-derstood, and must soon terminate fatally if the proper treatment is not adopted – is he at all justified in interfering; and if so, in what matter and to what extent?

Ans – In this delicate and disagreeable position . . . the utmost caution and good faith are necessary. As a general rule he should altogether discountenance what is a too common practice among the ill-informed and lower classes, – that gossiping criticism to which the practice of medical men is subjected . . . but there may be circumstances in which he cannot avoid listening to the appeals which may be made to him. 'When artful ignorance,' says Dr. Percival,[7] 'grossly imposes on credulity; when neglect puts to hazard an important life, or rashness threatens

---

[7] Thomas Percival (1740–1804), author of *Medical Ethics* (1803), one of the first and most influential works on the subject.

it with still more imminent danger – a medical neighbour, friend or relative . . . will justly regard his interference as a duty. But he ought to be careful that the information on which he acts is well founded; that his motives are pure and honourable; and that his judgement of the measures pursued is built on experience and practical knowledge, – not on speculative or theoretical differences of opinion . . .'

In opposition to this view . . . a friend . . . remarks – 'I really cannot see the propriety of assuming that, in any instance whatever, where he is not professionally consulted by friend or legal authority . . . a practitioner may or ought to give judgment regarding the treatment pursued. . . . In my view, a physician *as such*, has no more title to become a public censor or reformer than what may be claimed by any other member of society; and that office . . . will almost infallibly be regarded with a suspicion of self-conceit, which . . . a right-minded man would avoid, as calculated to injure his character and impair his usefulness'.

[. . .]

Query 23. – In cases where a surgical operation is indicated, which the medical man in attendance does not feel himself warranted or inclined to undertake, what is the proper course to adopt, and what the proper etiquette to be observed between or among the medical men concerned in the treatment of the case?

Ans – As the great majority of medical practitioners very properly eschew the performance of the more serious and capital operations in surgery, when the necessity for such an operation is clear and undoubted . . . the medical attendant should, with the acquiescence of the patient, select the person in whose judgement, experience, dexterity and other requisite qualifications he has most confidence. . . . The surgeon, however, should not assume any charge of the case beyond what his responsibility as the operator *pro tempore*[8] requires of him, and should no more lay himself out for continued employment or general consultation by the patient, than would a dentist . . . whose services might happen to be required in similar circumstances.

Query 24. – What is the proper frame of mind for the practitioner when engaged in the active duties of his profession?

Ans – To lay down a specific rule on this head were almost impossible. . . . But one thing is plain. . . . [k]indness, firmness, self-possession, circumspection, fidelity, candour and intelligence, ought . . . to form prominent features in his demeanour. The chief qualities necessary in a

---

[8] At the time, for the time being.

medical man are . . . unshaken fidelity and devotion to the interests of his patients, and gentleness and harmlessness in his dealings with them, combined with wisdom and caution in the treatment of their maladies.

But in his medical attendance generally . . . every practitioner . . . will frequently raise his soul to the great disposer of events – the ever flowing fountain, as well as the great terminal ocean of life and health – the only source of all true wisdom and consolation.

Science alone, particularly when accompanied by the inexperience of youth, and unbridled by the higher principles of religion and morality, is as powerful for evil as for good, and tends, moreover, to make its professors presumptuous, pedantic and arrogant.

5.5

Mesmerism *vs* ether: a professional battle

Alison Winter, 'Ethereal Epidemic: Mesmerism and the Introduction of Inhalation Anaesthesia to Early Victorian London', *Social History of Medicine*, 4, 1991, pp. 6–11, 13–14, 17–23, 25–6. [pp. 1–27].

Alison Winter has made an extensive study of mesmerism – the practice we now call hypnosis. In the nineteenth century, practitioners experimented with mesmerism both as a diagnostic tool and as a method of anaesthetising patients. This extract shows how the adoption of one of the great inventions of nineteenth-century medical practice – ether anaesthesia – over mesmeric anaesthesia was not due to its technical superiority, but was wrapped up in professional politics.

Mesmerism, or animal magnetism, was first popularized in late eighteenth-century France as a therapy for all diseases. There were several forms of 'animal magnetism', and purveyors of different therapies saw themselves as offering very distinct products in the medical marketplace. . . .

Mesmerism eventually became a vehicle for revolutionary political views during the French Revolution and was imported into Britain as one of many new 'democratic' physiologies. Hence when a few radical reformers of the late 1830s took up mesmerism, they had to work hard to exorcize its revolutionary reputation. The first and most prominent of these radicals was John Elliotson, Professor of Practical Medicine at the newly founded medical school at University College Hospital (UCH). Elliotson had a record of allegiance to unproven new therapies, such as the stethoscope and phrenology.[9] During the early 1830s he became a highly popular and controversial figure in London medicine. . . . The most controversial project Elliotson took up during these years, and the one of most personal consequence to him, was medical mesmerism.

In May 1838, Elliotson staged the first mesmeric experiments to be performed within a London hospital. Wakley[10] initially supported the demonstrations and provided *The Lancet* as a platform for reports of the proceedings. During the early demonstrations Elliotson demonstrated various trance phenomena exhibited by his subject, the young domestic servant Elizabeth O'Key. Elliotson's displays were taken very seriously, and the London medical journals took sides on what conclusions to draw from his work. But as the demonstrations progressed, Elliotson's subject was seen to play an increasingly active role in the mesmeric proceedings. She spoke rudely to Elliotson, calling him a 'foolish man', and mocked the various medical and aristocratic gentlemen in the audience. Eventually, she began to dictate instructions regarding how she might be placed in the mesmeric trance and retrieved from it. Wakley's support waned. Eventually he claimed that Elliotson was no longer in control of his mesmeric experiments, and that his conclusions could not be trusted.

[. . .]

The last straw, as far as the [UCH medical school] council were concerned, was a shocking subversion of authority of the physician over the patient, and of the experimenter over the subject: the mesmerized O'Key guided Elliotson through the male ward of the hospital 'at twilight', pronouncing life and death prognoses on the patients there. At one point she fell back in horror, crying out that she had seen 'Great Jackie', the angel of death, hovering over a man's bed. He died during the night. Elliotson was compelled to resign.

Whatever relief the London medical community may have felt at Elliotson's resignation, it was short-lived. In 1843 Elliotson launched his own forum for mesmeric research, *The Zoist: A Journal of Cerebral Physiology and Mesmerism*. *The Zoist* signalled a new campaign to

[9] Phrenology suggested that specific character traits were associated with particular areas of the brain: a person's character could be read from the shape and contours of the skull.

[10] Thomas Wakley (1795–1862), editor of the *Lancet*.

gain mesmerism entry into British hospitals via public demand for a service which it alone could offer: surgical anaesthesia.

From 1843 onward, members of the London mesmeric community launched an attempt to gain accreditation for mesmerism on two fronts, by simultaneously wooing the public and the surgical community with mesmeric anaesthesia. It is not clear why a community of researchers led by a physician—John Elliotson—should have chosen surgery as the focus of their campaign. However, the rising prestige of surgery may have seemed to offer the hope of carrying mesmeric anaesthesia along with it. . . . Moreover, the kinds of phenomena involved in mesmeric anaesthesia promised to avoid several of the problems which mesmerism had traditionally posed for its advocates.

Mesmerists represented their craft to the public as a broadly useful social tool. Mesmerism would subject 'pain' to medical discipline, therefore becoming a force (albeit a theatrical one) for public order. To do this, anaesthetists had to portray pain, as one physician wrote retrospectively of his own leg amputation. as:

> the black whirlwind of emotion, the horror of darkness, and the sense of desertion by God and man, bordering upon despair . . . which overwhelmed my heart.

Some mesmerists actually claimed that mesmerism would restore the presence of God to the surgical theatre—along with the 'solace' and 'peace' that that entailed. As part of the campaign to market mesmerism as a tool to restore peace and morality to the existing surgical theatre, mesmerists had to depict the unmesmerized surgical subject as being wild. Pain then became a sign of the surgeon's helplessness, rather than a necessary adjunct of his power. Mesmerists therefore painted a picture of the surgical theatre as the scene of chaos or revolution; and of mesmerism, in the hands of surgeons (or their mesmeric assistants), as the restorer of discipline and civilization.

With respect to the medical profession, mastery of the patient and of the theatre was a key issue: an insensible subject would be demonstrably under the control of the surgeon or mesmerist, and could not take over proceedings in the manner so abhorred in the case of Elizabeth O'Key. And in mastering the behaviour of the patient, mesmerists could claim that they had subjected surgical pain to a medical reform. Mesmerism could tame the surgical patient, whose insensibility became a sign of the surgeon's power. . . . But if the patients were to be subjected to medical 'discipline', the practice which subdued them would be disciplined as well. For mesmeric anaesthesia could only succeed if it could be marketed as a stable technique which could be restricted to specific medical purposes and to the use of licensed medical practitioners. Once under the control of the surgeons, mesmeric anaesthesia could be presented to the medical profession as an indispensable tool for reform.

[. . .]

In late 1842 the first British surgical operation under mesmeric anaesthesia was performed by a mesmerist and barrister, W. Topham and the surgeon W. Squire Ward. . . . James Wombell, 'a labouring man, of calm and quiet temperament' was placed into a state of complete insensibility, in which he felt none of the usual pain of the amputation of the hip, which was successful. The 'placid look of his countenance never changed for an instant' during the operation. When he awoke, he stated that he had felt no pain, though he had 'once felt, as if I heard a kind of crunching'.

The paper came under attack on two counts. The objection offered by Sir Benjamin Collins Brodie, President of the Royal College of Surgeons, was that the only proof of the effects of anaesthesia was the patient's testimony. In other words, he might be faking, for pride or for money. And since someone who would involve himself in mesmerism was untrustworthy, the whole question of mesmeric anaesthesia was unanswerable. Brodie accepted neither the credentials of Topham, as a barrister, nor of Wombell, as a straightforward man, as assurances of their honesty. According to Brodie, the issue of mesmerism rendered invalid all the normal credentials of a good witness. The other objection was raised by Marshall Hall, founder of the controversial theory of the 'excitomotory' reflex arc. . . . According to the doctrine of reflexes, Wombell's leg should have jumped when the sciatic nerve was cut. That it did not indicated that he had purposefully held his leg still throughout the operation, in collusion with his mesmerists and surgeon. . . .

Elliotson described and fought both objections in a pamphlet circulated publicly. In opposing Brodie's claims, he cited the many incidents in which a patient had pretended not to have felt surgical pain, but had been foiled by the surgeon. This approach emphasized the surgeon's ability to see through deceit, and stressed that the power of diagnosis and adjudication lay with him—not with the patient. In response to the 'reflex movement' Elliotson cited a discrepancy in Hall's work, which he claimed to be evidence undermining the validity of using the excitomotory system as an index of the reality of medical phenomena.

Both Brodie's and Hall's 'conspiracy theory' arguments against mesmerism must be understood in the context of mesmerism's reputation as an aid to dishonest patients like O'Key, and as a tool of subversion from revolutionary days. In the tumultuous years of the 1840s, when the medical profession was struggling with its own issues of 'mastery' and order, and when the middle class public were, more generally, in constant trepidation of the threat from working-class agitation, such claims were strong ammunition against a candidate therapy.

[. . .]

The campaign [for mesmeric anaesthesia] was at first moderately successful. By 1844, research into mesmeric anaesthesia had won cautious encouragement from various sectors of the medical community. Indeed, one mesmeric tract which emphasized the 'household' benefits of mesmerism and mesmeric anaesthesia and defined patients as wild animals whose cries resembled the 'bellowing of a wild animal [rather] than the intonation of a human voice' was especially well-received.

[. . .]

The pamphlets of John Forbes, founder and editor of the *British and Foreign Medical Review*, give some indication of the ambivalence felt by the medical profession in the face of the mesmeric campaign. Forbes consented . . . that the 'simple' mesmeric phenomena—those which he felt resembled sleep and other naturally-occurring phenomena—were unfeigned. He anticipated that mesmeric anaesthesia might become a great boon to medicine, though he claimed to find it equally possible that mesmerism might be proved false. His two books on the subject, *Mesmerism True—Mesmerism False* and *Illustrations of Modern Mesmerism*, were published in 1845. Their purpose was to present the medical and philosophical issues raised by mesmerism in a 'more calm and scientific' manner than had dominated previous discussion. Forbes condemned the pretence and exaggeration he felt produced the 'extraordinary effects', and described incidents in which he had exposed fraudulent exhibitions of 'extraordinary' mesmerism. Before they could deserve any respect, therefore, 'mesmerists, even those of the highest class, the members of the medical profession', needed drastically to alter their practice. Forbes's aim was not to drive mesmerism beyond the fringe of scientific enquiry, where he felt it existed at the moment, but rather to pull it into the mainstream of scientific attention where its merits could be appraised. . . .

[. . .]

The most successul work in mesmeric anaesthesia, and the most palatable to the medical profession, was performed by James Esdaile. Esdaile, a British surgeon, was the governor of the Native Hospital in Hooghly, India. He first heard of mesmerism in early 1845, and by April had performed almost a hundred quite serious operations on mesmerized subjects. These included amputations of large tumours, cataracts, and experiments including the 'racking of the electromagnetic machine', during which his mesmerized patients (all native Indians) were insensible. Esdaile's method in adapting mesmerism to surgery was the antithesis of Elliotson's research on mesmerism's medical effects. He took his patient into a darkened room, where he carried out the mesmerism in private. For Esdaile, the process of mesmeric anaesthesia was just a means to an end, and the presence of an audience was a distraction rather than a stimulus to that process.

Esdaile's own power as administrator of the hospital had helped him greatly in his efforts to gain credibility for mesmerism in India. . . . The power relations between the English doctor and native subject were secure, and the geography of the process, in which a specific room was allocated for mesmerism, was well-accepted within the hospital. . . .

Esdaile's version of mesmeric therapy was . . . well-received in Britain. One British medical journal decided, in considering Esdaile's claims, that Indian patients were 'scarcely intelligent enough' to have been able to pretend their invulnerability to pain. On these grounds Esdaile's patients' testimonies were believed. The editor concluded that:

> This claim of mesmerism admits of easy testing, and we repeat if its validity is proved, that of the various monstrous pretensions of this art will not be brought in anywise nearer admission, while a vast boon will have been secured to suffering mankind.

Most important in Esdaile's success to this point was the role he sought for mesmeric anaesthesia. He kept the process of mesmerism as a preparative stage only, such that the effect of suspended animation was the important aspect of the practice. Moreover, Esdaile's credentials as surgeon, as head of a native hospital, and more generally as a local administrator of the Empire, made him a natural master of the medical arena. . . .

Unfortunately for Esdaile, most of the support for his anaesthetic techniques . . . evaporated in 1847. Previous supporters decided that there was no longer any need to develop mesmeric anaesthesia. Ether anaesthesia would be perfectly sufficient.

The practice of inhalating the vapour of sulphuric ether for medical or recreational purposes was widely popularized during the early nineteenth century as a substitute for nitrous oxide in pneumatic medicine and in popular science demonstrations. Ether's pedigree was very similar to mesmerism's. It was a late enlightenment practice, developed by political radicals . . . which seemed to imply that mental processes were fundamentally physical. And during the first decades of the nineteenth century, the two shared an identity as recreational practices which drew crowds at popular science demonstrations. They were stock tools for travelling science lecturers, and both were put on display at the Adelaide Gallery, London's main forum for popular science lectures. In such contexts, the livelihoods of itinerant showmen depended on the variety and spectacular nature of ethereal (and mesmeric) effects.

[. . .]

It was largely through the ineffectiveness of a Boston dentist, Horace Wells, both in mesmerism and in the administration of nitrous oxide, that inhalation anaesthesia was developed in 1846. Wells had been experimenting for some time with mesmerism in the hope of anaesthetizing his dental patients. . . . Every attempt to mesmerize his dental patients was an abysmal failure. When he noticed, during a popular science demonstration in 1845, that subjects 'drunk' on nitrous oxide appeared to feel no pain, he immediately arranged a public demonstration, and administered the nitrous oxide himself.' . . . Unfortunately, the inhalation did not anaesthetize the patient—Wells found to his dismay that practice and skill were necessary for success. He retired in humiliation and later committed suicide when his ex-dental partner, William Morton, received the credit for discovering inhalation anaesthesia (using ether) only one year later.

Morton had been present for Wells' disastrous performance, and eventually decided to try ether instead. After much practice . . . Morton carefully arranged his public demonstration of ether on 19 October 1846. Morton administered the ether and Dr John Collins Warren performed the surgery. The operation involved a small incision to the jaw, followed by some minor dental work. According to several accounts, the patient moaned and moved restlessly during the operation. Ether had not made him insensible to the knife, he later testified, though his pain had been somewhat dulled. The incision had felt to him like a 'hoe' had been 'scraped' across his skin. When Warren had finished the surgery, the audience went wild. 'Gentlemen', proclaimed Warren, 'this is no humbug'.

News quickly spread through Boston and America, and almost as quickly to England. The first (by one historian's account) announcement of ether anaesthesia in the medical press stressed the 'medicalness' of ether by defining it as mesmerism's alter ego:

a remarkable discovery has been made. Unlike the trickery and farce of mesmerism, this is based on scientific principles, and is solely in the hands of gentlemen of high professional attainment, who make no secret of the matter or manner. To prevent it from being abused or falling into the power of low, evil minded, irresponsible persons, we are informed that the discoverer has secured a patent.

In this passage, ether is defined as being what mesmerism is not: a scientific practice, based on scientific principles, and restricted from the start to qualified practitioners.

[. . .]

The spread of anaesthesia to Britain was portrayed by a contemporary author as an 'epidemic'. The alacrity with which . . . ether was taken up by the medical profession, demonstrates the fact that since surgeons embraced the practice before they had any strong evidence of its effectiveness, other reasons must have prevailed in its acceptance. . . . [A]t every point in the brief 'epidemic' of popularity, ether was entirely defined as a substitute for mesmerism. Indeed, if a 'discovery' was made during ether's reign in Britain in 1847, it was the realization that ether could not easily be made to look sufficiently different from mesmerism to become a reputable anaesthetic agent.

When Francis Boott, the first to learn of the anaesthetic technique, wrote to Robert Liston . . . Professor of Surgery at University College Hospital, Liston moved quickly. He sent invitations to various medical and lay acquaintances, informing them of the time and place of his operation two days later. He consulted Peter Squire, an instrument maker, about the best techniques for effective administration of ether, and practised several times in the interim. He selected as his patient a butler—perhaps the best compromise in the search for a good witness who was simultaneously low on the social ladder.

Liston's operation was clearly an attempt to rival mesmeric demonstrations that had gone before. The operation, an amputation of the thigh, was identical to the Topham/Ward operation four years earlier and University College Hospital was again the setting of the events. After the operation, in which the patient moaned and stirred restlessly, but did not cry out, Liston was said to declare, 'This Yankee dodge beats mesmerism hollow'. Later that day he wrote to his friend, Professor James Miller of Edinburgh, exulting,

HURRAH! Rejoice! Mesmerism, and its professors, have met with a 'heavy blow, and great discouragement.' An American dentist has used ether (inhalation of it) to destroy sensation in his operations, and the plan has succeeded in the hands of Warren, Hayward, and others in Boston . . . Rejoice!

[. . .]

The next stage in the battle for control of anaesthesia was extensive coverage in the medical and general journals. In the first six months of 1847, *The Lancet* is said to have published 112 articles on ether anaesthesia. Wakley represented the 'ethereal' phenomenon as having 'a remarkable perfection' about it, especially since it would destroy, he felt, 'one limb of the mesmeric quackery'. . . .

One of the most important aspects of the campaign was the attempt to restrict the use of ether to the medical profession, and to limit the range of phenomena it produced to insensibility. Those who responded cautiously to ether warned that it would be difficult for British hospitals to restrict it to their own use. Editorials abounded in medical journals discussing how etherization might be controlled by licensing schemes. The physiologist William B. Carpenter, writing as editor of the *Medico-Chirurgical Review*, claimed that the public and the medical community had been 'spellbound' by ether. Carpenter condemned the fact that anaesthesia had transformed surgical theatres into fashionable 'scenes of operative display', and worried that it was being used 'too indiscriminately' by non-professionals and professionals alike in what his friend John Forbes had described as an 'ethereal epidemic'. . . .

[. . .]

Elliotson's rage at the hijacking of anaesthesia by the etherists is evident in the *Zoist* editorials of 1847. He was particularly furious at what he saw as a campaign of silence by the medical journals, which devoted little space to anti-mesmeric editorials after the first months of 1847. Elliotson interpreted this as an attempt to freeze mesmerism out of medical fora altogether, and to represent to the reading public that mesmeric research had been abandoned in the wake of ether anaesthesia.

[. . .]

The defeat of mesmeric anaesthesia was widely perceived to spell the end of mesmerism's chance of legitimacy. Mesmeric anaesthesia was not taken into hospitals as a preparation for surgery during these years, even when ether was deemed an unsuitable anaesthetic agent and exchanged for others.

5.6
A squabble between doctors

Anthony Trollope, *Dr Thorne* (London, Wordsworth Classics,
1996 [originally published 1859]), pp. 25–8.

Anthony Trollope (1815–82) was one of the most popular and accurate recorders of Victorian social life. Doctors regularly feature in
his novels, usually caricatured as pompous caricatures with ludi-
crous names such as Dr Omnicrom Pie and Dr Mewdew. However,
Trollope, like most novelists of his day, produced much more sympathetic portraits of the family doctor – the general practitioner
who might not be a brilliant clinician but faithfully and generously
served the community. This extract from *Dr Thorne* (1859) faithfully represents one of the many acrimonious disputes over status
between different types of practitioners.

And thus Dr Thorne became settled for life in the little village of
Greshamsbury. As was then the wont with many country practitioners,
and as should be the wont with them all if they consulted their own dignity a little less and the comforts of their customers somewhat more, he
added the business of a dispensing apothecary to that of physician. In
doing so, he was of course much reviled. Many people around him
declared that he could not truly be a doctor, or, at any rate, a doctor to
be so called; and his brethren in the art living around him, though they
knew that his diplomas, degrees, and certificates were all *en règle*,[11]
rather countenanced the report. There was much about this new-comer
which did not endear him to his own profession. In the first place he
was a new-comer, and, as such, was of course to be regarded by other
doctors as being *de trop*.[12] Greshamsbury was only fifteen miles from
Barchester, where there was a regular depot of medical skill, and but
eight from Silverbridge, where a properly established physician had
been in residence for the last forty years. Dr Thorne's predecessor at
Greshamsbury had been a humble-minded general practitioner, gifted
with a due respect for the physicians of the county; and he, though he
had been allowed to physic[13] the servants, and sometimes the children

[11] *en règle*: correct, literally by the rules.
[12] *de trop*: one too many.
[13] *physic*: literally, to dose the servants with medicine or more generally to provide all
forms of treatment.

at Greshamsbury, had never had the presumption to put himself on a par with his betters.

Then, also, Dr Thorne, though a graduated physician, though entitled beyond all dispute to call himself a doctor, according to all the laws of all the colleges, made it known to the East Barsetshire world, very soon after he had seated himself at Greshamsbury, that his rate of pay was to be seven-and-sixpence a visit within a circuit of five miles, with a proportionally increased charge at proportionally increased distances. Now there was something low, mean, unprofessional, and democratic in this; so, at least, said the children of Æsculapius[14] gathered together in conclave at Barchester. In the first place, it showed that this Thorne was always thinking of his money, like an apothecary, as he was; whereas, it would have behoved him, as a physician, had he had the feelings of a physician under his hat, to have regarded his own pursuits in a purely philosophical spirit, and to have taken any gain which might have accrued as an accidental adjunct to his station in life. A physician should take his fee without letting his left hand know what his right hand was doing; it should be taken without a thought, without a look, without a move of the facial muscles; the true physician should hardly be aware that the last friendly grasp of the hand had been made more precious by the touch of gold. Whereas, that fellow Thorne would lug out half a crown from his breeches pocket and give it in change for a ten-shilling piece. And then it was clear that this man had no appreciation of the dignity of a learned profession. He might constantly be seen compounding medicines in the shop, at the left hand of his front door; not making experiments philosophically in materia medica for the benefit of coming ages – which, if he did, he should have done in the seclusion of his study, far from profane eyes – but positively putting together common powders for rural bowels, or spreading vulgar ointments for agricultural ailments.

A man of this sort was not fit society for Dr Fillgrave of Barchester. That must be admitted. And yet he had been found to be fit society for the old squire of Greshamsbury, whose shoe-ribbons Dr Fillgrave would not have objected to tie; so high did the old squire stand in the county just previous to his death. But the spirit of the Lady Arabella was known by the medical profession of Barsetshire, and when that good man died it was felt that Thorne's short tenure of Greshamsbury favour was already over. The Barsetshire regulars were, however, doomed to disappointment. Our doctor had already contrived to endear himself to the heir; and though there was not even then much personal love between

---

[14] Medical practitioners – Aesculapius was the Greek god of healing.

him and the Lady Arabella, he kept his place at the great house unmoved, not only in the nursery and in the bedrooms, but also at the squire's dining-table.

Now there was in this, it must be admitted, quite enough to make him unpopular among his brethren; and this feeling was soon shown in a marked and dignified manner. Dr Fillgrave, who had certainly the most respectable professional connexion in the county, who had a reputation to maintain, and who was accustomed to meet, on almost equal terms, the great medical baronets from the metropolis at the houses of the nobility – Dr Fillgrave declined to meet Dr Thorne in consultation. He exceedingly regretted, he said most exceedingly, the necessity which he felt of doing so: he had never before had to perform so painful a duty; but, as a duty which he owed to his profession, he must perform it. With every feeling of respect for Lady —, – a sick guest at Greshamsbury – and for Mr Gresham, he must decline to attend in conjunction with Dr Thorne. If his services could be made available under any other circumstances, he would go to Greshamsbury as fast as post-horses could carry him.

[. . .]

It will therefore be understood, that when such a gauntlet was thus thrown in his very teeth by Dr Fillgrave, he was not slow to take it up. He addressed a letter to the Barsetshire Conservative *Standard*, in which he attacked Dr Fillgrave with some considerable acerbity. Dr Fillgrave responded in four lines, saying, that on mature consideration he had made up his mind not to notice any remarks that might be made on him by Dr Thorne in the public press. The Greshamsbury doctor then wrote another letter, more witty and much more severe than the last; and as this was copied into the Bristol, Exeter, and Gloucester papers, Dr Fillgrave found it very difficult to maintain the magnanimity of his reticence. It is sometimes becoming enough for a man to wrap himself in the dignified toga of silence, and proclaim himself indifferent to public attacks; but it is a sort of dignity which it is very difficult to maintain. As well might a man, when stung to madness by wasps, endeavour to sit in his chair without moving a muscle, as endure with patience and without reply the courtesies of a newspaper opponent. Dr Thorne wrote a third letter, which was too much for medical flesh and blood to bear. Dr Fillgrave answered it, not, indeed, in his own name, but in that of a brother doctor; and then the war raged merrily. It is hardly too much to say that Dr Fillgrave never knew another happy hour. Had he dreamed of what materials was made that young compounder of doses at Greshamsbury he would have met him in consultation, morning, noon, and night, without objection; but having begun the war, he was

113

constrained to go on with it: his brethren would allow him no alternative. Thus he was continually being brought up to the fight, as a prizefighter may be seen to be, who is carried up round after round, without any hope on his own part, and who, in each round, drops to the ground before the very wind of his opponent's blows.

But Dr Fillgrave, though thus weak himself, was backed in practice and in countenance by nearly all his brethren in the county. The guinea fee, the principle of *giving* advice and of selling no medicine, the great resolve to keep a distinct barrier between the physician and the apothecary, and, above all, the hatred of the contamination of a bill, were strong in the medical mind of Barsetshire. Dr Thorne had the provincial medical world against him, and so he appealed to the metropolis. The *Lancet* took the matter up in his favour, but the *Journal of Medical Science* was against him; the *Weekly Chirurgeon*, noted for its medical democracy, upheld him as a medical prophet, but the *Scalping Knife*, a monthly periodical got up in dead opposition to the *Lancet*, showed him no mercy. So the war went on, and our doctor, to a certain extent, became a noted character.

Part six
Women in medicine

6.1
The biological destiny of women

Michael Ryan, *A Manual of Midwifery*, in *Women from
Birth to Death. The Female Life Cycle in Britain
1830–1914*, eds Pat Jalland and John Hooper (Atlantic
Highlands, NJ, Humanities Press International, Inc., 1986),
pp. 20–1.

Michael Ryan, a physician, practised in London in the early nineteenth century. He published and lectured on obstetrics and edited
the *London Medical and Surgical Journal* from 1832–38. His
Manual of Midwifery, published in 1828, was written for medical
students and went through several editions.

The character of a woman's mind is chiefly determined by the part she
bears in relation to generation. Her destiny to be united to a husband,
and to become a mother, is perceived in the plays of her infancy, and
afterwards becomes manifest in the commencing struggle in her
bosom, between her modesty and her inclination for the other sex, as is
seen in her lovely blushes, often united with a noble feminine pride and
reserve, until she meets the man of her heart, when all these feelings are
succeeded by a full and unlimited abandonment to the object of her
affection. Conjugal love has speedily, however, to submit itself to the
stronger feeling of maternal affection, of the power of which we have
many and the most extraordinary examples. . . .

It has long been a medical axiom, that women are more sensitive,
weak, more influenced by moral and physical causes, and more liable to
diseases than the other sex. The constitution is more feeble, and is

peculiarly influenced by the mysterious process of reproduction, pregnancy, parturition,[1] the puerperal[2] state, and lactation[3] as well as by the other function peculiar to it. I have also to observe, that want of exercise in the open air, tight lacing[4] and constipation are among the more common causes of female disorders and diseases. The natural sensibility is increased during menstruation . . .

These facts being admitted, the treatment of diseases of women cannot be so active, as those of the stronger sex; and we must never forget that indescribable, or perhaps mysterious influence on the female system, which predominates during the performance of any function peculiar to the sex, and is subservient to reproduction. It always guides a scientific practitioner and causes him to be less active in his treatment of the ordinary diseases of women than of men.

6.2
Women as doctors and women as nurses

Editorial, 17 August 1878, *The Lancet*, II, pp. 226–7.

The Lancet was founded in 1823 by Thomas Wakley. Unlike earlier medical journals, which published research or clinical cases of note, *The Lancet* carried a mix of medical knowledge – lectures, research papers – plus professional politics – editorials on matters affecting the profession, letters, news of institutions. From its founding, *The Lancet* stood up for the ordinary practitioner against the elite, and campaigned for improvements to the incomes, conditions of work and status of general practitioners. In the late 1860s and 1870s, under the editorship of James G. Wakley, son of the founder, it consistently opposed the movement for women doctors. This editorial appeared in response to a decision by the British Medical Association to continue to exclude women from its ranks, even though some women had been registered with the General Medical Council by virtue of foreign licences.

[1] Childbirth.
[2] Post-natal.
[3] Breast feeding.
[4] Wearing corsets which pulled in the waist to make it smaller. An eighteen-inch waist was the desirable standard.

Again, 'the woman question' in relation to the practice of physic and surgery, is forced upon us by the wise decision of the British Medical Association to exclude female practitioners; and, by a curious coincidence, we are, at the same moment, invited, by an able article in the last number of the *Spectator*,[5] to consider the peculiar physical state and mental susceptibilities of 'Invalids'. The two topics, thrown together, not inopportunely, suggest the comparison, or contrast, as it will be found, of woman as doctor and woman as nurse. In the one character she is as awkward, unfit, and untrustworthy, as she is at home, capable, and thoroughly worthy of confidence in the other.

Setting aside the anomalies and, as we believe, the gracelessness, of the position which a well-meaning but misguided young woman assumes when she undertakes the practical study of medicine, and waiving the question of feminine personal and social disabilities for the vocation of physician and surgeon, there is the all-important issue of natural and constitutional fitness. In the economy of nature – whether expounded by the Oracular utterance,[6] or evolved by experience – the ministry of woman is one of help and sympathy. The essential principle, the key-note of her work in the world, is *aid*; to sustain, succour, revive and even sometimes shelter, man in the struggle and duty of life, is her peculiar function. The moment she affects the first or leading *role* in any vocation she is out of place, and the secondary, but essential, part of helpmate cannot be filled. A more womanly sister may nominally assume the position of *help*, but, however willing, she cannot sustain the part, because the lead is out of natural concord, and harmony is impossible.

This is not a mere sentimental view of the facts. If women undertake the duties of physicians and surgeons, we shall presently feel the want of nurses. It is opposed to the genius of woman's nature to act as helpmate to her own sex. Men may tend men, and women women, in sickness, but, except in cases where the ties of blood or friendship hold nurse and patient together in sympathy, the service rendered is that of 'hospital orderly', a thing to be tolerated in the absence of something better, rather than valued for its intrinsic fitness and excellence. The heartlessness of such a ministry will be still colder and less genial when all that pertains to the harmony of woman as nurse acting as the helpmeet of man as doctor in the sick room is sacrificed. The superiority asserted and the deference claimed by the woman doctor will not readily be conceded by her less favoured but not less ambitious sister. The unsuitability of men as nurses is not due to any want of power or tact

[5] A popular periodical, written for a general middle-class audience.
[6] The Bible.

117

on their part; they are stronger, and, therefore, able to perform many services for the sick with less fatigue to the patient than woman-nurses, and when feeling and interest inspire the touch of a man's hand, it is steadier, more precise, and not less gentle than that of a woman; but, unless under exceptional circumstances, man's nature rebels against the complete surrender of his own judgement and that implicit obedience in spirit, as well as letter, which are the first essentials of a good nurse. In the same way women will, unconsciously, perhaps, but effectually, cease to play the subordinate part required of them as nurses when their own sex is elevated to the control of the sick chamber and the treatment of disease. Already, since the craze of women to become physicians and surgeons has attained proportions promising success to the movement, we recognise an evil influence on the training and work of female nurses. Subjects of purely medical and surgical concern are beginning to be included in the 'studies' of the *nurse*, while other matters, on which mainly the success of treatment must always depend, are regarded as menial, and relegated to the care of servants told off to wait on the 'skilled'. This is a small but significant sign of the condition of matters to which the 'woman-doctor' movement is progressing. In the end there will be no nurses, because the female sick-tenders will not yield docile obedience to their feminine medical superiors, and because the craft of 'skilled nurse' will be so developed that it must jostle the profession of woman-physicians. Ultimately the evil will probably cure itself; the women-doctors will find it necessary to nurse their own patients, and in the school of experience they will at length become convinced that this ministry is their personal and best vocation, which no intruder can occupy, because none save themselves can fulfil.

The needs of the sick are in part physical, and in part mental, and so far as the constant and immediate associations of the sick chamber are concerned, they are all of a nature which women alone can effectively satisfy. It is a woman's prerogative to nurse, whether the helpless being at her mercy be an infant, or an adult reduced to the level of childhood by disease. Women cannot desert the position of nurses of the sick unless they also abandon the rearing and tending of the young. The sympathies and graces called out by the one function are those which must be enlisted in the service of the other. It is our contention that by becoming doctors women virtually, and – so far as the vast influence always exerted by strong-minded individuals on their order is concerned – in a representative sense, cease to be nurses. The influence will, in this case, be, and is in truth becoming, especially disastrous socially, because the omen of the movement is held to mark an advance of the sex to higher ground, and this too certainly implies the contemptuous abandonment of every sphere of action conceived to be less elevated. There is only one natural safeguard as regards the spread of this revolt against the reign of natural law. Confidence in man is an integral part of the instinct which has constituted woman his helpmeet in life, and however exceptional women may disport themselves in the new sphere unwisely, as we believe, thrown open to them, the great body of sensible females must, in the more critical moments of peril from sickness, whether in their own cases, or those of persons dear to them, recur to the counsel of their natural leaders. We have no misgiving as to the ultimate issue of this weak exploit. There will probably be always a few 'women doctors' for those of their own sex who care to seek their services; but for the aid of the many, and in the more serious maladies, the services of the profession will be required. We say 'the profession' advisedly. The law may recognise the qualifications obtained by women, but the profession must, in self-respect, and we will not scruple to add in common decency, decline to accept them as titles of admission to the general body of practitioners. The confraternity of physicians and surgeons will not, we apprehend, either consult or hold professional intercourse with those who have assumed a position, and now desire to exercise functions, opposed to the instincts of their sex.

<hr />

6.3
Elizabeth Blackwell, a medical pioneer

Margaret Foster, *Significant Sisters. The Grassroots of Active Feminism 1839–1939* (London, Penguin, 1984), pp. 70–4.

Elizabeth Blackwell was the first woman to be registered with the General Medical Council in Britain. She had graduated from Geneva College in New York State in 1849 and she registered in England in 1858, as the holder of a foreign medical degree. Blackwell served as a role model for other pioneering women doctors, but gave little support to the early Women's Rights movement. She thought that women had a particular place in humanising medicine, especially through midwifery, preventative medicine and treatment of the poor. Here we see Blackwell in 1849, soon after graduation, attempting to gain clinical training in order to become fully qualified as a doctor. This stage was to prove a stumbling block for many other medical women.

In January 1849 Elizabeth graduated from Geneva medical school, the acknowledged leader of the class. . . . But, in spite of this success and in spite of the solid qualification she had gained, Elizabeth appreciated only too well that she had yet another beginning to make. The problem now was to gain hospital experience, to become a practically qualified doctor as well as a theoretically qualified one.

Immediately after graduation she returned to Philadelphia. [S]he had been prepared for this and did not in fact let it worry her because she had already decided that Paris was her destination. Everyone told her that Paris was the medical centre of the world so there she would go and somehow obtain experience. After that, no American institution would dare to keep her out. . . . She docked in Liverpool, then went on to London where to her amazement and delight she was warmly received. The medical profession showered her with invitations and although not used to socializing she found she greatly enjoyed being fêted (and developed a taste for iced champagne which she pronounced 'really good'). But in Paris, where she arrived at the end of May, her reception was rather different. There were no dinners or other invitations and she was lucky to have her sister Anna with whom to share a flat. Her French was poor, she had little money and her introductions to medical people were few. Her fame had not preceded her and she had instead some difficulty establishing her identity. Nobody seemed the slightest bit impressed by her degree. She was rapidly forced to face the fact that a degree, said to be vital before it was won, suddenly became, in the case of women, of no importance once it was. The question changed to one of experience and it looked as though the chance to gain that was not to be given to her.

But Elizabeth had come a long way and had no intention of returning empty-handed. Luckily, she had learned to be thick-skinned and to persevere. To all suggestions that she should just be content and perhaps start a *women's* medical career she turned a deaf ear. She was not going to be caught on that one. Women had to become qualified in exactly the same way as men or they would always be inferior. So she went on seeking out medical men who might help her and finally hit on one – a man called Pierre Louis[7] who advised her to enter La Maternité, the major lying-in hospital in France, and said he would back her application. Elizabeth promptly took his advice and accepted his help even though she was not immediately attracted to La Maternité, a grim old convent of

---

[7] Pierre Louis (1787–1872) was one of the most eminent practitioners working in the Paris hospitals at the beginning of the nineteenth century. He pioneered the use of statistics to prove the effectiveness of therapeutics.

little appeal. Nor was she attracted by the conditions of admission when they were presented to her. No concessions were to be made to her doctor's degree. She would enter with the same status as all the other young girls who came to train as midwives, would live communally with them and be subjected, as they were, to the same schoolgirl discipline. She accepted because she had no alternative. On June 30, 1849, aged twenty-eight, she entered La Maternité, but privately hoped only to use it as a stepping stone to greater things – she intended only to stay three months and then use her experience there to gain entry to another more general hospital.

It was a strange experience for her. She slept in a huge dormitory, took a bath with six others, was served poor food and had not a moment to herself. Most of the girls were around eighteen and naturally behaved quite differently from Elizabeth who felt ancient beside them. They came from all over France so there was every variety of accent for her to learn. The day was extremely long – fourteen hours at a stretch was common – and the work hard. La Maternité delivered 3,000 babies a year and the students were present for all 'interesting' cases which happened at the most inconvenient times. But Elizabeth, in spite of what she always called her 'hermit-like tendencies', settled in well. She felt more camaraderie among those young girls than among her colleagues in either Geneva or Blockley[8] and enjoyed helping and mothering them. And she came to have enormous respect for some of the staff who were efficient and as hardworking as the students. She learned so much in her first three months that she realized she would be stupid to leave and ought instead to complete the course. So she decided to stay on. What also influenced her was the attitude of some of the staff who were helpful and interested in her (she was disgusted by the immorality of others) and encouraged her to believe she would make a good obstetric surgeon. . . .

By November Elizabeth was being given more responsibility. On November 4th she got up early, after snatching a few hours' sleep at the end of a particularly exhausting day, and made her way along the cold corridors to the ward where she was to syringe a baby who had purulent ophthalmia.[9] The light was poor, she was still sleepy, and as she injected warm water into the baby's tiny eye she was aware of her own clumsiness. What she thought was some of the water she was using spurted up into her own eyes as she bent over the baby. She dashed it out and went on with the job. By the afternoon she was uneasily admitting to herself that she had a prickling sensation in her

[8] The hospital in Philadelphia where she had earlier worked.

[9] An infection of the newborn, often the result of the mother suffering from gonorrhoea.

121

right eye. By the evening there was no pretending – both eyes were visibly swollen and closed and even before she went to be examined she had no doubt that she had contracted the dreaded disease for which she had been treating the baby. Every possible treatment was instantly resorted to. Her eyelids were cauterized, leeches applied to her temples, her eyes syringed every hour with scrupulous care . . . She lay for weeks in bed with both eyes closed, in an agony of apprehension, remembering the words of Dr Webster in Geneva – 'Your fingers are useless without your eyes.' After three weeks her left eye finally opened. She had a split second's clarity and then total blackness. She was blind in one eye and her vision was impaired in the other.

[. . .]

She could not be a surgeon. The realization that this had to be admitted brought her as near to collapse as she was ever to be. What had all her struggles been for if she was now forced to abandon medicine? She simply could not bear it and out of her misery and rage at the gross unfairness of it came a new determination. There was more to medicine than surgery. Why should she not turn now to general doctoring?

This is what she did. With superhuman courage she once more began seeking out people who would help her to complete a practical training as a doctor. Not only did she have her sex against her but she also had her disablement. A one-eyed woman was not exactly going to be a prime candidate for an arduous hospital training. But thanks to the endeavours of a cousin and the genuine sympathy her accident had awakened St Bartholomew's Hospital in London agreed to let her enter as a student.

<hr>

6.4
Motives for medical training

Hope Malleson, *A Woman Doctor. Mary Murdoch of Hull*
(London, Sidgwick & Jackson, 1919), pp. 16–17, 36–7.

Mary Murdoch was one of the first woman doctors, qualifying in 1892 from the London Medical School for Women. She then worked in hospitals until her own poor health encouraged her to set up her own practice in Kingston upon Hull in East Yorkshire in 1896. She remained there until her death in 1916. She had a strong Catholic faith. She supported the feminist movement and drove a car at a time when women drivers were a rarity (to the peril of local pedestrians). Her biography provides details of her radical views and public opinions.

[In] 1883, Mary Murdoch finally left school and returned to Elgin. . . . [C]hanges had taken place in her home. Her two sisters had married, and the three brothers had scattered to different parts of the world. One was a doctor, another a planter in Ceylon, the third . . . a naval surgeon.

There followed four uneventful years, but Mary Murdoch made the best of them. She read much, she practised singing, the piano, and the violin. She made friends and shared in the interests of the town; she indulged in her favourite amusements of fishing and dancing. Occasionally she and her mother journeyed south to Moffat to visit her married sister. But her letters grew infrequent, and showed that 'her spirit was chafing at the limitations of her home life and at the small activities of the country town'. Afterward she would refer to this time as 'wasted years'.

In 1885, the youngest son died in Malta of malaria. Mrs. Murdoch never recovered from the shock; her health began to fail, and she grew to need her daughter's constant care. Eighteen months later she died, and the family home was broken up.

The idea of studying medicine seems to have been suggested to Mary Murdoch by an article in one of the 'monthlies',[10] on the need for women doctors in India; but whether this was before or after her mother's death is uncertain. It was through the old family physician, Dr. Adams, that the idea took definite shape. He had seen Mary Murdoch grow up, and with rare penetration recognised her aptitude for the work. It was by his advice that she decided to devote the small legacy her mother left her to her medical training.

[. . .]

The following extract from a letter . . . shows Mary Murdoch's attitude towards her profession:

'When I first took the great love of my life – Medicine – to my heart, I said to her: "You shall change what you like; you shall take everything the world calls pleasure from me; you shall take real joys from me, and still I shall love and serve you." She has been an exacting mistress, and has taken thing after thing from me; tethered me down, taken my

[10] Monthly magazines.

freedom and liberty; upset my own and everyone else's plans a thousand times a year, and yet I love her and serve her with the same passion as I did twenty years ago.'

6.5
The impact of women doctors

Editorial, 2 August 1873, *The Lancet*, II, pp. 159–60.

This editorial, also by James G. Wakley, was prompted by the vigorous campaign from 1869–74 by a determined group of women, led by Sophia Jex-Blake, to be trained in medicine at Edinburgh University. At varying times they were denied access to lectures and to clinical training, but having overcome many obstacles, admittance to the degree exam still eluded them. In Edinburgh in July 1872, Lord Gifford ruled that the women were entitled to all the rights and privileges of the university and could therefore proceed to exams for medical degrees. This decision was overturned by appeal the following year. The women students stayed in Edinburgh taking advantage of training opportunities, but were barred from graduation. During this time *The Lancet* constantly attacked the efforts of women to become doctors.

It is no part of our task to explain or account for the redundancy of women, nor to point out in what particular departments of the business of life they may best devote their energies; but shall confine ourselves to the task of endeavouring to show that, contrary to a widely-spread popular opinion, they are neither by nature nor habit adapted to the multifarious duties of a medical practitioner. It is asserted by the advocates for female doctors that there is a field for the usefulness of women in the medical treatment of diseases of women and children, and that women themselves would rather be attended in their labours and various ailments by members of their own sex than by men. We must demur to this, for from an extended experience we are convinced that the mothers of England prefer to be attended in their labours by medical men, and that, in fact, the idea of female medical attendants is positively repulsive to the more thoughtful women of this country. Judging from the mental, moral, and emotional characteristics of the female organisation,[11] we should say that women are not well fitted to regard calmly and philosophically the pains and agonies of their sisters, nor are they constituted to battle seriously and determinedly with many of the dangerous and alarming accidents of parturition, which always require prompt and vigorous action. Moreover, it is the result of ignorance or oversight to imagine that anyone can comprehend the details of obstetrics and gynaecology without a thorough knowledge of all the departments of medical science, or that they can become skilful and successful practitioners of the art without adequate acquaintance with the general manifestations of disease. We ought not, with the empiric specialist,[12] to divide the body into separate organs and systems, and treat only this or that; but we must take the body as a whole, and learn the intimate relationship and sympathy which one part bears to another. The opinions we have stigmatised have, unfortunately, too long held men's minds in bondage, and have resulted only in a retrogressive quackery. The best specialist is he who, thoroughly conversant with the general working of the complicated machinery of the human body, has yet an intimate acquaintance with all its individual parts, and is therefore able to comprehend it in its entirety. Obstretrics has only comparatively recently been rescued from the midwives and the *sages-femmes*,[13] and is just beginning to enjoy a scientific reputation as the result of the labour of many intelligent and enlightened observers. Shall we, then, again consign it to the dark regions from which it has just been snatched?

Further, women are neither physically nor morally qualified for many of the onerous, important, and confidential duties of the general practitioner; nor capable of the prolonged exertions or severe exposures to all kinds of weather which a professional life entails; nor capable of keeping the social secrets of patients, which are often dearer than life, and are second only to the claims of justice; nor ought they to be able to give instruction on many points of worldly wisdom which serve often to save many from temptation, or even to reclaim them from actual sin or impending ruin.

It has been foolishly asserted that the difference between the mental constitution of a man and a woman is the result of education, and that

[11] i.e. the female mind and body.

[12] A quack or untrained practitioner, who relied on experience and often offered a very narrow range of treatments, such as operations for the removal of cataracts. Educated practitioners, by definition, possessed a body of theoretical knowledge. At this time, a small proportion of practitioners chose to spend some of their time focusing on some specific aspect of medicine, but would also work as general practitioners.

[13] Literally 'wise women' – untrained women who helped at births.

if a girl were brought up under the same conditions as a boy, the difference would not exist, or would be reduced to a minimum. This is erroneous in the highest degree, for there is a fundamental and structural difference which shows anatomically and physiologically in early life, and declares itself most emphatically at puberty. It cannot be doubted that it is possible to make women more *man-like*, but it is not possible to produce in them the characteristics of man without destroying many of their feminine attractions and possibly also their feminine functions. It is probable that, by careful selection, we might succeed in producing a race of strong-minded, masculine women, who might be capable of sitting on our school boards, or in the Houses of Parliament, or engaging in the active work of the learned professions; but by that time men might have become reconciled to the gentler occupations of domestic life, and capable, mentally, morally, and perhaps physiologically, of staying at home to nurse the baby.

We must now turn to examine another phase of this subject. From what we have stated it is evident that the only justification for the present movement in favour of female doctors can be that the work is not properly done at present; and if this be so, it remains to be proved that women possess in a high degree all the qualifications necessary to the scientific and practical physician and surgeon. If it cannot be shown that women are better, or at least as well fitted for medical practice as men, it is surely opposed to all the principles of political and social economy to urge females into the field to the necessary exclusion of many men, for already the profession is overstocked. It may be replied, however, that by competition the product is supplied to the public at a smaller cost; but the result of this will be that the labour will become too unremunerative to engage the energies of the higher intellects, who will turn their attention to more profitable pursuits; and therefore unless women can be produced who are able to grapple with the profound problems of scientific medicine, the subject must necessarily lapse into charlatanism, to the ultimate prejudice of mankind.

6.6

Nurses and servants

Robert Dingwall, Anne Marie Rafferty and Charles Webster,
An Introduction to the Social History of Nursing (London,
Routledge, 1998), pp. 9–18.

This study was part of a move to bring nursing history out of the
long shadow cast by Florence Nightingale. *Introduction to the
Social History of Nursing* explores the work of nurses since the
beginning of the nineteenth century, and the development of their
role. It shows the impact of social, medical and technological
change on nursing practice and on the image of the nurse.

[T]he provision of nursing care by village women, and, we might add,
by working-class women in towns or cities, has been largely ignored by
historians of the occupation. The position has not changed greatly
since so that any account inevitably depends upon scraps of information in the margins of other studies, although, in fairness, the lack of
documentation would make it hard to write a full historical treatment.
Nevertheless, 'handywomen' were probably the largest group of paid
carers operating throughout the nineteenth century and well into
the twentieth.

Much of the conventional image of the handywomen is formed by
fictional accounts, which can be treated as evidence of characters
whom readers were expected to recognize from life. Perhaps the
most celebrated is Sarah Gamp, from Charles Dickens's 1844 novel,
Martin Chuzzlewit.

[. . .]

[N]ursing at this level was a very basic form of domestic service. The
following descriptions are from St Thomas's and Guy's Hospitals,
respectively, in the 1850s.

> As regards the nurses or ward-maids, these are much in the condition of
> housemaids and require little teaching beyond that of poultice-making
> which is easily acquired, and the enforcement of cleanliness and attention
> to patients' wants. They need not be of the class of people required for
> sisters, not having such responsibility . . .[14]

[14] J. South, *Facts relating to Hospitals* (London, 1857).

For the more subordinate appointment of nurse, which at the time referred to included not only attendance on the more immediate wants of the sick but the cleaning and scrubbing of ward floors and of the staircases of the hospital, it was necessary to select from a class of inferior grade to the others ... preference is given to a good class of domestic servants between the age of 20 and 40 years. After a woman has taken to the work it rarely happens that she leaves it.[15]

But it does not necessarily follow from this that patients were badly treated. A hundred years earlier, the 1752 regulations of the Manchester Infirmary had run together these two types of work but emphasized their common duties in requiring 'That the Nurses and Servants obey the Matron as their Mistress and that they behave with Tenderness to the Patients, and Civility and Respect to Strangers'. Early in the nineteenth century, the matron of the Radcliffe Infirmary in Oxford would simply advertise for a 'careful woman' or promote one of the existing servants if a nurse were required. Part of the attraction of the work seems to have been the acquisition of skills which would be useful in seeking positions in private households upon marriage. The Salisbury Infirmary in 1796 advertised the value of nursing to 'young respectable women who would be taught how to look after sick people'. Whatever the realities of the situation, statements like these do indicate at least an aspiration to create a caring environment. The extent to which this was achieved in practice is underlined by the independent report of the Charity Commissioners on St Thomas's Hospital in 1836 which documents a disciplined and responsible system.

Conditions were undeniably more problematic under the Poor Law[16] which was coming to provide most of the institutional care of the sick.

[. . .]

[In workhouses m]ost of the direct care was provided by other pauper inmates. This was preferred because it was a form of work that did not compete with outside trades, it was unpleasant enough to discourage people from staying in the workhouse for longer than necessary and it was cheap, since the pauper nurses did not have to be paid market wages. They simply received extra privileges in the form of food or

---

[15] Dr. Steele, 'Report on the Nursing Arrangements of the London Hospitals', *British Medical Journal*, 1874, p. 285.

[16] The 1834 Poor Law Amendment Act (often called the New Poor Law) established a system of workhouses where people unable to support themselves – paupers, the elderly, orphans and the sick – were housed. The regime was deliberately designed to be unattractive, in order to discourage applicants for relief. Assistance, including medical care, was also offered to paupers in their own homes, and was referred to as 'outdoor relief'.

liquor or token cash payments. At the Strand workhouse in the 1860s, for instance, pauper nurses were given a glass of gin 'for laying out the dead and other specially repulsive duties'. As a result able-bodied nurses left as soon as they could get other employment and the burden of care fell on the least infirm of those who remained. Pauper nurses tended to be elderly women with little prospect of employment outside the workhouse, except when the guardians allowed them out to nurse poor people receiving outdoor relief. At the Strand, 14 out of 18 pauper nurses were over 60 and 4 were over 70. Only 8 could read the labels on the medicines. Two trembled and coughed all day and were too frail to lift any patient. But it is also clear that some workhouses did manage to make the system work. The *Lancet* commission, whose report was a key text for reformers in the 1860s, singled out the pauper nurses in Islington as 'well-conducted, zealous and well managed'.

Both before and after 1834, however, a good deal of nursing care was provided as outdoor relief. This included both midwifery and assistance with sickness. The picture which emerges is one of relatively poor women, perhaps widows or deserted wives, providing a service to other poor people. Their payments from the Poor Law might well have functioned, in effect, as a form of outdoor relief for themselves. Sometimes they would work for paupers, sometimes for people who were simply poor but not so impoverished as to qualify for relief. Again, though, there are hints of a concern for standards which belies the simple chronicle of abuse. Acland's memoirs of the 1854 cholera outbreak in Oxford record that the Poor Law guardians kept a list of 'respectable women' who were willing to do home nursing. Patients could either hire nurses from this list or be nursed by one of them at the guardians' expense. The existence of such lists presupposes criteria of respectability and a desire to encourage it.

Although we have questioned the suggestion that Sarah Gamp's character is typical of handywoman nurses, her duties probably were: nursing the sick, delivering babies, and laying out the dead. To these one might well add procuring abortions and disposing of unwanted infants. Out of these various tasks, some handywomen might have developed a particular reputation as counsellors on the health problems of women and children, which were of little interest to doctors in general until the twentieth century. Not all handywomen would necessarily have taken on all these tasks and it is doubtful whether more than a few made a full-time living from them. It may be better to see nursing as an interlude in their work as cleaners or laundresses.

The handywomen had no consciousness of themselves as an occupational group: indeed this is one of the reasons why so little documentary evidence is readily available. They simply filled a traditional social and economic role in their locality. This was an important factor in their survival in community-based work. . . . [H]andywomen remained serious competitors to certified midwives and district nurses until the 1930s and 1940s.

If the handywoman was part of the traditional organization of care among the poor, the private duty nurse was equally well-established among the middle and upper classes. However, whereas the handywoman was working essentially with clients of her own class, the private duty nurse was a servant of her social superiors. Jane Austen describes one such woman, Nurse Rooke, in *Persuasion* (1818).

> (Mrs Smith) could not call herself an invalid now compared with her state on first reaching Bath. Then, she had indeed been a pitiable object – for she had caught a cold on the journey and had hardly taken possession of her lodgings, before she was again confined to her bed, and suffering under severe and constant pain; and all this amongst strangers with the absolute necessity of having a regular nurse, and finances at that moment particularly unfit to meet any extraordinary expense . . . she had been particularly fortunate in her nurse, as a sister of her landlady, a nurse by profession, and who had always a home in that house when unemployed, chanced to be at liberty just in time to attend her . . . 'Every body's heart is open, you know, when they have recently escaped from severe pain, or are recovering the blessing of health, and nurse Rooke thoroughly understands when to speak. She is a shrewd, intelligent, sensible woman . . . call it gossip if you will; but when nurse Rooke has half an hour's leisure to bestow on me, she is sure to have something to relate that is entertaining and profitable, something that makes one know one's species better . . .' Anne . . . replied 'I can easily believe it. Women of that class have great opportunities and if they are intelligent may be well worth listening to.'

Nurse Rooke may sound indiscreet by modern standards but her behaviour probably reflects the problems of making a living as a freelance nurse. Gossiping with someone like Mrs Smith would be one way of finding out who else was ill and securing recommendations to her friends. But Nurse Rooke's behaviour may also indicate a sensitivity to the importance of nurses' amusing or entertaining their patients, of raising their spirits as well as caring for their physical needs, at a period when carers may have had little else to offer. She is clearly well liked by Mrs Smith.

Nurse Rooke was employed as a live-in servant for particular episodes of illness. When she was not working, she stayed with her sister who kept lodgings for the better-off classes. From the way Anne Elliott and

Mrs Smith talk about her, she was obviously thought of as a social inferior, a paid companion rather than an equal. At the same time, she is clearly a superior class of person to Sarah Gamp. This ambiguous status is a marked feature of private duty nurses, who seem to have occupied a marginal role between their employers and the rest of the household staff, rather like that of the governesses. Her work was supported by other servants but, as an employee, she was not the equal of the family members. [Jean] Donnison refers to the uncertainty at a later period about whether she should dine with the family or with the servants and [Christopher] Maggs has noted the questions over her eligibility as a marriage partner for the son of a middle-class household which formed a potent theme in late Victorian popular fiction.[17] Was this a legitimate aspiration or would it merely lead to her seduction and abandonment?

What is perhaps more important is that these structural conditions made the private duty nurse a more specialized care provider than the handywoman. She was also more likely to be working for a client with the resources to purchase medical services so that her work was at least partly defined by whatever passed as orthodox medicine.

These women had their counterparts in the voluntary hospitals. Although there was some internal promotion, sisters and the matron tended to be separately recruited from more elevated social backgrounds than the ordinary nurses. Sisters at St Bartholomew's in the 1830s were described as 'widows in reduced circumstances' and 'persons who have lived in a respectable rank of life'. At St Thomas's in the 1850s they had often been head servants in gentlemen's families. Their status is caught by this later memoir of Guy's Hospital at the same period.

> It appears to have been the custom at all times for each ward to have the benefit of supervision by a separate sister who, in addition to the care of the sick should have the charge of the ward stores and also be the medium of communication between the patients and the medical staff. It . . . was the practice to select for this office respectable females who, previous to their appointment had experience of household work, been upper servants in private families, or been engaged in the capacity of nursing the sick out of doors, and not unfrequently the post was filled by one of the ordinary nurses whose promotion was merited from length of service and presumed suitability.[18]

[17] Jean Donnison, *Midwives and Medical Men: A History of Inter-professional Rivalries and Women's Rights* (London, Heinemann, 1977); Christopher Maggs, 'Sarey Gamp's Daughters: the English Nurse in Fiction', paper presented to Nursing and Anthropology workshop, Oxford, 26–7 April 1986.

[18] *Guy's Hospital Reports* 1871, pp. 541–3, quoted in K. Williams, 'From Sarah Gamp to Florence Nightingale: A Critical Survey of Hospital Nursing Systems from 1840 to 1897', in C. Davies (ed.), *Rewriting Nursing History* (London, Croom Helm, 1980).

The matron was a senior administrative officer in most hospitals. This advertisement is for a post at Leeds General Infirmary in 1852.

> Candidates for this office are required to be free from the care of a family, of middle age, active, and of good address, qualified to keep an account of the disbursements and other matters in the house department; it is necessary that she be staid, sober, and discreet, mild, and humane disposition [sic], at the same time possessed of firmness to rule the household; it is also desirable that she be experienced in the management of a family and the duties of a sick room.[19]

This is the sort of position that might attract the widow of a marginal member of the middle classes, such as a clergyman or an army officer, with the experience of managing a large Victorian household rather than necessarily of nursing the sick.

In most workhouses, the nurses were supervised by the matron. She was usually the master's wife and his official deputy. Workhouse masters were commonly drawn from the ranks of retired non-commissioned officers in the Army so that one is here dealing with people of rather more humble origins. The matron, as in the voluntary hospitals, was primarily an administrator. This description of her work is from the Workhouse Infirmaries Report of 1866.

> The matron's duties are varied and multiplied. She superintends the whole internal working of the establishment, the cleaning, the linen, the food, the cooking, the distribution of food, the stores, etc. and in the discharge of these duties has as much as an active person can properly do. But in many workhouses she is expected to superintend the nursing and bedding and other questions relating to the sick.[20]

Notice the order of priority.

It would probably be a mistake to draw too strong a distinction between handywomen and private nurses. Some handywomen would certainly have had middle-class clients for midwifery and very possibly for services like the laying-out of the dead. There was clearly some mobility both socially and sectorally, between employment and self-employment. A young woman might plausibly begin as a hospital servant, become a hospital nurse, leave on marriage, work as a handywoman to support her family, go into private nursing as a

---

[19] John Woodward, *To Do the Sick No Harm. A Study of the British Hospital System to 1875* (London, Routledge Kegan Paul, 1974), p. 30.

[20] Brian Abel Smith, *A History of the Nursing Profession* (London, Heinemann, 1960), pp. 15–16.

young widow and finish as a hospital sister. But the social distinctions are important: private nurses were integrated into the service of the affluent while handywomen were autonomous workers among the poor. Private nurses were likely to command other servants while handywomen laboured on their own or in partnership with other family members.

We have seen that, in the first half of the nineteenth century, the boundary between nursing and domestic service was less clear-cut than it was to become later. But nursing was also to acquire a technical component to its work, as an administrator of medically prescribed treatments. To understand this aspect of the process we need to examine the other side of the occupation's territory, its frontier with medicine. We must in particular consider the work of the apothecary and his assistants and of the apprentice physicians and surgeons.

The apothecaries were often the only salaried medical attendants in a voluntary hospital. Since the early seventeenth century, their guild had successfully enlarged the scope of its work from compounding and supplying medications to advice, prescription and diagnosis. They were an important source of medical care to the middle classes, who were looking for a reasonably reliable practitioner but could not afford the fees of a physician. With the passage of the Apothecaries Act 1815, they became the first of the medical occupations to establish a recognizably modern form of education and registration. Although regarded as social inferiors, they were ultimately to be united with the physicians and surgeons when the medical profession acquired its current shape under the Medical Act 1858, which created the predecessors of the General Medical Council. In the hospitals the apothecary would be responsible for the daily bleedings, scarifyings, cuppings, and blisterings, for the supervision of baths and electrical treatment, and for the maintenance of the surgical instruments, in addition to making up, dispensing and administering the prescribed medications.

During the 1820s, the hospitals also began to be peopled by medical students and junior medical attendants. This resulted from new examination requirements by the College of Surgeons and the Society of Apothecaries. . . . [P]art of the consequence was that these new grades of hospital staff came to supplement and eventually take over much of the apothecary's work. At the Royal Devon and Exeter Hospital, for instance, a nurse would help

> with dressings, but only in fetching tins of warm water with which the doctor cleaned the wounds. She was allowed to apply either a bread or linseed poultice but 'as soon as dressings of lotion or lint were ordered, the

pupil will take charge' . . . if the state of the patient was such that someone had to sit up all night, it was not the nurse who did so but a pupil.[21]

The pupils here were apprenticed to the physicians, surgeons or apothecary. In effect, the forerunners of modern nurses were more like domestic servants because the precursors of modern doctors were performing what would now be regarded as relatively low-level technical procedures and routine treatments, although, at the time, many of them may have been thought to be highly innovative.

How should we assess the quality of nursing care in the early years of the nineteenth century? By modern standards much of it seems basic, primitive and unsophisticated. It may be fairer, however, to judge this care by the standards of its own time. Much of the critical comment on early nineteenth century nursing comes from the writings of reformers like Charles Dickens, Louisa Twining and Florence Nightingale. Some of their descriptions still have an undeniable power to shock and appal. At the same time their judgements would not have been possible without some conception of how nursing care could be given in a more humane fashion. If one relies on hospital records as evidence, then it is important to remember that complaints leave more traces. When a hospital dismissed a nurse for drunkenness, this would generate a series of documents while good work went unreported. It may be just as significant to observe that nurses were dismissed at all, which suggests that hospital administrators were trying to set a positive standard for their staff.

The greatest problem in summarizing early nineteenth century health care is breaking the constraints of present-day assumptions about nursing and medicine. Sick people were nursed by a wide variety of attendants, paid and unpaid, women and men, skilled and unskilled. These attendants provided a range of care which covered basic physical needs, the moral welfare of the patient and some rudimentary treatments. Within this spectrum, the paid nurse, whether at home or in hospital, would mostly have given the elementary physical care that a patient in other circumstances might have received from an amateur family member or personal servant. There was very little technical content. Nurses were drawn from the classes in domestic service and their work was of little interest to anyone other than their immediate employer. While contemporaries were unhappy about the standards of some of the care provided by nurses, especially in the workhouses, it is far from clear that abuse was either systematic or widespread. Nursing care reflected the expectations of the society in which it was given and

---

[21] R. Hawker, 'A Day in the Life of a Patient', *Nursing Times*, 12 June 1985, pp. 43–4.

the limited technology available. The indeterminacy of the occupation's boundaries reflected the limited degree of specialization in the general organization of pre-industrial and early industrial employment.

<hr>

6.7
Florence Nightingale on nurse training

Monica E. Baly, *Florence Nightingale and the Nursing Legacy*
(London, Croom Helm, 1986), pp. 23–5.

Baly's study is one of a group of biographical studies of Florence Nightingale that look beyond the heroic image of the 'lady with the lamp', an image constructed originally by the War Office in response to public criticism of conditions in the Crimean War. In contrast to the usual image of Nightingale as a forward-looking innovator, this excerpt shows her as conservative both in her belief in the sanitary approach and that nursing should be separate and different to medicine.

Miss Nightingale increasingly believed, and rightly, that proper sanitation, ventilation and the right food would banish much current sickness. Writing to Dr Pattison Walker in 1886 she said that the purpose of medicine should be to 'make the public care for its own health'.

For this reason she saw nursing as more than a mere handicraft but rather as a sanitary mission. In a curious way, and by the same reasoning, Miss Nightingale was blindly and fanatically against the germ theory of infection. 'There are no specific diseases', she reiterated, even when men like Koch[22] had demonstrated that there were. This attitude coloured her views on nurse training and made her fearful that the new scientific training and lectures from medical men like Bernays at St Thomas's would turn nurses into 'medical women' and deflect them from their proper task of being sanitary missioners. . . .

Miss Nightingale was still ambivalent about how hospital nursing should, or could, be developed. This uncertainty is important because it is reflected in Miss Nightingale's changing attitudes to nursing as a 'profession' and who should be selected as nurses, what their tasks

[22] Robert Koch (1843–1910) identified a number of disease-causing bacteria, including those responsible for cholera and tuberculosis.

should be and, above all, how they should be prepared to meet those tasks. The fears about nurses becoming imbued with ideas about bacteria made her suspicious of doctors' lectures and what was later to be described as 'the medical model'. Her fears in this respect were often justified — but for the wrong reason. However, she was soon to find out that if 'tradesmen's and farmers' daughters' were to be trained even in the handicraft of nursing they needed educated women to teach them. Furthermore, educated women were necessary to teach the public 'to care for its own health'. Miss Nightingale's difficulty was that she had no body of nursing knowledge or educational theories in order to substitute 'nursing matters' for medical knowledge, and the educated women brought in to teach the less educated all too soon absorbed medical knowledge.

No doubt part of the difference in Miss Nightingale's attitude to what was necessary for nurse education arose from purely pragmatic considerations: the need for medical education was already established, the need for nurse training was not, and it would be necessary to proceed slowly and experimentally. However, there was a more fundamental reason; Miss Nightingale saw the main object of nurse training as being the development of character and of self-discipline with moral training being more important than mere academic education — 'you cannot be a good nurse without being a good woman' she was fond of saying, though she acknowledged that goodness without intelligence and training was the path to disaster.

Part seven

Disease in populations

7.1

An early account of public health history

Erwin Ackerknecht, *A Short History of Medicine*
(Baltimore and London, Johns Hopkins University Press,
1968), pp. 210–17.

Erwin Ackerknecht (1906–88) was one of the founders of the discipline of the history of medicine. He trained in medicine then in history of medicine under Henry E. Sigerist. From 1947–57 he was professor of the history of medicine at the University of Wisconsin-Madison, and later held a similar post at the University of Zurich. During his long career, Ackerknecht published on a wide range of topics, including the history of therapeutics, pathology and medical ethnology.

Both individual hygiene and public hygiene owe an enormous debt to bacteriology. But this should not obscure the fact that preventive medicine . . . is as old as human societies. We have encountered it among primitives, in Egypt, in Babylonia, among the ancient Jews, in Rome, and in the Middle Ages. We have observed the great preventive medicine movement of the eighteenth century, the fruit of the philosophical Enlightenment. We have seen that this movement was much rather the consequence of the will and necessity to do something about public health than the result of new scientific insight. And we have seen that this approach achieved results and led to new discoveries. The same approach characterises the first of the preventive medicine movements of the nineteenth century, the sanitary movement.

The sanitary movement was well under way before the great discoveries of bacteriology. It received its stimulus from the utilitarian philosophy of such thinkers as Jeremy Bentham,[1] and it grew out of the needs of the new industrial society. Plague, leprosy, scurvy, and smallpox had receded from Western and Central Europe before their true nature was known. But the health situation was still appalling. Malaria prevailed in the country slums; typhus, typhoid fever, and tuberculosis were rife in the slums of the cities. A particularly strong incentive to the development of preventive medicine was given by the four great cholera pandemics which after 1830 swept Europe and the whole world, sparing neither rich nor poor. Cholera was once called by Robert Koch 'our best ally' in the fight for better hygiene. Its dramatic effects frightened legislators into taking progressive measures far more rapidly than the creeping death resulting from tuberculosis or typhoid.

. . . In the big cities the death rate had reached such levels by the middle of the nineteenth century that there were serious doubts whether sufficient hands would be available for the factories, and whether enough able-bodied recruits could be found for the general draft armies of the Continent. The big-city slums represented reservoirs of infectious diseases and epidemics, menacing not only the poor, but the life and health of the upper classes as well.

In England and Germany, the hygiene movement of the Enlightenment seems to have experienced a decline at the end of the eighteenth and beginning of the nineteenth century. But it was vigorously promoted in France. In fact, France assumed the lead in hygiene at this time, as it had done in most other branches of medicine. The work of the French hygienists, particularly of René Louis Villerme (1782–1863), was an inspiration to German, British, and American authors. This French movement was overshadowed by the large-scale practical achievements in England after the passage of the General Health Act of 1848.

The driving spirit of the new English sanitary movement was, typically enough, an outsider, the lawyer Edwin Chadwick (1800–1890). He was a pupil and former secretary of Jeremy Bentham, the philosopher who strove for the greatest good for the greatest number. Chadwick's 1842 report on the health of the labouring classes revealed an ugly and dangerous situation. . . . Chadwick's statistical evidence was based to a large extent on the outstanding statistical work of Dr. William Farr (1807–1883), who in 1839 entered the Registrar General's office and started publishing his classic letters on the causes of death in England.

---

[1] Jeremy Bentham (1748–1832), a philosopher and social reformer, best known for his idea that governments should strive for the greatest happiness of the greatest number.

Of the other outstanding English public health men of the period, Sir John Simon (1816–1904) was perhaps the most influential. He was the first medical officer of health of London, and later was medical officer to the General Board of Health. Although the General Board of Health operated on the erroneous 'filth' theory of disease, its successes were striking. According to the filth theory, miasmatic hazes rising from decaying matter, rather than contagion and micro-organisms, were supposed to cause epidemics. But cleaning filth from the slums helped, whatever the underlying theory.

A much deeper understanding of the spread of infectious diseases was contributed by the English epidemiologists John Snow (1813–1858), also an outstanding anaesthetist, and William Budd (1811–1880). Snow showed in 1849 that cholera was a water-borne disease, and in 1854 he proved his point conclusively in his classic treatise on the Broad Street pump. Budd demonstrated in 1856 that typhoid was also water-borne. . . .

A strong hygiene movement arose at this time in Germany under the leadership of Max von Pettenkofer (1818–1901). Pettenkofer, father of the ground-water level theory[2] operated under erroneous assumptions with regard to contagion and was unsympathetic to bacteriology – to the extent of swallowing a virulent cholera culture in 1892 without evil effects. (An earlier, mild attack had probably made him immune). But his practical achievements were considerable. He made Munich a healthy city, as [Rudolph] Virchow[3] had done for Berlin. Pettenkofer went beyond the application of such ordinary measures as the improvement of water supply and sewage disposal; a trained physiologist and chemist, he was the first to submit all aspects of hygiene to experimental analysis, systematically investigating the effects of such factors as food, clothing and housing. He was thus the father of modern scientific hygiene. He occupied the first chair of experimental hygiene in Munich in 1865.

The prebacteriological hygienists fought against 'filth and stench'. While this was insufficient, it went far toward eliminating many disease causes and disease carriers such as rats and lice. The prebacteriological hygiene movement concentrated on the fight against overcrowded housing, polluted water supplies, bad sewage, adulterated food, and child labour. It fought for the isolation of those suffering from infectious diseases. It urged control of dangerous trades involving occupational

[2] Max von Pettenkofer (1818–1901) developed the theory that cholera germs only become infectious once 'activated' in damp soil, where the ground water level had fallen.

[3] Rudolf Virchow (1821–1902), a distinguished German researcher into cell pathology, who discovered that all cells arose from other cells. He also took a keen interest in public health and oversaw improvements to the Berlin sewage system.

intoxications from contact with lead or phosphorus. Under the leadership of Virchow and Hermann Cohn, school hygiene was vigorously developed. Better sewers and water supplies appeared in Western Europe after 1850. Pure food laws were introduced in the 1870s. Chairs of hygiene had been founded in the sixties.

Bacteriology led to unprecedented advances in preventive medicine. Direct attack against certain diseases could now replace haphazard measures. The incidence of typhoid fever and diphtheria could be rapidly reduced through control of water and milk supplies, through control of [human] carriers, and through immunization.

7.2
Unhealthy environments

(i) 'Report of Mr Gilbert on the sanitary condition of Tiverton, Devon, in Edwin Chadwick, *Report on the Sanitary Condition of the Labouring Population*, ed. M.W. Flinn (Edinburgh, Edinburgh University Press, 1965), pp. 80–1.

(ii) [Henry Mayhew], 'A Visit to the Cholera Districts of Bermondsey', *Morning Chronicle*, 24 September 1849, p. 4. Reprinted in Kate Flint (ed.), *The Victorian Novelist: Social Problems and Social Change* (London, Croom Helm, 1987), pp. 165–8.

(iii) Charles Dickens, *Bleak House* (Oxford, Oxford University Press, 1998), pp. 235–6, 654–7 (first published 1852–53).

(iv) Editorial, *The Times*, 1 December, p. 6, 1865, col. d.

(i)

The *Report on the Sanitary Condition of the Labouring Population*, compiled by Edwin Chadwick, is one of the classic documents on the insanitary living conditions found in nineteenth-century Britain. Although urban areas were usually singled out for condemnation, this extract on Tiverton, Devon shows that housing in rural towns was also in a very poor condition.

The land is nearly on a level with the water, the ground is marshy, and the sewers all open. Before reaching the district, I was assailed by a most disagreeable smell; and it was clear to the sense that the air was full of most injurious malaria.[4] The inhabitants, easily distinguishable from the inhabitants of the other parts of the town, had all a sickly, miserable appearance. The open drains in some cases ran immediately before the doors of the houses, and some of the houses were surrounded by wide open drains, full of all the animal and vegetable refuse not only of the houses in that part, but of those in other parts of Tiverton. In many of the houses, persons were confined with fever and different diseases, and all I talked to either were ill or had been so: and the whole community presented a melancholy spectacle of disease and misery.

[. . .]

It is not these unfortunate creatures only who choose this centre of disease for their living-place who are affected; but the whole town is more or less deteriorated by its vicinity to this pestilential mass, where the generation of those elements of disease and death is constantly going on.

'Another cause of disease is to be found in the state of the cottages. Many are built on the ground without flooring, or against a damp hill. Some have neither windows nor doors sufficient to keep out the weather, or to let in the rays of the sun, or supply the means of ventilation; and in others the roof is so constructed or so worn as not to be weather tight. The thatch roof frequently is saturated with wet, rotten, and in a state of decay, giving out malaria, as other decaying vegetable matter.'

(ii)

Jacob's Island, a part of Bermondsey, was one of the most notorious of London's slums in the mid-nineteenth century. It had once been part of Bermondsey Abbey and was still surrounded by a ditch connected to the Thames. Its inhabitants suffered badly during the cholera epidemics of 1832 and 1849. The area attracted the attention of Victorian writers on social conditions: Charles Dickens set part of *Oliver Twist* here. Henry Mayhew was a campaigning journalist, famous for his *London Labour and the London Poor*, describing the life and work of the working classes.

---

[4] *malaria*: literally, bad air, believed to cause disease.

On entering the precincts of the pest island, the air has literally the smell of a graveyard, and a feeling of nausea and heaviness comes over any one unaccustomed to imbibe the musty atmosphere. It is not only the nose, but the stomach, that tells how heavily the air is loaded with sulphuretted hydrogen;[5] and as soon as you cross one of the crazy and rotting bridges over the reeking ditch, you know, as surely as if you had chemically tested it, by the black colour of what was once the white-lead paint upon the door-posts and window-sills, that the air is thickly charged with this deadly gas. The heavy bubbles which now and then rise up in the water show you whence at least a portion of the mephitic[6] compound comes, while the open doorless privies that hang over the water side on one of the banks, and the dark streaks of filth down the walls where the drains from each house discharge themselves into the ditch on the opposite side, tell you how the pollution of the ditch is supplied.

The water is covered with a scum almost like a cobweb, and prismatic with grease. In it float large masses of green rotting weed, and against the posts of the bridges are swollen carcasses of dead animals, almost bursting with the gases of putrefaction. Along its shores are heaps of indescribable filth, the phosphoretted smell from which tells you of the rotting fish there, while the oyster shells are like pieces of slate from their coating of mud and filth. In some parts the fluid is almost as red as blood from the colouring matter that pours into it from the reeking leather-dressers' close by.

[. . .]

The inhabitants themselves show in their faces the poisonous influence of the mephitic air they breathe. Either their skins are white, like parchment, telling of the impaired digestion, the languid circulation, and the coldness of the skin peculiar to persons suffering from chronic poisoning, or else their cheeks are flushed hectically, and their eyes are glassy, showing the wasting fever and general decline of the bodily functions. The brown, earthlike complexion of some, and their sunk eyes, with the dark areolae round them, tell you that the sulphuretted hydrogen of the atmosphere in which they live has been absorbed into the blood; while others are remarkable for the watery eye exhibiting the increased secretion of tears so peculiar to those who are exposed to the exhalations of hydrosulphate of ammonia.

[. . .]

On approaching the tidal ditch from the Neckinger-road, the shutters of

---

[5] hydrogen sulphide, which has a characteristic smell of rotten eggs.

[6] *mephitic*: foul-smelling.

the house at the corner were shut from top to bottom. Our intelligent and obliging guide, Dr Martin, informed us that a girl was then lying dead there from cholera, and that but very recently another victim had fallen in the house adjoining it. . . . As we walked down George-row, our informant told us that at the corner of London-street he could see, a short time back, as many as nine houses in which there were one or two persons lying dead of the cholera at the same time; and yet there could not have been more than a dozen tenements visible from the spot.

(iii)

Through his novels Charles Dickens both described and demanded action to improve the social conditions of the poor in London. Although rather melodramatic, this account of another London slum – the curiously-named Tom-all-Alone's – was based on fact.

Jo lives—that is to say, Jo has not yet died—in a ruinous place, known to the like of him by the name of Tom-all-Alone's. It is a black, dilapi-dated street, avoided by all decent people; where the crazy houses were seized upon, when their decay was far advanced, by some bold vagrants, who, after establishing their own possession, took to letting them out in lodgings. Now, these tumbling tenements contain, by night, a swarm of misery. As, on the ruined human wretch, vermin parasites appear, so, these ruined shelters have bred a crowd of foul existence that crawls in and out of gaps in walls and boards; and coils itself to sleep, in maggot numbers, where the rain drips in; and comes and goes, fetching and carrying fever, and sowing more evil in its every footprint than Lord Coodle, and Sir Thomas Doodle, and the Duke of Foodle, and all the fine gentlemen in office, down to Zoodle, shall set right in five hundred years—though born expressly to do it.

Twice, lately, there has been a crash and a cloud of dust, like the springing of a mine, in Tom-all-Alone's; and, each time, a house has fallen. These accidents have made a paragraph in the newspapers, and have filled a bed or two in the nearest hospital. The gaps remain, and there are not unpopular lodgings among the rubbish. As several more houses are nearly ready to go, the next crash in Tom-all-Alone's may be expected to be a good one.

[. . .]

But [Tom-all-Alone's] has his revenge. Even the winds are his messen-gers, and they serve him in these hours of darkness. There is not a drop

143

of Tom's corrupted blood but propagates infection and contagion some-where. It shall pollute, this very night, the choice stream (in which chemists on analysis would find the genuine nobility) of a Norman house, and his Grace shall not be able to say Nay to the infamous alliance. There is not an atom of Tom's slime, not a cubic inch of any pestilential gas in which he lives, not one obscenity or degradation about him, not an ignorance, not a wickedness, not a brutality of his commit-ting, but shall work its retribution, through every order of society, up to the proudest of the proud, and to the highest of the high. Verily, what with tainting, plundering, and spoiling, Tom has his revenge.

(iv)

By the mid-nineteenth century, the London-based *Times* news-paper had acquired a reputation as an authoritative source of information. Its editors consistently supported the movement for sanitary reform. This account of an inquest was part of an editorial urging the need to enforce the laws against insanitary conditions.

An inquest was held on Wednesday in Spitalfields upon the bodies of a man and his wife, each 38 years of age, who died within two days of each other of typhoid fever; in other words, of that particular class of fever which is generated by the effluvia of decaying animal and vegetable matter. It is evident how the fever was produced in this case – that is, how these two poor persons were brought to a premature death – when we learn the state of the house in which they lived. The doctor said that 'he found them both delirious in one bed. There was an accumulation of animal and vegetable refuse outside the door; the passage and stairs were extremely dirty, the walls dilapidated and filthy; the closet[6] was in a disgraceful state, and the flooring was partly destroyed. The water, which was kept in an old tar barrel, was quite unfit to drink, through the foul exhalations from the drain and closet.' Indeed the two sufferers were so surrounded by unhealthy influences that he considered that they had not a chance of recovery if they remained there. He advised that they should be removed to the Fever Hospital. This was not done, and they died. From one of the inmates, who lived on the ground floor, we learn further that there is a stable

---

[6] Privy or lavatory – which would not be a flush lavatory at this date.

next door, the nuisance[7] from which had only been lately been abated through the interference of the inspectors. Before that time 'her sleeping room was below the level of the back yard, and the drainage from the stable in question flowed over her yard and past her window.' Again, by the same witness, we are told that 'the flooring of her room lay level on the earth; there were no rafters.' Lastly, Dr Letheby, who also testified to the 'filthy and insalubrious condition of the place', was informed by the inmates that the water could only be used for washing purposes,[8] that there was no tap to the old tar barrels in which it was kept, and that these they had supplied themselves.

7.3

Reassessing Chadwick's *Sanitary Report*

Christopher Hamlin, 'Edwin Chadwick, "Mutton Medicine", and the Fever Question', *Bulletin of the History of Medicine*, vol. 70, 1996, pp. 237–60 [pp. 233–61].

Christopher Hamlin has written some of the most interesting and important works on Victorian sanitary improvement in Britain. In this article, he challenges the prevailing belief that Chadwick's *Report on the Sanitary Condition of the Labouring Population* (1842) was an objective account of the urban environment, and represented the views of the medical profession.

When, in the spring of 1838, Edwin Chadwick and the Poor Law Commissioners initiated investigations into the 'physical causes' of disease, the new poor law they administered was not even four years old. It remained controversial, and was vigorously resisted. . . . Its main premise, and the source of much opposition, was the famous principle of 'less eligibility,' the attempt to discourage the election of pauper status by making sure that the pauper's life would be clearly less desirable—in liberty, diet, and other 'necessaries of life'—than that of the person who remained independent. In principle, the pauper would be required

---

[7] A nuisance was an accumulation of dirt or material which was both unpleasant and thought to be a possible cause of disease.

[8] i.e. that it was not suitable for drinking.

to move into a local workhouse administered by a union of neighboring parishes. Family members would be sent to men's, women's, or children's wards, hard work would be required, and a minimal and tedious diet imposed.

To Chadwick, chief architect of the new law, the unpleasantness of the workhouse was to be a dam of disincentive, holding back the current of lazy people who would otherwise drift naturally into demoralizing (and costly) dependency. The provision of medical relief represented a hole in this dam . . .

[I]t seemed both practically and morally inappropriate to treat in the same way both the able-bodied laborer temporarily unable to work due to illness and the indolent laborer who would not do his utmost to find work to support self and family. Practically, it seemed wasteful to institutionalize an entire family whenever the breadwinner became ill; morally, it seemed wrong to treat the innocent disease victim in the same way as the wanton deviant. Accordingly the law had provisions for providing emergency aid, in the form of both medical care and the 'necessaries,' to those who normally maintained their independence but who could neither pay for medical care nor sustain a loss of income for any significant period. . . .

The deterrent principle required that the workhouse diet sustain life and (at some level) health, and yet be at best no more desirable than that available outside. So long as the independent poor had enough to eat the approach might be viable, but during a depression (as in the late 1830s) maintaining credible deterrence became difficult as wages and diet (and access to medical care) fell. . . .

Chadwick and the PLC took the view that starvation was an acute condition, quickly manifesting itself in the absence of food. They rejected the idea of a chronic exhaustion and malnutrition that slowly damaged health, eventually manifesting itself in some disease. . . . Similarly, Chadwick assumed a clear demarcation between health and disease, in which disease, whether acute or chronic, had a clear beginning and end and struck more or less randomly. It might be that certain *places* were especially prone to disease, but this could be ascribed to exposure to environmental poisons rather than to the prevailing social and economic conditions. Thus both malnutrition and disease had to be seen as binary phenomena: a person was either healthy and adequately fed, or obviously ill and starving. For Chadwick, to have admitted a concept of disease as the product of slow decline under the totality of debilitating conditions would have been to portray the new poor law as ridiculous and unconscionable, as causing disease in the name of lowering costs and increasing efficiency.

146

For a number of reasons many medical men took the opposite view on these questions. They did so, first, because it was a prominent axiom of most contemporary medical theories that overwork, poor diet, and bad living conditions did continually undermine health and thus led ultimately to disease. Health and disease . . . were not binary opposites, but different areas of a continuum. One's place on this continuum was not the result of some random exposure to a poison but the product of an initial constitution, modified by place, occupation, passions, ingesta, and so forth—and it was always changing. Accordingly, many poor-law medical men found reason to sympathize with those applicants for medical relief whom Chadwick suspected of malingering. Equally, they recognized that the effects of overwork, cold, and hunger were manifest even in 'normal times': the supposedly 'healthy' workhouse inmate or independent laborer might not be very healthy at all . . .

In attending the very poor, medical men frequently found that what was really needed was food, and . . . that was what they prescribed— sometimes in substantial quantities, such as two to three pounds of mutton per week, along with bread and wine . . . Edward Evans, medical officer of St. George the Martyr, in Southwark [London] . . . acquired such a reputation for prescribing food that people applied to him when they really wanted general relief. Initially, Evans's board had supported his orders in an effort to 'subdue typhus.' But as the cost of the 'extras' seemed poised to rise indefinitely high, they found a need for restraint—he was 'ruining half the ratepayers of the parish'; Evans's response was that 'nearly every patient required support and nourishment. Whatever the disease, a large proportion of the illnesses he had to treat would never have arisen had the poor enjoyed a better diet.'

[. . .]

To Chadwick and the PLC, prescription of the basic commodities of life was unacceptable, a violation of the laws of political economy. Hunger was to spur work; here, under the ruse of illness, it was . . . being relieved by union medical officers. The very provision of good medical care seemed incompatible with the deterrence principle; the inclusion of nourishment for the convalescing laborer (and family) was, according to Assistant Commissioner Edward Tufnell, 'the avenue to all pauperism.'

[. . .]

Thus there are strong reasons to think that what Chadwick sought from the Sanitary Inquiry was the basis to make a case for [the] claim, that

147

hunger did not cause disease and death. Fever was the key disease here because it, even more than consumption, was seen as the disease of misery. Many saw it as a general systemic response to debilitating forces. Such a view did not preclude fever's being a contagious or a miasmatic disease: 'debility' simply identified those likeliest to succumb. Chadwick claimed in the *Report* that few still took this 'debilitationist' view. This is not the case. With regard to the circumstances in which fever arose, most contemporary authorities . . . agreed that fever was usually a contagious disease, though one in which predisposing factors were more important . . . than in the classic contagious disease, smallpox. Crucial predisposers were dirt, damp, lack of ventilation, vitiated air, poor nutrition, cold, exhaustion, and anxiety. . . .

Chadwick and his associates . . . continued to recognize the influence of debilitating causes, but focused only on a subset of the usual list of predisposers: on vitiated air (including poisonous emanations), poor ventilation, damp, and dirt—but not on hunger, exhaustion, or anxiety, and only rarely on cold. Via the ancient concept of 'malaria' they elevated emanations from the status of being one of many debilitating predisposers to that of replacing contagia as the exciting cause . . . In this move other causal factors, . . . were relegated to insignificance.

[. . .]

The great Sanitary Inquiry launched in autumn 1839 would determine 'the extent to which the causes of disease stated . . . to prevail amongst the labouring classes in the metropolis prevail also amongst the labouring classes in other parts of England and Wales.' . . .

[T]he questionnaire [sent to medical men read:]

> The Poor Law Commission have been informed that within many districts chiefly inhabited by the labouring classes fever and other diseases occur at regular intervals or are never absent.
>
> It has also been stated that such diseases arise in places where there is no drainage; where filth is allowed to accumulate, or where there are other physical causes of disease which are removable if steps be taken.
>
> It is further stated that where such causes exist the suffering of disease, often fatal, is extensively inflicted on the inhabitants, mostly of the labouring classes, and very heavy burthens are cast upon the ratepayers.— Instances have been given to the commissioners where setting aside the higher consideration, even regarding only the expenditure of the rates, it would be good economy to remove the causes in question at public expense if there were no other means for their removal.

148

You will . . . describe to them the nature of any such places it may have been your duty to visit, and specify the number of cases of illness ascribable to such causes, which have become chargeable to the parish.[9]

In no sense, then, was the inquiry an attempt to test rival hypotheses—namely, that filth causes fever, or that destitution causes fever. The questionnaire assumes what the study is usually taken to demonstrate, a causal relationship between filth and fever.

[. . .]

[D]espite Chadwick's attempts to deflect the inquiry from embarrassing matters of exhaustion and starvation, several informants made a point of giving these factors a greater role than they gave to bad drains and so on. Moreover, unlike Chadwick and most laissez-faire political economists, they held that wages and prices, these key determinants of health, did not lie outside the sphere of matters properly remediable through legislation.

[. . .]

Despite fever's being the ostensible rationale of the *Report*, there is relatively little in it on fever . . . Chadwick's most focused treatment is in the third section: 'Domestic Mismanagement, a Predisposing Cause of Disease.' There he argues that medical men are often deceived by rogues, who feign sickness to get relief in cash or exchangeable commodities like food and fuel (with which they then buy drink); that there is no causal relation between either destitution or depressing passions and fever; that medical men spend too much time squabbling about causal questions when they could be out stopping epidemics; and that even if privation does cause fever it does so not through gradual debilitation, but through the inability to purchase things like soap, 'and in various ways by inducing lax habits of life, [so as to] . . . increase the amount of exposure to and loss from the all-pervading cause [the malaria from filth].' Finally, even if deprivation is a cause, it is not within the scope of the inquiry, which is the effect of 'sanitary conditions,' a domain that Chadwick is himself arbitrarily defining in the *Report*. He also builds straw-man arguments, making the destitution-fever hypothesis appear a stronger claim (i.e., that fever is a *necessary consequence* of privation, or that privation *alone* produces fever) than were most contemporaries (the common view

---

[9] Circular to Greater London vestries, April 27 1838, Public Record Office, MH3/1.

was that when fever occurs destitution is often, even usually, a chief predisposing factor, and that one of the most practical ways to prevent fever or end an epidemic was to deal directly with privation through the provision of food, fuel, and shelter). Further, he simply asserts epidemiological generalizations without citing evidence for them. He ignored the many investigations of epidemics that had reached the latter conclusion, and ignored theoretical discussions of what fever was and how it was linked to both contagious and constitutional factors.

[. . .]

What I am suggesting in this article is the reverse of what is often entertained, which is that Chadwick rejected hunger, overwork, contagion, and other possible causes of fever in the process of building a case for the malarial cause of disease, which, he believed, could alone warrant sanitary improvement. A belief in these other supposed causes would at best distract attention from sanitary improvement—and at worst, would subvert it entirely. On the contrary, I have argued that the *Sanitary Report* came about not as an opportunity to take on the new and useful project of urban improvement, but to meet the immediate political need of discrediting powerful enemies. For Chadwick and the PLC, the *Sanitary Report* was to be an ideological document, not a blueprint for sanitary engineering: it was less important that people actually build sanitary works than that they believe that in works, not mutton, was to be found the appropriate domain for the humanitarian's charity and the true path of progress.

7.4

The problems of sanitary reform in Islington

Gerry Kearns, 'Cholera, Nuisances, and Environmental Management in Islington 1830–1855', in W.F. Bynum and Roy Porter (eds), *Living and Dying in London* (London, Wellcome Institute for the History of Medicine, 1991), pp. 118–23 [pp. 94–125].

Gerry Kearns's research has explored issues of nineteenth-century public health including the impact of urban living and the clashes of public and private interests provoked by sanitary reforms. In this article, he provides a detailed study of how sanitary reforms were implemented (or not) in one district of London.

The provision of water and sewerage services by private companies was a prominent concern of the public health movement. . . . However, it is also clear that the local authority was unable to take matters into its own hands and contract on behalf of all parishioners for an improved supply. The Board of Trustees felt powerless to do more than await legislative intervention. Under the exceptional circumstances of 1832, the Islington Board of Health asked 'the New River Company to afford a supply of water which was readily granted in abundance'. Each year the Board of Trustees purchased a supply of water for cleaning the streets. In 1846, the Highways Surveyor highlighted the insufficient supply of water in fifty of the poorer courts and alleys of the parish. The Trustees set up a 'committee to inquire into the most effectual and economical means of obtaining a supply of water in the localities referred to in the Surveyor's Report'. This committee reported that, although only one court was completely without water, there was a need for a better provision in many others 'to improve the sanitary conditions of the poorer districts of the parish'. . . . [T]he committee recommended that a constant supply be established, but noted that the cost would be very high and doubted whether the Board of Trustees was entitled to assume such a liability. It warned that 'if it were to undertake to purchase water, the expenditure under that head would be liable to objection, and might possibly be successfully resisted before the Auditor, or by an appeal to the Quarter Sessions', and concluded, with regret, that: 'The great desideratum is a constant supply introduced into all houses so as to be available for use at any time day or night, but this is the case in all parishes and is one which the powers of the Board will not reach and which nothing short of a general legislative enactment will remedy.' . . .

The Board of Trustees' efforts to secure a comprehensive improvement in the drainage of the parish through the Commissions of Sewers reached a similar impasse. This is exemplified by the efforts the Board made to improve the drainage of Holloway, a district in centre of the parish. The subject was first raised by C.H. Hill in 'a survey and report made and published gratuitously by me in July 1825' . . . in which he suggested straightening the drainage lines and putting some larger drains in. Nothing was done. In 1832, Hill, then Surveyor to the Highways Committee, referred the matter to it, but again nothing was done. On 23 December 1833, 'houses in Holloway Place, Loraine Terrace, Camden

Place and the neighbourhood were from two to three feet deep [in drainage water] in their kitchens and gardens' and in January 1834, Hill produced another report for the Highways Committee. This report was referred to the Board of Trustees and the Highways Committee urged the Board to encourage the inhabitants of Holloway to pay for the necessary improvements 'as they [the Highways Committee members] are of the opinion that the parties to be benefitted ought to provide the money before any of the works are commenced'. Hill estimated that the improvements might cost £4,000. The Trustees did nothing since the question appeared 'to be taken up by the House of Commons' and government measures might render it unnecessary for the parish to spend any money in this area; it might be better if the parish acquired no further interests in sewerage and if the control of all sewers in the parish rested with the Commissions of Sewers; and, finally, since the Trustees did not have the necessary approval from the Vestry for such expenditure. The question of the drainage of Holloway was repeatedly raised by the Committee of the Board of Trustees, and in 1848 the Board wrote to the new Metropolitan Commission of Sewers which had been given reponsibility for the sewerage of the whole of London, on the subject. No reply to this is recorded. In 1849, one of the District Sanitary Committees made a special report to the Metropolitan Commission of Sewers. The Surveyor to the Commission replied that 'there is at present no drainage for this place and it will be provided for in the general plans for drainage', but in 1850 the Trustees again complained of the Metropolitan Commission of Sewers' inactivity and asked for 'immediate steps to provide a remedy for the evil'.

In its dealings with the water companies and commissions of sewers, the local authority of Islington found that neither set of bodies was willing to make exceptions to the general rule of providing services only for payment. If these private enterprises were to continue to serve paying customers it was inconceivable that they should behave in a benevolent fashion, which might depress prices and implicitly commit them to a very broad view of their duties. The Trustees were unable to step in as effective consumers on behalf of the poor because the expense would be politically unacceptable. . . .

In raising the question of the political acceptability of sanitary measures, one is broaching that of the responsibility of the Board of Trustees. The Trustees were answerable to the Vestry. The Vestry jealously watched all parish expenditure and would, through its assessors and auditors, disallow expenditure . . . This reluctance on the part of their masters lay behind the Trustees' nervousness in contemplating extensive environmental works.

... In general, however, the Vestry did not query the few hundred pounds spent annually on sanitary measures, but a particularly intransigent Vestry could paralyse the Trustees. This was a serious problem in the 1850s: between March 1851 and July 1851 all sanitary works were suspended, and in 1854 many of the Committees of the Board of Trustees ran up large overdrafts in the absence of Vestry funds.

... Finer wrote of the tradesmen and shopkeepers of London vestrydom as 'the narrowest and meanest class that England ever produced' and claimed they smashed the Public Health Act of 1848. However, in Islington with its Vestry packed with builders and tradesmen, particularly associated with the noxious trades, the Trustees did not fall victim to any concerted opposition to their use of public health legislation. ... [T]he Trustees were not censured for co-operating with central authorities in improving the environment. The constitution of the parish proved an obstacle to sanitary improvements insofar as the Vestry's veto of large-scale schemes of improvement confined the Trustees to the piecemeal removal of particular nuisances. They had no power to prevent nuisances from recurring or from being established. Thus they were unable to interfere when they received a letter 'complaining that a person of the name of Martin has built a shed at Belle Isle which he intends for horse slaughtering purposes, and requesting the Board to prevent it'. The Trustees tried to keep the parish clean by responding to complaints. But the large-scale engineering and water works they recognized as necessary were placed beyond them by the organization of local government finance. The ratepayers felt unable to raise the money among themselves and looked to the national purse. Thus the Vestry, keen for Parliament to take these matters under consideration, was not disposed to give the Trustees their head.

... The most serious obstacle to their efforts at improving the environment in Islington came from the rights of private property owners. Under the Local Act, the Trustees could only act where nuisances threatened the parishioners' enjoyment of the public area of the parish. In general, the Board was reluctant to interfere if 'the cause of the complaint appears to be on private property' ...

The rights of property extended to many small businesses producing unpleasant smells. A Mr Cork who processed dung and had done so in south Islington for 'upwards of forty years' replied to one complaint that his:

> Dung is worth to me from 15/– to 20/– per week and as the annoyance (if any) is only felt during the hot weather, I do hope my neighbours will not make an attempt under the circumstances, to deprive me of this source of

income, . . . should such an attempt be made, I shall feel it my duty to resist it.[10]

The Lamp committee agreed that 'the nuisance complained of if any is a private one' . . .

It is difficult to resist the conclusion that legal officials went out of their way to make sanitary legislation unworkable. For example, in 1840, the Trustees complained to Mr Flight that 'in consequence of the defective state of his dung carts the solid drops from them in transit through the parish'. In fact, the carts belonged to a Mr Dodd and one of his drivers was taken into custody by the streetkeeper and brought before the Magistrate, but 'it being the first offence the Magistrate discharged him with a reprimand'. Another symptomatic case concerned a dust-shoot certified by two medical practitioners to be 'an accumulation of offensive or noxious matter on the said premises . . . likely to be prejudicial to the health of the persons whose habitations are in the neighbourhood of the above mentioned premises'. A month later, the Magistrate ordered its removal but the owner 'threatened to resist the execution of the order'. The Trustees sought the opinion of counsel, and Mr Bodkin QC advised that, under the Nuisances Removal and Diseases Prevention Act, 'The matter removed must be the identical matter referred to by the order. It is now I apprehend impossible to show that the matter adjudicated upon on the 11th February still remains, there may be similar matter emitting effusions equally offensive but this is not I think sufficient.' The delay caused by legal proceedings was frequently noted and the Inspector of Nuisances once bemoaned the 'dangerous delay' occasioned by his having to bring medical certificates or notices from aggrieved parties before the Board of Trustees in advance of serving a notice or a summons in the offenders 'where a prompt abatement is most urgently needed and essential for the prevention of disease'. Yet the 'nice' interpretation of Mr Bodkin meant that delays not only endangered health, they basically prejudiced any access to legal sanctions. Given the scope for obstruction by those against whom proceedings were being taken, this opinion effectively made it impossible to deal with any but fossilized nuisances.

---

[10] St Mary's, Islington, Lamp and Watch Committee Minutes, 1772–1856, 21 August 1840. Islington Public Library, YL 385/98422–8.

7.5

The problems of sewering Farnham

Anthony S. Wohl, *Endangered Lives. Public Health in Victorian Britain* (London, J.M. Dent & Sons, 1983), pp. 105–7.

Anthony Wohl's book was one of the first, and remains one of the best social histories of public health, exploring the urban environment and its impact on urban life. This extract reveals the difficulties faced by local authorities when implementing sanitary improvements.

Throughout the 1850s the sanitary condition of Farnham had been a cause of dispute between the local Board of Guardians and the vestry, and when in 1866 Farnham finally established a local board of health the town's excrement removal was still an unwholesome mixture of open sewers and cesspits. The new Board decided that the proper sewering of the district was its most important and immediate responsibility, and it placed advertisements in *The Times*, the *Engineering Journal*, and the *County Chronicle* for plans to be submitted by qualified engineers. Prizes of £100 and £50 for the two best plans were offered. This was, no doubt, as good a way as any of going about the task, but when the replies, in a bewildering variety, started to come in, the local Board found itself faced with the daunting task, for which it was unqualified, of judging the entries. It soon realized that it had ventured into something well beyond its competence, and hired a civil engineer, at forty guineas, to evaluate the plans. Unfortunately his report was, like the plans, too technical for the Board to act upon with any confidence, and so they turned to a local farmer who had some practical knowledge of drainage and who, presumably, could communicate in terms comprehensible to laymen. Had they turned instead to the Privy Council they would have received excellent free advice, for Simon's[11] team was building up considerable expertise in sewage disposal and was only too happy to travel to local communities to help. Perhaps Farnham thought that it was too small, or, more probably, it simply wished to handle its own problems without government

---

[11] John Simon (1816–1904), Medical Officer of the Privy Council, led a group of medical men investigating into a range of public health problems.

interference. In any case, faced with conflicting advice and a variety of possible schemes, the local Board dithered, then lost interest. In 1877, some two years after Farnham appointed its first medical officer, there was another show of interest, and again a civil engineer was hired, this time for ten guineas; but, again, no action was taken. Then in 1879 an influential landowner, a Mr Potter, through whose land the polluted river Wey flowed, threatened under the recently passed Rivers Pollution Act (1876) to restrain the Board from using the river for its untreated sewage. Alarmed by the spectre of litigation, the Board was thrown into confusion, and then at last acted, travelling to Taunton and Chiswick to examine their sewage systems, and it showed its good faith by taking the plunge and writing to the Local Government Board for advice. Presented with the alternative of precipitation or irrigation and filtration methods, the Board was again indecisive, and nothing was done until another local landowner, a Mr Bateman, brought suit against the Board under the Rivers Pollution Act. Although the Board argued in its defence that it now had under serious consideration some fifteen drainage schemes, the judgment in Bateman *versus* Farnham (1883) went against it, and it was at last compelled to act. Again an engineer was appointed to draw up plans and at last work began, only to be accompanied almost immediately by numerous problems – construction difficulties, disputes over the site of the sewage farm, haggling over the cost of the land and over the injury which the sewage site (against which, understandably, there was much prejudice) might cause local farmers, squabbles with house-owners who fought to preserve the integrity of their gardens against the upheaval of sewers and connecting drains. In all, some nine months elapsed between the initial drafting of the engineer's plans and their approval by the Local Government Board and accompanying sanctions of a loan of £14,000 payable over thirty years. Once the plans were put out to bid they attracted thirty-six engineering firms, mostly located in the Midlands, for the boilers and pumping engines, ranging from a low of £1,119 to a high of £2,270, and for the laying of sewers a further twenty bids, from £9,342 to £14,888. In both cases the lowest bids were accepted. The problems of Farnham must, however, have struck the local Board as just beginning, for the contractor for the sewer went bankrupt, local inhabitants somehow managed to fall into unfinished sewers, and compensation costs for damage done to property by the laying of sewers and legal costs of arbitration began to soar.

Finally in 1887 the sewer lines were completed and in the summer of 1888, when the total costs were all in, the Board discovered that the scheme had cost £18,000 and it was forced to go to the Public Works

Loan Commissioners for an additional loan. Unfortunately, its difficulties did not end there, for several leaks appeared in the sewers, the sewage farm smelled, and the wash from the local breweries caused the sewage to ferment. The Board discovered also that in several cases where householders had made connections into the main sewers they had failed to install flushing toilets. Although the Board could compel the connection, it had no power to force landlords to install w.cs, and since hand flushing rarely had the force to cleanse the pipes fully, the whole new system did not work quite as efficiently as the Farnham authorities hoped. At the beginning of this century there were still many houses in Farnham which were connected to the main sewers but were without w.cs.

7.6
Popular health education

Something Homely. A Fireside Chat (London, Jarrold & Sons, n.d. [c. 1872]), pp. 11–12.

This extract is from one of many pamphlets issued by the Ladies' Sanitary Association. The Association campaigned on many fronts, educating the poor on health matters through pamphlets and home visiting (techniques copied from religious evangelising), running lecture courses aimed at the middle classes, and campaigning for more comfortable dress for women. This extract features a dialogue between two working men, Eden Williams and John Smith. Eden wants to know why John's home is so much more comfortable when they both earn similar wages.

'Ever since I joined the evening classes[11] I have been waked up more to learning things from books. My brains are none of the best; but still, I have picked up more than one good notion through these classes. About health, now – two winters ago, one of the great doctors from the West-end gave us six lectures about fresh air, food and drink, washing and such-like. He talked real good stuff, such as all of us understood – none of your crack-jaw. See that square of zinc with tiny holes in that

---

[11] At his local Working Men's Association. These associations provided a forum for education, mainly through lectures on a wide range of subjects.

window? Well, I put that up the next day I heard the first lecture. That lets the fresh air in, lad, without draughts enough to hurt a fly; that's for ventilation. Then, too, I bought half a butter firkin for a bath, and now I have a good wash down every morning from top to toe, that takes off all the perspiration which chokes up the skin; nothing so good for the preservation of health . . .'

'Why, you will wash all the goodness out of you,' said Williams, laughing.

'Ah, nay; there's little to wash. But, without laughing, Williams, I do believe some things I heard at the lectures have done a deal to keep me off the sick list. I never knew till then the harm it does a man to breathe hot, dirty air or to go about day by day with his skin choked with dirt. Nothing, I do believe, so bad for health as dirty air, and dirty clothes and skin, except it is' – and John paused thoughtfully – 'dirt at one's heart.'

'Well,' said Williams, 'I must say as you tells it like a book, but it ain't no way clear to me but what there's a deal of gammon[12] in this fuss about air, and washing, and such-like, as we hears so much on now-a-days. Anyway, you look well enough, though.'

Truly, John *did* 'look well'. Just as that man looks to whom has been given the inward purity and peace which lead to all outward order and cleanliness, and comfort; just as he looks, who earns his bread honestly, and eats it in temperance and thankfulness; just as he looks who sleeps the sleep of God's beloved – whose pillow is a good conscience, whose curtains are angels' wings. Just as such a one looks – and no other.

'Thank God, I am well,' John replied; 'and so far as the things said about health being gammon, I believe they are some of the truest things going. Why, ask my Mary, she will tell you; our second, our little Benny – him as lies under the daisies at Highgate[13] . . . well, he might have been here to-day, if she had known then what she knows now about health. Mary's a good scholar . . . and she takes on these notions about health wonderfully. The lady at her mother's meetings, has given her some little books about them, and so we have learnt many a good thing.'

[. . .]

[John explains how he helps around the house – to Williams's surprise.]

'Whatever time do you turn out, then?' asked Williams.

'Six, this time of year. We always get up early, else all gets wrong of a morning; get up early, and there's time for everything. While Mary gets breakfast, I trim myself a bit, and we all sit down comfortably together.

---

[12] i.e. nonsense.
[13] Highgate Cemetery in London.

Our fare's plain enough . . . yet I dare say few men get more comfort. Mary knows how to make a little go a long way, she does. When I get home at night, I always know there will be a nice bit of fire and supper ready for me, and the little ones all eager for the first kiss. You should see them flattening their noses against the window, looking for me, and cutting about when I come in, one setting my chair, one bringing my dry shoes. Then we have a bit of supper and when the children are put to bed, there's a spare hour or so. This I pass in a different way. Mondays and Tuesdays, generally at home, reading and talking to my wife, as you found us tonight. Wednesdays we both go to the week-evening service. Thursdays and Fridays I go to the classes or lecture at the Working Men's Association . . . Saturdays I find plenty to do getting ready for Sunday.'

Part eight
Colonial and Imperial medicine

8.1
Health, race and nation

David Arnold, *Colonizing the Body. State Medicine and Epidemic Disease in Nineteenth-Century India* (London and Berkeley, University of California Press, 1993), pp. 280–8.

Arnold has published widely on culture, imperialism and environmental history of South Asia. This book is concerned with the way in which a state-centred scientific medical system was created in colonial India between 1800 and 1914. It describes the negotiations and complexities that accompanied the varied readings of the body by both colonizers and the colonized. Arnold demonstrates these readings and their effects by looking at epidemic disease and Indian responses to Western medical ideas.

Just as there were few doctors among the municipal councilors of early twentieth-century India, so were they few among the Indian political leaders of the time. But while it may be true to say, as Roger Jeffery has done, that medical practitioners exercised little influence on Indian politics and on the development of the Indian National Congress, Western medical ideas had a far greater impact on political movements and social ideas than such a comment suggests. This is not to say that Western medical ideas held undisputed sway even over the Western-educated middle class, but they had begun to infiltrate and inform public debate and political language to a quite remarkable degree.

The discussion of race and nation points up this trend. It was not surprising that imperial ideas of race and latterly of social Darwinism had a profound impact on India in the late nineteenth and early twentieth

160

centuries. Not only were they part of an assertive ideology of imperial expansion and domination but they were also extensively used in social and political discourse within India itself. On the one hand, there was the praise lavished by the British on the 'martial races' of India for their fighting prowess and 'manly physique,' juxtaposed with descriptions of the weak, cowardly 'effeminate babu.' On the other, there was a renewed assault on Indian social institutions, particularly child marriage. Although the government itself was reluctant to act in such a controversial matter, British doctors contributed their own strong and seemingly authoritative opinions about the resulting enfeeblement and degeneracy of the Indian people. . . . Edith Pechey's address to the Hindus of Bombay in 1890, roundly denounced the practice of child marriage in medical and racial terms and concluded that Hindus' attachment to it was 'one important factor in the predominance of the Anglo-Saxon race.' This was by no means an isolated example. 'As regards race,' declared Dr. Kenneth McLeod of the IMS in the same year, 'there can be little doubt that the marriage of children, often with aged males, tends to physical deterioration of the human stock, and physical deterioration implies effeminacy, mental imperfection, and moral debility.'[1]

In an address given at Madras Medical College later in the year, Surgeon John Smyth asked why the medical profession should interfere in this sensitive issue. His reply was that

> we know more about it than anybody else; that we are the recognised and responsible protectors of the persons of our neighbours; that our unique relations with our neighbours have unfolded to us a state of affairs hostile to the welfare of our race, and we feel morally responsible to do our best to remove this source of danger to the persons of our neighbours as we do to run and arrest a haemorrhage that would otherwise prove fatal.

He impressed upon his audience the seriousness of the 'canker of child-marriage' which affected the health not only of individuals but of an entire race. And he ridiculed a Hindu who had told him that India's climate would forever keep it 'in the rear of the rest of the nations of the earth.' Environmentalist explanations might have been acceptable in the 1830s, but they were not to Surgeon Smyth in the 1890s:

> Poor fellow! His small rotund figure and childish prattle were clearly incompatible with the accomplishment of much in this 'struggle for existence'; but these conditions were by no means attributable to climate. His mother was 13 years old at the time of his birth and his father 17! His little mother and little father and himself prattled away happily enough

[1] *Indian Medical Record* 1890, I, p. 249.

maybe—but it was impossible that a man should be the outcome of it all. The impossibility was intensified . . . by the fact that childishness was to him a hereditary condition transmitted through many ages.[2]

It was not surprising that this racial assault, at its height in the 1880s and 1890s and backed with all the confident authority of medical science, found its reflection and response in Indian debate and polemic. When the Parsi social reformer Behramji Malabari launched his crusade against Hindu child marriage in the mid 1880s, many local organizations endorsed the view that the institution was, as the doctors claimed, a cause of physical and moral degeneracy. The Indian Association of Jessore, for instance, held that 'early marriage weakens the physical strength of the nation; it stunts full growth and development, it affects the courage and energy of the individuals, and brings forth a race of people weak in strength and wanting in hardihood.' As president-elect of the Indian Social Conference in 1889, Dr. Mahendra Lal Sarkar of Calcutta told his audience that 'the Hindu race consists at the present day . . . by virtue of this very blessed custom [of child marriage], of abortions and premature births.' It was not surprising, he added, that the people of such a weak nation had fallen victim to every tyrant that had chosen to trample on them. Fifteen years later, when G.K. Gokhale addressed the National Liberal Club in London, he spoke of the 'continuous dwarfing or stunting of our race that is taking place under your [British] rule,' and though his immediate reference was to the spiritual and moral diminishment of Indians through the denial of political rights and responsibilities, his earlier remarks about the 'frightful sum of human misery' evinced by India's high death rate and the physical frailty of its people, gave his remarks a literal as well as metaphorical meaning.

This sense of racial decay seems to have been particularly powerful in Bengal. Speaking in November 1912, at the Second All-India Sanitary Conference, Motilal Ghosh, editor of the Calcutta newspaper *Amrita Bazar Patrika*, gave an extended account of Bengal's decline under British rule, an account in which disease and race were again closely linked. He claimed, on the basis of his own childhood in Jessore, that sixty years earlier the Bengali countryside had been remarkably free from disease. After the autumn rains people might have been attacked by fever, but by fasting or following a 'low diet' they were quickly cured. Enteric fever was rare; cholera practically unknown. Smallpox occurred intermittently, but the *tikadars*[3] treated it 'with wonderful success.' 'What a pity,' lamented Ghosh before an audience of doctors

---

[2] *Indian Medical Record* 1890, I, pp. 328–32.
[3] *tikadars*: inoculators.

for whom the battle against variolation was barely over, 'that this race of specialists has now become extinct and that their treatment is lost to the world.' In those days, he continued, the 'pick of the nation' lived in the countryside. Villages had 'an excellent system of drainage' and tanks were full of clean drinking water. No people on earth 'were more cleanly: they rubbed their bodies with mustard oil and bathed at least once during the day.' Food was abundant, and villages 'teemed with healthy, happy and robust people, who spent their days in manly sports,' untroubled by 'the bread question or the fear of being visited by any deadly pestilence.'

But those idyllic days were over, and 'those fine specimens of humanity are now rarely to be found in Bengal.' Citing official reports and statistics, Ghosh dated the 'deterioration of the race' to the outbreak of 'Burdwan fever' (malaria) in the 1860s. 'Within the last sixty years malaria and cholera have swept away tens of millions of people from Bengal. Those who have been left behind, generally speaking, are more dead than alive.' Where once prosperity, health, and happiness had reigned, now there were deserted villages, chronic malaria, and common misery. To stop the people from 'dying like flies from malaria' the state must confront the problems of poverty and disease through a comprehensive program of rural sanitation before it was too late. Reminding his audience that the recorded birth-rate for Bengal had sunk below the death rate, Ghosh concluded: the 'Bengali race is . . . dying out, and it must ultimately disappear like the old Greeks, who also fell a prey to this fell disease [malaria], unless vigorous steps of the right sort are promptly taken to save them from extinction.'[4]

Not all contemporary commentators drew such extreme contrasts between an idyllic past and current misery, but there was much in common between this account of Motilal Ghosh and many others written by Bengalis at the time, stressing the weakness of the race and internalizing many of the brutal judgments the British had made about them over the course of the past half-century and more. Ghosh looked to the British government in India, and more especially to Western sanitation and science, to provide answers to this problem of physical and moral decline. But others among his contemporaries looked to Indians themselves to recover their physical prowess or reassert the value of their own cultural traditions as a way of reversing their decline and re-creating pride in their own race.

Swami Vivekananda, one of the most influential Hindu reformers of the period and again a Bengali, provides an interesting illustration of

[4] *Proceedings of the Second All-India Sanitary Conference* 1913, vol. 2, pp. 514–23.

this latter trend, for he showed in his speeches and writings a familiarity with Western medical science, while at the same time seeking to contrast the crass materialism of Western civilization with the virtues of India's spiritual legacy. In an article entitled 'The East and the West,' first published in 1901, Vivekananda began with a striking description of the way Westerners saw India, in which disease played a significantly conspicuous part.

> Devastation by violent plague and cholera; malaria eating the very vitals of the nation; starvation and semi-starvation as second nature; death-like famine often dancing its tragic dance; the Kurukshetra of malady and misery; the huge cremation ground, strewn with the dead bones of her lost hope, activity, joy and courage . . . —this is what meets the eye of the European traveller in India.

Similarly:

> A conglomeration of three hundred million souls, resembling men only in appearance; crushed out of life by being down-trodden by their own people and foreign nations, by people professing their own religion, and by others of foreign faiths; patient in labour and suffering, and devoid of an initiative, like the slave; without any hope, without any past, without any future; . . . full of ugly, diabolical superstitions which come naturally to those who are weak and hopeless of the future; without any standard of morality as their backbone; three hundred millions of souls such as these are swarming on the body of India, like so many worms on a rotten, stinking carcase,—this is the picture concerning us, which naturally presents itself to the English official!

Against this unrelenting picture of vice and misery, of disease and oppression, Vivekananda contrasted the Indian's view of the Westerner as the 'veriest demon':

> lustful; drenched in liquor, having no idea of chastity or purity, and of cleanly ways and habits; believing in matter only; . . . addicted to the aggrandisement of self by exploiting others' countries, others' wealth by force, trick and treachery; having no faith in the life hereafter, whose Atman [soul] is the body, whose whole life is only in the senses and creature comforts.

Vivekananda saw error and ignorance on both sides. Europeans judged India only on the basis of their contacts with the servant class, just as Indians judged Westerners by superficial impressions—their neglect of caste distinctions, their fondness for liquor, their brazen attitudes toward women. Vivekananda conceded that in some areas, such as health, 'westerners are far superior to us' and that there were many things Indians could learn from them. Westerners lived longer: they

164

lived in a better climate, but also they did not marry at an early age like Hindus. 'In point of longevity and physical and mental strength,' therefore, 'there is a great difference between the Westerners and ourselves.' But he also asked why it was that, despite so much 'misery, distress, poverty and oppression,' the Hindu race had not died out centuries ago: 'If our customs and manners are so very bad, how is it that we have not been effaced from off the face of the earth by this time?' His answer was that India had a 'national idea, which is yet necessary for the preservation of the world.' India was 'still living' because 'she has her own quota yet to give to the general store of the world's civilisation.'

Vivekananda met the assertive universalizing of Western materialism and science with an equally universalistic but, in his view, superior notion of spirituality. The two ideas were represented in opposing (but to Vivekanada not entirely irreconcilable) concepts of cleanliness and purity. Westerners might have a scientific and medical understanding of what constituted pure or clean water. This was not invalid, but Indians possessed, and could give to the world, a sense of spiritual health and purity which transcended any strictly medical or materialist definition.

In the early years of the twentieth century, M.K. Gandhi went even further than Vivekananda in seeking to detach Indians from what he saw to be the harmful influence of Western civilization and to link ideas of health with India's *swaraj* (literally 'self-rule'). In his youth Gandhi appears to have been attracted to the medical profession. At one stage he wanted to go to England to train as a doctor but was stopped from doing so by his brother, who said that 'we Vaishnavas should have nothing to do with dissection of dead bodies.' Nonetheless, as Bhikhu Parekh has aptly observed, the adult Gandhi's language and thought were 'suffused with medical images. He thought that the Indian "body politic" had become "weak" and "diseased" and unable to resist the attack of "foreign bodies." ' It was the self-appointed task of 'Dr Gandhi,' as Parekh dubs him, to be India's 'national physician' who diagnosed his country's ills and 'knew how to restore it to health and build up its strength.'

Gandhi's medical and sanitary 'experiments' began during his years in South Africa. In a series of gestures which on a personal level rolled back the swelling tide of Western medicine and, like the successive changes in his dress from English suits to homespun *khadi*,[5] marked stages in an individual but highly emblematic decolonization of the body, Gandhi acted as midwife for his last child and refused to allow Western doctors to attend his son Manilal when he was close to death

---

[5] *khadi*: homespun cotton cloth.

from typhoid and pneumonia. At Tolstoy Farm, the community he established near Johannesburg in 1910, medicinal drugs and doctors were banned, and Gandhi pursued various health cures of his own. Unlike some Indian nationalists, he found no inspiration in Ayurveda and the traditional healing arts of India, developing instead his own eclectic ideas and practices. But above all, Gandhi saw health as an integral part of his spiritual and physical quest for self-discipline, for *swaraj*[6] in its widest, as well as most intimate, sense. For Gandhi, good health did not mean having the services of a good doctor but rather, by being able to control bodily desires, to prevent disease and nurture one's spiritual well-being.

Perhaps Gandhi became so obsessed with health and sanitation because he recognized the extraordinary authority Western medicine had acquired by the 1890s, an authority which had to be confronted and contested if India were ever to free itself from its colonial bondage. Possibly health and sanitation assumed such importance for Gandhi in South Africa because of the accusations made by whites that Indians were 'filthy in habit and a menace to the public health.' These accusations seem to have stung Gandhi's growing pride in his own race and civilization, a civilization which, after all, regarded purity and cleanliness as supremely important values. He seems to have internalized these racist jibes by assuming a scrupulous attention to personal sanitation and hygiene, while hurling back at the West a biting critique of its spiritually corrupting and physically deleterious civilization.

The clearest statement of Gandhi's linkage of health with nationhood was made in *Hind Swaraj* ('Indian Home Rule'), first published in 1909. In the course of a rather cumbersome dialogue between the Editor, whom one takes to represent Gandhi's views, and the Reader, doctors are implicated along with lawyers and railways as being responsible for the decline of India under British rule. In a familiar simile, Western civilization is likened to consumption, a disease that does not seem to cause much 'apparent hurt' but which, below the surface, progressively undermines health and strength. When the Editor turns to doctors in the course of his diagnosis of the 'condition of India,' Gandhi reveals that, although he had once been 'a great lover of the medical profession' and had intended 'to become a doctor for the sake of the country,' he now sees doctors in an unfavourable light and understands why traditionally India's *vaidyas*[7] did 'not occupy a very honourable status.'

[6] *swaraj*: home rule or self-government.
[7] *vaidyas*: Ayurvedic practitioners.

But it is Western doctors and Western medicine that are the main target of Gandhi's attack. 'The English,' he declares, 'have certainly effectively used the medical profession for holding us.' They have done this in a literal sense by using their professional position with 'Asiatic potentates' for political gain, but in a more general sense they have done so by undermining Indians' capacity to rule their bodies as well as their country. Disease is the result of indulgence, of overeating or 'vice.' Doctors cure their patients, but take a fee for themselves (exploiting suffering for material gain) and allow the patients to return unrepentant to their old vices and indulgences. 'A continuance of a course of medicine must, therefore, result in loss of control over the mind' as well as the body. If the doctor did not intervene, the Editor insists, 'nature would have done its work, and I would have acquired mastery over myself, would have been freed from vice and would have become happy.' Hospitals, the principal temples of this vicious cult, are 'institutions for propagating sin. Men take less care of their bodies and immorality increases.' European doctors are 'worst of all.' In a deft inversion of Western medical claims and racial stereotypes, Gandhi declares that doctors 'induce us to indulge,' with the result that 'we have become deprived of self-control and have become effeminate. In these circumstances, we are unfit to serve the country. To study European medicine,' he concludes in a memorable phrase, 'is to deepen our slavery.'

Gandhi's critique was as rare as it was radical. Not many Indians of his time were prepared to go so far in rejecting not just British rule but also Western civilization as a whole. Some, like Vivekananda, looked for a way in which the East could both learn from and subsume the West; others, like Dr. T.M. Nair, wholly endorsed Western medicine but were critical of the British for not doing more to give—or allow—India the benefits of science and sanitation. But if Gandhi's views were far from being representative, they were nonetheless, by the very ferocity of their exposition, a demonstration of the hold which Western medical ideas and practices had begun to exert on Indian society and the extent to which what had once been the hallmark of an alien presence was fast becoming part of India's own ideology and leadership.

8.2

La lutte: the campaign against sleeping sickness

Maryinez Lyons, 'Sleeping Sickness Epidemics and Public
Health in the Belgian Congo', in David Arnold (ed.), *Imperial
Medicine and Indigenous Societies: Disease, Medicine and
Empire in the Nineteenth and Twentieth Centuries*
(Manchester, Manchester University Press, 1988),
pp. 105–13 [pp. 105–24].

Lyons's work is concerned with the study of public health issues in
Africa. This work on sleeping sickness was extended to a book
published in 1992. Lyons considers that historical analysis of past
epidemics, and the response to them, has relevance today for those
involved in dealing with Aids/HIV. She has also co-edited a study of
responses to sexually-transmitted disease in Uganda. This book
was based on a Social History of Medicine conference in 1986. In
this article, Lyons shows how responses to the sleeping sickness
epidemic in the Belgian Congo was integral to the creation of the
medical services, and thus, to the 'civilising mission'. Public health
measures often meant the reorganisation and restructuring of
African society itself. The epidemic was fought as a military campaign; native peoples were controlled 'for their own good' and
indigenous notions of disease control were ignored.

Colonial powers commonly regarded their medical and public health
programmes as a form of compensation for the hardships caused by
their colonisation of African peoples. By the early 1940s the Belgians
were proud of their colonial medical services in the Congo which they
considered to be an outstanding feature of their 'civilising mission'. The
history of medical services in the Congo is intimately linked to the
special campaign to fight epidemic sleeping sickness early this century.
That campaign formed the basis both for a public health programme
and for the creation of a medical service, since it was, as in many
African colonies, the first real effort made by the Europeans to deal
with the health of Africans.

Following the British discovery in 1901 of a major sleeping sickness
epidemic in Uganda, King Leopold of Belgium invited the recently
established Liverpool School of Tropical Medicine to examine his

Congo Free State. Alarmed at the high mortality rate in neighbouring Uganda, Leopold feared a demographic collapse in the Congo Free State which would frustrate its economic exploitation. By 1902, the year of his invitation to the Liverpool School, the violent practices of Congo Free State agents had aroused international indignation and condemnation. Leopold was much concerned about his tarnished image and he realised that prompt response to a possible epidemic of sleeping sickness in the territory might help to improve his reputation. From the outset, medical provision for the Congolese was related to economic and political considerations. While the Belgian government, which subsequently took over the running of the Congo from Leopold, tried to avoid further administrative mismanagement, medical provision remained closely related to economic and political objectives.

[. . .]

La lutte: the campaign against sleeping sickness

The sleeping sickness campaign operated on two fronts which the Belgians referred to as the *médicamenteuse* and the *biologique*. The former included all the more purely medical aspects such as development and training of staff, European and African; the creation of the annual, itinerant medical missions which by 1930 were examining nearly three million people; the gradual evolution of a network of hospitals and rural clinics, especially in Province Orientale; and research into the disease and possible cures. The second front, *biologique*, was primarily administrative and involved public health measures intended to control the incidence and spread of the disease. The measures within this front were often early attempts at 'social engineering' through the reorganisation, restructuring and control of African societies. Features of this front were the identification and mapping of infected and non-infected zones and the creation of a *cordon sanitaire* to protect mainly non-infected regions such as large portions of the northeast; isolation of infected individuals in one of the special lazarets, or isolation camps, located on the fringes of uninfected zones, the regrouping and re-siting of African populations as part of the overall programme with which the Belgians hoped simultaneously to solve public health, political and economic problems, and, finally, a score of administrative measures designed to regulate various African activities in order to control the incidence and spread of sleeping sickness.

Disease was regarded as an enemy agent against which the Belgian colonial administration fought on these two fronts. The predominantly military administration of the Congo Free State, which was only gradually altered after Leopold's state became a Belgian colony in 1908, quite naturally conceptualised the battle against sleeping sickness as a military campaign, *la lutte*. Sleeping sickness, the foe, had to be isolated, cordoned off, contained and eliminated. After 1903–4 when the aetiology of the disease was discovered, those factors believed by the Europeans to cause the disease – trypanosomes and tsetse-flies – could be targeted for the attack. Supported by the assumption that European science with its superior technology and medicine would succeed where primitive African societies simply floundered, the colonial authorities had no doubts about their methods. After all, said a medical administrator in 1943, 'we know how primitive and futile was the knowledge of the natives in matters of hygiene'.

Diseases, like recalcitrant Africans, were to be forced into submission. In protecting from infection their future labourers and tax-payers, the new colonial authorities felt fully justified in attempting to assert total control. The major feature of the early campaign against sleeping sickness, the *cordon sanitaire*, reflected the paternalistic nature of Belgian colonial policy in which health priorities formed a part of the justification for the methods of the social engineer. African societies, like the labouring classes in Europe, had, it was felt, to be controlled for their own protection. There was a crucial difference, however, in the scope of measures possible in a colonial setting, where social control could sometimes be exercised to a degree unimaginable in the metropole. A growing profusion of legislation from both Brussels and Boma, the capital of the Congo, was sanctioned by the judiciary and enforced by the military and the police. At the same time, an evolving medical infrastructure of personnel, facilities and procedures was directed at locating, isolating and dealing with all those infected with the trypanosome.

Cordon sanitaire and isolation: 1903–9

The sleeping sickness campaign began officially on 5 May 1903 when the Vice Governor-General announced that isolation of victims was the 'principal precaution to take in order to check the spread of the disease'. One doctor raised the 'delicate question' of what to do about victims' families. Should they also be isolated? But, he added, considering the 'insouciance and negligence of hygiene of the Africans', how could effective surveillance be achieved? Reminding the Governor-General that during the recent cholera and plague epidemics in Asia

Minor and Arabia more than one port in the Mediterranean had become infected in spite of the *cordon sanitaire*, the doctor explained that he feared the Congolese manifested the same 'hatred of all hygiene measures conceived of by Western civilisation' as did the oriental populations, and that would prevent a successful *cordon* being established.

Local officials as well as all religious and philanthropic organisations, in the state were instructed to investigate villages in their localities and alert the chiefs of the measures they were to take. These included, naturally, the isolation of victims at a distance from the village and the burning of their huts, as well as the destruction of all the clothing and daily utensils of those who had died of the disease. There were no instructions on how these aims were to be achieved (even when suitable language translators were available), and there was no discussion of the possible relevance of cultural differences between African societies, especially how these affected indigenous ideas of disease management.

[. . .]

There were no significant policy changes between 1903 and mid-1906 because there was no available cure and, as sleeping sickness was always fatal, the only feasible measure was the total isolation of all suspected victims. But the situation was greatly changed in December 1906 when new sleeping sickness regulations were issued as a result of the development of the arsenical compound, atoxyl. This drug was valuable for victims in the first stage of the disease while parasites were present in the peripheral circulatory system. It was mistakenly believed that it could effect a cure in four to six weeks, thus regular screening was undertaken to identify suspect cases. Some doctors, however, were reluctant to use atoxyl which they considered to be dangerous even in the hands of specialists.

[. . .]

The cordoned 'triangle'

Perhaps the most significant feature of the act of 5 December 1906 was the *cordon sanitaire* it placed around Uele District in the northern Congo, a territory some 300,000 square kilometres in extent. This was achieved by means of a series of lazarets[8] located on the periphery of the district. Between 1907 and 1910 the key lazarets and observation posts

---

[8] lazarets: isolation camps.

were established at the state posts of Ibembo, Barumbu, Stanleyville, Aba and Yakoma. By 1912, there were fourteen observation posts throughout the whole colony, with the major epidemic areas designated as the Semliki basin, Kivu, the Kwilu basin, and Kwango, all lying to the south and west of Province Orientale.

The main principles of the lazaret system were described by Inge Heiberg, the first director of the principal lazaret for the north, located at Ibembo. He advised that isolation camps should be located at the limits of contaminated areas, rather than inside them, and stressed that the traffic caused by labour recruitment from infected areas was highly instrumental in the spread of the disease. All recruitment should be accompanied by thorough medical examinations which should be repeated along the transit routes, and, in effect, constitute a 'sieve' to catch sleeping sickness victims. Heiberg also described how a search tour should be conducted to trap all suspects. The doctor should begin at a point furthest from the centre of the area and in that way 'brush ahead of him like the hunter' all suspects and expel them through the observation post, or 'key' to the district.

Once inside the lazaret, victims would receive atoxyl injections and periodic examinations which were to be carefully recorded in registers. Isolation would vary from complete 'lock-up' to relatively unrestrained surveillance. Heiberg felt that prison-style confinement was administratively preferable for both Europeans and Africans. The boundaries and tasks were clear and public order was not disrupted, 'except, perhaps, at the moment of internment of a sleeping sickness victim'. No meeting could occur between victim and African soldiers or natives and more significantly, no arms would find their way inside the lazaret. 'After all,' the doctor added, 'it is isolation which makes a lazaret.' He saw, however, some disadvantages to the prison-style system, which required, 'energetic and firm surveillance' and other stringent measures. The major problem was the ever-present threat of rebellion, and Heiberg consequently favoured more liberal and open lazarets, keeping strict isolation for the really obstinate or advanced cases.

[. . .]

Heiberg warned that it was of paramount importance to treat the patients with kindness, goodwill and indulgence. They must be carefully fed. He advised that it was best to allow people to live in culturally similar, small groups – 'village style' – with a former sergeant or corporal of the *Force Publique* appointed as the headman. Doctors and administrators should interfere as little as possible in the people's internal disputes.

Lazarets in trouble

By 1910 the prison-style, total isolation system was clearly in difficulties although serious problems had arisen almost immediately with the policy of 1905–6. Lazaret doctors very soon realised that, contrary to earlier hopes, atoxyl cured very few patients in the early stages of the disease, with some relapses, while it had no effect on those in the advanced stages. Africans were very quick to observe the poor results, The mortality rates were appalling – at Ibembo lazaret, nearly one-third of those admitted had died by 1911. Furthermore, there was a dreadful side effect of atoxyl injections – up to thirty per cent of those treated became blind as the drug atrophied the optic nerve. Africans were terrified of *la lutte* and the lazarets became popularly known as 'death camps'. Wild rumours circulated that the colonial officials were not only causing the disease, but were rounding up people in order to eat them. A missionary's advice of 1902 that the state should establish 'colonies of incurables' had been made a reality.

[. . .]

The sleeping sickness campaign, like other Belgian colonial policies, was highly centralised with most instructions issued directly from Brussels. There was no separate colonial medical department until December 1922. A medical service had functioned from Brussels since December 1909, but doctors in the colony remained strictly subordinated to the authority of their local territorial administrators. Before December 1910 and the first medical department for the Congo, there was no true 'medical authority which made sanitation regulations'. All such regulations were issued by civil and military authorities. Thus measures such as medical passports and the epidemiological maps upon which the *cordon sanitaire* was based emanated from non-medical administrators. Ordinances controlling African life – village siting, fishing, salt-production, travel, kin relations – were all drafted by non-medical staff.

[. . .]

In 1909 the major features of *la lutte* were the *cordon sanitaire* and isolation in lazarets, considered by one doctor as being together 'the great panacea for public health in the Congo'. But, as he acknowledged, combined with the ineffective, even dangerous, chemotherapy, the campaign evoked intense distrust from the people. Furthermore, he said, the sporadic surveys for victims in African villages were viewed as 'little more than man hunts' and the result was that 'people fled [from] the doctors more quickly than they did the tax collectors!' Often the army was required to assist doctors to examine Africans and then to effect their isolation. Clearly, the combination of a complicated and blundering bureaucracy with an isolation system from which the only exit was escape or death and in which one third of those treated became blind was a failure.

African responses to the early period of *la lutte* made it apparent to the colonial administration that no public health programme could be really effective unless everyone involved, African and European, co-operated. Slowly, the realisation dawned that medical and administrative staff would have to co-operate in order to implement sleeping sickness measures. There had been calls previously for the understanding and support of African authorities in the campaign to examine all of the people and to isolate infected individuals, but by late 1909 it had become clear that the understanding and support of all Africans affected by the campaign would be necessary if it were to stand any chance of success. The responses of the people to the Belgian sleeping sickness campaign were indeed a significant factor which shaped the future development of public health in the colony.

8.3
The madman and the medicine men

Megan Vaughan, *Curing Their Ills. Colonial Power and African Illness* (Cambridge, Polity Press, 1991), pp. 100–23.

Vaughan's research concerns social and economic history, including studies of gender, nutrition and famine in Malawi and Zambia and the history of colonial medicine in Africa. This book analyses the encounter between Western medicine and disease among the indigenous population in Africa. In this chapter, she discusses the problematic categorisation and definition of Africans by Western psychiatry.

In 1935 Drs Shelley and Watson, two Nyasaland[9] Government medical officers, appointed to investigate 'mental disorder in Nyasaland natives', reported on their findings. In the territory's one lunatic asylum

---

[9] *Nyasaland*: modern Malawi.

they found a high percentage of inmates suffering from 'schizophrenic delusions' which, they wrote, could be divided into two categories – the 'European type' and the 'Native type'. Examples of the 'European' type of delusion were given as follows:

> Very rich man and built asylum at his own expense.
> Heaven and earth are separated and he wants to join them.
> Owns Port Herald and is married to a white girl.
> Owns a silver mine, is son of a king, an Englishman.
> Thinks himself God and Principal Headman of the sky.
> Thinks himself very wealthy.
> Lives at Government House, which a previous governor gave him.
> Is commander of a great army.

'Native type' schizophrenic delusions were apparently less common, but Shelley and Watson gave the following as examples:

> Is a lion, wants to kill people and eat them.
> Thought he was a barking dog and tried to bite people.
> His wife is always committing adultery.

As is the case with many other colonial documents on African insanity, Shelley and Watson's report reveals a great deal more about colonial categories than it does about madness. In order to define the mad, it was necessary first to define the 'normal' African. This exercise, as we shall see, preoccupied many a colonial psychologist. Having defined the 'normal' workings of the African mind, it was then possible to identify a 'normal' African delusion ('I am a lion and I want to eat people' or 'My wife is always committing adultery'), as against those apparently very unAfrican delusions of power and control ('I am wealthy'; 'I am God'; 'I am married to a white girl').

The history of madness in colonial Africa is not a simple one. Though there are many parallels with the now well documented history of the defining and the confining of the mad in modern Europe, there are times when the specificities of a colonial situation seem to stand out in relief. To put it simply, whilst the history of insanity in Europe is the history of the definition of the mad as 'Other', in colonial Africa the 'Other' already existed in the form of the colonial subject, the African. The category of the mad African, then, more often included the colonial subject who was insufficiently 'Other' – who spoke of being rich, of hearing voices through radio sets, of being powerful, who imitated the white man in dress and behaviour and who therefore threatened to disrupt the ordered non-communication between ruler and ruled. I should make it clear, however, that the history of the creation of these colonial categories and their articulation is not synonymous with the history of psychiatry in colonial Africa. Theory and practice, colonial thought and colonial policy, only rarely meshed. There was no 'great confinement' in colonial Africa to match that of nineteenth-century Europe, and colonial psychiatric institutions, as we shall see, have their own, rather separate history.

[. . .]

If madness, in Porter's words, is 'a foreign country', what of madness in a colony? If 'normal' communication between ruler and ruled was no more than a 'stammered dialogue', and one which was, for most of the colonial period, purposively so, how were the utterances of the mad interpreted? For the most part, of course, the voices of the mad cannot be heard by us at all. Historians of Africa search constantly for the authentic 'African voice' in the colonial archives, and find it hard to uncover. Hearing the authentic voice of the mad African in written documentation really does involve straining the ears. However, many colonial governments adopted some form of legislation for the control and care of 'lunatics', and this legislation produced its own historical record, notably in the form of enquiries and court cases.

[. . .]

Many a case heard in the early colonial courts of Central Africa involved the murder of a wife by her husband, and the subsequent suicide, or attempted suicide, of the murderer. In 1924 one Njoromola was sentenced to death in the Dedza district of Nyasaland for the murder of one of his wives and her child. The magistrate (and later the High Court judge) was faced as always with the problem of defining whether the man had been legally insane at the time of the crime. Arriving at a view on this involved a prior understanding of many things, including the nature and meaning of relationships between husbands and wives, their emotional and symbolic significance. This was not easy. No evidence was provided for a motive, except that provided by Njoromola himself: 'People believed me impotent and wanted to kill me so that my wife could marry someone else. So I decided to kill my wife and child and then be hanged myself.'

The magistrate will have known, through his hearing of the hundreds of marriage cases which came to his court at this time, that impotence and infertility were frequently the cause of great anguish, of much friction between spouses and their families, and of divorce. With this in mind, he had asserted that there was a distinction between insanity and what he described as a 'fit of passion due to perverted imagination',

176

and had sentenced the accused to death. But when the case reopened other evidence was brought forward to indicate that Njoromola had been suffering from more than a 'perverted imagination'. People in his village, it was said, looked upon him as mad. In 1923 he had attacked his other wife with a knife, for no apparent reason, and on the way to the Boma (the local colonial government headquarters) he had fallen over a cliff ('though that may have been an accident'). For two years he had not visited friends 'as is the native custom', and after the murder he went to the house of his aunt and 'sat naked inside the fence, and attempted to kill himself'.

As a result of such evidence, Njoromola's sentence was commuted to life imprisonment with hard labour, and he was confined in the Central Prison at Zomba. By late 1926 his mental condition had begun to deteriorate. He assaulted other prisoners and warders, believing that the warders wanted to kill him. He was found 'digging up the ground near B-block, and when asked why he was digging he replied "I am digging for tobacco", and when told there was none there he replied "I am making a Boma".' Njoromola, who by now was recognized by all as 'very far from normal', was transferred from prison to asylum to live out the rest of his life.

If colonial officials had problems interpreting the rationality or otherwise of murder in this cultural context, things were further complicated by witchcraft beliefs and the legislation designed to eradicate these. With both a Witchcraft Ordinance and a Lunacy Ordinance on the statute books in Nyasaland by the First World War, it was essential to distinguish not only between the mad and the bad but between the mad person and the person who thought himself or herself bewitched. The confusing part of this was that whilst insanity was held to be a real and definable condition (despite all the problems of understanding local behavioural norms), bewitchment was held not to exist in reality but to be evidence of malice. Denial was the basic approach of colonial authorities to the phenomenon of witchcraft, and if you believed yourself to be bewitched you were just as culpable as the person who purported to have bewitched you. But if insanity was real and witchcraft not, what was to be done with the woman whose children had died in quick succession, who went 'berserk' and assaulted her mother-in-law in the belief that she had caused these deaths? Was she mad, and therefore ill and to be pitied, or was to be charged under the Witchcraft Ordinance for accusing another of being a witch? It was 'normal' (if punishable) for an African to believe in witchcraft – it was not 'normal', however, to suffer from paranoid delusions. Unsurprisingly, the distinctions were very often blurred, and magistrates relied heavily on the opinions of 'native court assessors' in such cases. Certainly in the Nyasaland asylum, as in other colonial African asylums, a fair proportion of inmates suffered from the peculiarly 'native' delusion that they were bewitched, or that they had offended against some 'custom'. Any attempt to classify and distinguish 'witchcraft' and 'insanity', then, largely broke down under the pressure of African realities, reminding us that colonial categories were not all-powerful.

However, African communities could sometimes pick up these categories and run with them. The idea that insanity was a condition sometimes calling for confinement in a distant institution, at no charge to the insane or their relatives, held some attractions. On occasions, individuals exhibiting slightly abnormal behaviour might be presented as 'insane' to the magistrate because there existed other grudges against them. In one Nyasaland case of 1934, headmen Mwamadi claimed that Chipendo was mad and should be confined. The case was suspicious from the beginning, Mwamadi making the following statement (presumably in response to the magistrate's prodding): 'I myself owe no money to Chipendo, nor have had any trouble with his women. His wife, Ellesi, cannot come in as she only gave birth to a child yesterday and is not in a fit state to attend. I am certainly not the father of the child.' Other evidence pointed rather conclusively to the fact that Chipendo was not insane at all but had differences with his headman. He was released into the custody of his brother, Kettle, who took him off to live in another village, and the case was closed.

[. . .]

The 'labelling' of the mad African as carried out in the colonial court room, then, was often a confused and hesitant business. It would be hard to read this record, incomplete as it is, as the process whereby . . . society creates the mad person, so that by invalidating her or him as evil, it may be confirmed as good. The colonial authorities had no need for such a scapegoat, such was the colonizers' belief in their innate superiority – the social distance between the European and the colonized African was sufficient to create the objectification . . . there was no need for the mad person to be invented for this role.

But the history of the colonial classification of insanity amongst Africans can be read in other ways. The writings of colonial psychiatrists and psychologists provided one language, and perhaps a potent one, in which to describe and define the 'African' in general and not just the 'mad African'. The changing nature of African insanity itself could stand for the more general problems of colonial rule – the social and economic upheavals of industrialization and the problems of social order. But the languages of psychology and psychiatry, as we shall see, described these problems largely in terms of cultural and 'racial' difference. 'The African' in the twentieth century, like the European woman in the nineteenth century, was simply not equipped to cope with 'civilization'.

We might begin to explore these aspects of the colonial history of African madness by returning to Shelley and Watson's report on insanity in Nyasaland. The two doctors had individually examined each of the eighty-six inmates of the Lunatic Asylum and had divided them into what were the current categories of psychiatric disorder. 'Schizophrenia' accounted for 35.7 per cent of the total, and 'affective psychoses' for another 21.4 per cent.

The doctors believed that the incidence of insanity was rising, especially amongst the educated, but the evidence they used to support this view was already determined by the theory that 'civilization' was sending Africans mad. Finding that 24 per cent of inmates of the asylum were from the Yao 'tribe' (whose representation in the population as a whole was only 14.5 per cent), they argued that this might be expected as 'the Yao form the intelligentsia of the indigenous peoples and have been in more intimate contact with European civilization than the members of other tribes'. Only 15 per cent of the inmates were female, and this could be easily explained because 'women do not come into intimate contact with Europeans and their minds lack the stimulation which the male mind encounters by such contact'.

Their argument would have been a familiar one to those with an interest in African psychiatry in the 1930s – the central cause of insanity was 'acculturation', brought about, in the main, by education. Just as the late nineteenth-century Social Darwinians warned European women of the profound dangers of education and self-fulfilment, so psychiatrists of the 1930s to 1950s warned that Africans would face similar consequences.

Shelley and Watson provided further evidence to support their thesis that 'deculturation' was the cause of rising insanity. It appeared to them that inmates of the asylum fell into two main categories – firstly, those whose illnesses could be explained by reference to the strains and injuries of 'traditional' society (in particular those driven mad by the fear of witchcraft) and secondly, the more numerous category of those driven mad by 'acculturation' and the strains of 'modern' society. These two groups could be distinguished not only by their educational backgrounds but, as we saw at the beginning of this chapter, by the content of their delusions, which were either 'European' or 'Native' in character. Their argument appeared to be that not only had contact with the colonizer's culture affected the content of the delusions (producing images of bicycles, radios, telephones and so on) but that such contact had actually caused the illness to come about in the first place. Shelley and Watson focused their attention on the group they had defined as schizophrenics. 'Native schizophrenics', they wrote 'with their sexual disturbances and European type of delusions, and their fondness for offence against property, seem to manifest a more European attitude of mind than the members of other groups.'

A preoccupation with sexual matters, along with visions of bicycles and 'motors', defined the 'native schizophrenic'. Missionaries were largely to blame for destroying the 'primitive innocence' of so many Africans, for they had 'encouraged the natives to clothe themselves and at the same time stimulate[d] the sex consciousness by causing to be hidden the natural functions of the body'. It seemed to the doctors that education and Christianity had had 'an obscure influence on the powers of copulation', for many of the 'Christian natives' in the asylum complained of impotence.

What was behind these theories of Shelley and Watson? The methods and reasoning of their investigation are of dubious 'scientific' value, yet there seems to be a real concern behind the pseudoscientific language. Though the Chief Secretary drew his red pen through large sections of this report (more especially the discussion of African sexuality), there is no doubt that Shelley and Watson's ideas had many familiar resonances for colonial administrators of the 1930s. This was the decade in which social and scientific research on the problems of African colonies really took off. In the Central African colonies there were investigations undertaken on many aspects of African life, which particularly focused on the changes which had been wrought by over thirty years of British rule. There were reports on nutrition, on health, on the fertility of the population, on the status of women, on education. There were anthropological studies of the effects of education and economic change on rural societies, on ritual and beliefs, and studies of 'traditional' political systems. Underlying all of this research was a deeply felt colonial fear, expressed more and more anxiously in the 1930s, that the 'disintegration' of the 'traditional' structures of African societies was endangering social control, that industrialization, education and urbanization contained within them the seeds of disaffection. The political solution devised to address this problem was the system of indirect rule. The disruptive changes wrought by colonialism and capitalism could, so it was argued, be contained if only people obeyed their 'traditional' leaders and followed 'traditional' norms. Africans would be ruled through 'custom' – one had only to identify such customs and to give them the new force of law. Of course some customs were unacceptable and would have to be discarded (it could not be denied that 'civilization' held some advantages), but in general customs were a good thing. It was especially important that Africans experiencing the upheavals of industrialization should know who they were, that they should retain a cultural identity (expressed in terms of belonging to a specific 'tribe' with its distinctive customs). Only by this means would the alienation and disorder of the nineteenth-century European experience of industrialization be avoided.

Part nine

From germ theory to social medicine

9.1
Responses to laboratory medicine

Bruno Latour, *The Pasteurization of France* (trans.
Alan Sheridan and John Law) (Cambridge, Mass. and
London, Harvard University Press, 1988), pp. 116–18.

Bruno Latour has published widely in the field of science studies.
His work explores how science, like medicine, is shaped by social
forces. Latour's early work drew on anthropological and sociological approaches to study the laboratory, using participant-observa-
tional techniques. This research has generated much debate over
the degree to which scientific knowledge can be seen as constructed, not discovered.

In *The Pasteurization of France* Latour argues that Louis
Pasteur did not simply discover the causes of disease – his work
had far wider implications, turning the laboratory into a 'passage
point' for disease problems. In future, all epidemiological problems had to be handed over to laboratory scientists, who would
analyse the situation and, possibly, devise a solution in the form of
a vaccine. Latour shows how Pasteur, an excellent propagandist,
enrolled allies into his bacteriological programme, and made the
laboratory indispensable for doctors, armies and the state. However, perceptions of the usefulness of Pasteur's ideas and of laboratory medicine varied between different groups of practitioners.

The ordinary civilian doctors . . . were out of step [with the hygenists] They were skeptics. Even more than skeptics, they would be called 'grumblers,' if that category were accepted in sociology. Those who were directly concerned with diseases and patients saw nothing extraordinary in Pasteurism, or even relevant, at least before 1894. When they at last made up their minds to use Pasteurism, they saw it not as a revolution in their own practices but as a way of *continuing* in strengthened ways *what they had always done*. Finally, when they had fully assimilated the interest of Pasteurism after the passing of the law of 1902 on the organization of public hygiene, the new medicine seemed to owe more to the old than to the Pasteurian strategy, which had in the meantime shifted toward tropical medicine.

What the other protagonists said about the hygienists, surgeons, or army doctors defined in absentia the reasons why private doctors did not budge an inch to make use of Pasteurism. In simpler terms, all the progress of Pasteurism amounted to for them was a dissolution of the medical profession. Others criticized private physicians for their obscurantism[1] whereas they were being asked to commit suicide. What group would do so willingly? The Pasteurian strategy amounted to attacking disease by a transversal[2] movement which never took the individual sick person as a unity. How could that bring joy to a doctor who knew nothing but the sick individual? What could he make of this vision, which was both too public and too biological, without ever focusing on the patient? What could he make of a few great infectious diseases, which amounted after all to a fraction of his daily work and which were of such a scope that they lay quite outside the capacity of the local physician? What could he do with all those pigs, chickens, dogs, horses, bulls, broods,[3] that had so little to do with medicine, with a human face? What could even be done with a cure, spectacular as it certainly was, like that of rabies which concerned a very rare disease and which, furthermore, required that a patient go to Paris to be cured by a product that was absolutely unavailable to ordinary physicians? In short, what could be done with all those doctrines and methods that were the negation of medical work? The answer is clear: nothing, or not much. And since there was nothing physicians could do with those doctrines, they expressed a polite but unenthusiastic interest,

[1] *obscurantism*: opposition to the spreading of knowledge.

[2] *transversal*: crossways or indirect.

[3] The animals used by Pasteur in his laboratory.

tinged even with a certain ironic condescension. This proves nothing about the obscurantism of the physicians; it proves simply that the Pasteurians had not yet learned to take those allies, unlike the other allies, the right way.

The *Concours Médical*, a corporate journal if ever there was one, speaks of Pasteur's work with a distance and prudence that contrasts starkly with the avidity of the hygienists, insisting that Pasteur be absolutely right and extend the implementation of his work at once. The 'conclusive' character of Pasteur's experiments can indeed not be attributed to their inherent qualities. The doctors found disputable what for the hygienists was indisputable. Of course the doctors showed 'good will'; they supported the subscription to the Institut Pasteur and were proud of him: 'We feel deep joy at the idea of fighting the good fight as obscure but willing soldiers'. But they were cautious: 'Of all that slowly accumulating work, a body of precise knowledge will certainly emerge one day; we can just about catch a glimpse of the way ahead and already a great many facts are piling up. But we should maintain a certain reserve for the time being and not see bacteria everywhere, after previously seeing them nowhere. The aseptic method in surgery has already given great service, not so much by its detailed applications as by the correct ideas of which it was often an exaggeration; it will no doubt serve the physician likewise'.[4]

Were they obscurantists? Did they resist? No, they took great care to separate what was exaggerated from what was useful from their own professional point of view. At the time when Pasteur was attempting his takeover of medicine and the hygienists were claiming to have conquered the state because of the added power offered by the Pasteurians, the physicians waited to see how they would get out of a very difficult situation in which they had everything to lose and preferred to maintain the state of affairs that they had set up with such difficulty: 'We believe that, despite the somewhat impassioned attacks of Monsieur Pasteur, clinical medicine is not quite dead'. They defended themselves, which was quite normal. They even took a certain delight in giving Pasteur lessons in scientific method: 'M. Pasteur ended his communication (on cholera among chickens) by deducing from those various facts applications to the general history of contagious diseases. We shall not follow the learned chemist in his generalizations: before deducing such conclusions from those facts, which are certainly very interesting, he should repeat and vary the experiments'. Like Koch and like Peter, the

---

[4] Dr Gosselin, Editorial, *Concours Médical*, 4 October 1879, p. 159.

physicians of the *Concours Médical* were of the opinion that Pasteur really was exaggerating. How can we deny that they were right?

9.2

A bacteriological approach to controlling typhoid

John Andrew Mendelsohn, 'Cultures of Bacteriology: Formation and Transformation of a Science in France and Germany, 1870–1914' (PhD dissertation, Princeton University, 1996), vol. I, pp. 589–94.

Andrew Mendelsohn's interests focus on the human and life sciences since the Enlightenment, especially the role of bacteriology. This excerpt explores the debates between a bacteriological approach to public health, centred on the laboratory, and older environmental initiatives. Mendelsohn shows how Robert Koch reinvigorated the campaign against typhoid as a way to enhance his public and government status at a time when typhoid had a low public profile and its treatment and prevention were seen to be questions of environmental public health. Koch argued that new measures against the disease should be directed against the typhoid bacillus not the environment.

If politics and passions flared around the diagnosis 'typhoid' in the Alsacian town of Ingweiler in 1900, elsewhere in the Reich it was often difficult to become excited about a disease at once familiar and not often fatal. Even a professional like Carl Flügge, longtime co-editor with Koch of the *Zeitschrift für Hygiene und Infektionskrankheiten*,[5] had more pressing business than to accompany Koch and his former student Martin Kirchner, a high medical official in the Kultusministerium, on yet another government 'hygienic excursion' to Upper Silesia. It was not just that Flügge needed a vacation and was overrun by his duties as university rector. As he wrote in a letter to Koch, he did not see anything new to learn, 'any sort of obscurities as to the spread' of the disease to be cleared up.

[5] *Zeitschrift für Hygiene und Infectionskrankheiten*: Journal of Hygiene and Infectious Diseases.

In Upper Silesia, a half century since Rudolf Virchow's famous investigations into epidemic typhus, which became an important model for progressive scientific hygiene, typhoid now prevailed. A different scientific theory of disease prevailed, too. Flügge granted that the region had deserved and received much attention from the Prussian medical department after a large epidemic in 1897 in Beuthen left 2,000 sick in a city of 36,000. But it was 1901 now, and the first three months of that year the population of 1.7 million had seen only scattered cases – four here, five there, a containable outbreak of 14 in the north. Meanwhile, in the environs of such cities as Breslau, Düsseldorf, and Trier, there were dozens, sometimes over a hundred cases during the same period. Besides, in Silesia as elsewhere, large city epidemics always proved traceable to infected water supplies; rural ones, to 'wide-spread contact infections' aided by the 'open uncleanliness' of ground-floor tenants in the region's towns and villages. In short, Flügge was bored by typhoid fever, its scientific case was basically closed, all was explainable without recourse to any 'hidden, sinister influences'.

Flügge's flagging interest aside, in 1900 Robert Koch needed a *Typhusbekämpfung*.[6] He needed a *Typhusbekämpfung* because he had devoted his life to gaining hegemony for bacteriology – for his kind of bacteriology – over public health, and because by 1900 other options for achieving that goal were gone. Koch had arrived at his model for public health bacteriology in the *Cholerabekämpfung* following the Hamburg epidemic of 1892. But now the cholera years appeared to be over. Meanwhile, diphtheria had been taken care of therapeutically, even miraculously, by the antiserum of Behring and Roux, and Koch was not involved in that miracle. Koch's tuberculin had brought scandal; attempts at a bacteriological tuberculosis campaign had come to frustration; and now, in July 1901 at the First British Tuberculosis Conference, Koch embroiled himself in international controversy by announcing that human and bovine tuberculosis were distinct diseases caused by different microorganisms and that all precautions against tuberculous meat and milk were superfluous. And finally, Ronald Ross, not Robert Koch despite his enormous contributions to malaria research, had just cracked the secret of the disease by identifying the *Anopheles* mosquito as the insect vector of the parasite. After several years of German malaria expeditions under his leadership, Koch needed a new basis for his relation with the state. What disease was left? [Chief medical adviser of Alsace-Lorraine, Dr Joseph] Krieger's estimate of what could and should be done in the application of bacteriology to

[6] *Typhusbekämpfung*: typhoid campaign.

hygiene was on the mark: test for typhoid. Still, typhoid was a difficult choice. . . . [U]nlike such scourges as cholera, tuberculosis, and diphtheria, typhoid was a disease with little or no public profile. The views Flügge expressed in his letter being typical, Koch would clearly have to reinvent typhoid fever if he wanted to have a typhoid campaign. It would not be enough to invent a new typhoid diagnostic technique, as two young bacteriologists at Koch's institute, Wilhelm von Drigalski and Heinrich Conradi (from Forster's Strassburg institute), had just done. What good would a new weapon be if the enemy was uninteresting? Koch would have to make a new unknown and sell a new danger.

Perhaps an old danger, typhoid in its explosive, urban water-borne form, would come to Koch's rescue. But the summer of 1901 came and nearly went without a large epidemic. Koch had no choice but to propose a typhoid campaign whilst appealing to his most notable success in bacteriological hygiene, the cholera campaign of 1892–94, and thus also clothing typhoid in the aura of that deadlier, more dramatic disease. On 14 August, Koch submitted to the Kultusminister a grant request for a bacteriological 'Bekämpfung des Typhus' along the lines of the *Cholerabekämpfung*. Ninety percent of typhoid outbreaks, he began, were caused by infected drinking water. Instead of calling on the government to help all-too-poor communities safeguard their water supplies, however, Koch recommended these remain entirely in local hands. Since it would thus be a long wait before the water 'of the whole monarchy' was safe, Koch proposed 'that we must go at the typhoid directly in the body, that is, search out and render harmless each person who harbors typhoid bacilli in his organism until he poses no more danger to his fellow creatures [*Mitmenschen*]. With the execution of this principle we reached the goal in the cholera campaign.' Koch gave no reason why the focus had to be the human body and why the effort had to be radical. He relied on the subtext that typhoid was as much a national emergency as cholera had been. 'Search out and render harmless each person who harbors typhoid bacilli in his organism': this was truly militant hygiene, medical police taken to an extreme. The human being began to be revisualized as a mere vehicle for infection.

Typhoid bacilluria studies and pathological investigations of the 1890s gave Koch other ways to suggest that typhoid was less known and more dangerous than it seemed. The usual discourse of epidemic typhoid was a discussion of waters and places, if not airs; little of this was to be found in Koch's grant request. Instead, the focus would be on the human body. . . .[P]athologists using bacteriological methods in the 1890s had revealed typhoid bacilli not only in the stools of the sick, but in the urine of convalescents, weeks or even months after the end of fever. 'This factor is still not at all appreciated in practical hygiene,' Koch counselled the Minister. Nor were 'light cases' given enough attention. Koch closed by requesting 30,000 Reichsmark to support a travelling team of four bacteriologists for a year-long trial campaign. He sat back to let his letter do its work.

9.3
Population and politics in Italy

Maria Sophia Quine, *Population Politics in Twentieth-Century Europe* (London, Routledge, 1996), pp. 34–7.

Maria Sophia Quine is a specialist in the history of modern Italy. She follows an interdisciplinary approach, with interests that cover European science and medicine, philosophy and politics. In this book she looks at debates concerning race and population in Fascist Italy, France during the Third Republic (1870–1945) and Germany in the time of the Third Reich. By this time, early nineteenth-century Malthusian fears of overpopulation had given way to anxieties concerning depopulation and degeneration in most industrialised nations. In *Population Politics in Twentieth-Century Europe* Quine discusses the fortunes of eugenics in the three different countries, demonstrating the common denominators and the differences under varying political systems. In this excerpt she discusses how the 'New Italy' was to be created on eugenic, racist foundations.

In his Ascension Day Speech on 26 May 1927, Mussolini defined the objectives of his regime, chief among which was the goal of population increase. He argued that a nation transformed by fascism could comfortably accommodate at least ten million more citizens. Reclamation projects to clear cultivable land and agrarian reforms to boost crop yields would make Italy self-sufficient in food production 'within ten years'. And a future empire would absorb any excess population in colonial settlements. In his 'Numbers as Force' essay, the Duce[7]

---

[7] *Duce*: The Duke, a commonly used nickname for Mussolini.

launched an attack against neo-Malthusianism[8] which borrowed heavily from earlier eugenic pronatalists. He specifically addressed the question of subsistence when criticizing advocates of birth control. Population increase, he argued, would not cause unemployment to rise or famine to ensue. He claimed that one of the most troubling weaknesses of the Italian economy, chronic under-consumption, did not derive from low wages and living standards. On the contrary, a falling birthrate stunted the growth of a home market and manufacturing productivity. Italy, in fact, was underpopulated and needed more workers and consumers to accelerate economic expansion.

The demographic campaign was central to fascist rule in Italy. The 'battle for the birthrate' was tied to the larger foreign policy and political aims of fascism. Because it was launched by a fascist dictatorship, the Italian pronatalist programme must be understood within the context of the ideology and practice of Mussolini's regime.

[. . .]

Fascist propaganda had an overwhelming presence in daily life under the dictatorship as the state seized control of the machinery of mass communication, the press, newsreels and the radio. During the twenty-one years of fascist governance, the drive to increase the birthrate figured prominently in the regime's unstinting efforts to portray a positive image of itself as a strong state with a mission. Ordinary Italians faced a constant barrage of claims about the many achievements of the first government in Italy to be committed to the health and welfare of its people. The dictatorship also implemented an authoritarian plan to alter Italian fertility. The numerous legislative and institutional initiatives which accompanied the birthrate campaign gave the state much leverage for social control and marked the inauguration of public intervention in private life as a form of fascist rule.

Secondly, population policy also became an integral part of the political mythology surrounding a party in power which was otherwise bereft of a systematic doctrine and ideology. Fascism depended on the propagation of certain political myths to give it credence with the public. Chief among these was the myth of itself as a revolutionary movement which stood for the creation of a powerful New Italy. What one historian has called fascism's 'palingenetic vision' became an indispensable instrument of dictatorial power. To capture the consciousness of the people,

[8] *Neo-Malthusianism*: the idea (based on the writings of Thomas Malthus, 1766–1834) that the growth of populations would inevitably outstrip potential sources of food. Populations could only be kept within the limits of food production by war, famine and disease.

the regime constructed an image of itself as the embodiment of a momentous 'national resurrection'. The fascist 'revolution' was a radical new beginning after a dark age of decline under liberalism. The language used in the dictatorship's pronatalist propaganda reflected fascism's claim to be a progressive and regenerative force in Italian politics. The Duce promised to 'heal, cure, and restore' a nation which had become 'sick, weak, and degenerate' under liberal parliamentary democracy. Mussolini's pronouncements on the birthrate included constant mention of a 'spiritual renewal' of the Italian people and the 'rebirth' of a 'young and fertile race'. The regime also presented its population policy as an ambitious form of social planning and engineering by a government determined to remake Italy into a proud, productive and prolific nation. As health reforms figured prominently in the demographic campaign, fascists spoke of a 'welfare revolution' which the caring and benevolent state had purportedly enacted.

9.4
Social hygiene in the Soviet Union

Susan Gross Solomon, 'Social Hygiene in Soviet Medical Education', *Journal of the History of Medicine and Allied Sciences*, 45 (1990), pp. 614–15 [pp. 607–43].

Susan Gross Solomon has published widely on Soviet public health and on relations between the Soviet Union, America and Europe with respect to medicine in the inter-war period. This paper concerns the attempt to create an academic discipline of social hygiene, and to place it within the medical curriculum in post-revolutionary Russia. Social hygienists saw disease as a social phenomenon, and this led to an increased focus on the occupational and social origins of disease and the creation of a healthy population through preventive measures. In their view, medicine should be oriented towards health rather than disease. This approach was seen as distinct and innovative, but died out in the early 1930s.

In 1923 the newly-founded journal of Soviet social hygiene, *Sotsial'naia gigiena,* carried a brief report of the creation in Germany of three academies of social medicine. The founding was something of a milestone.

Although the leading figures in German social medicine had been con-
ducting pioneering research on the social aspects of public health
before the turn of the century, the field of social medicine had been
slow to gain acceptance in the academic mainstream in Germany. The
first full professor (*Ordinarius*) of social hygiene, Alfred Grotjahn, was
not appointed until 1920. The academies in Charlottenburg, Dusseldorf,
and Breslau whose creation was heralded in the Soviet report were
specialized institutions, designed for graduate physicians who elected
to work in communal hygiene, school hygiene, or regional hygiene.

The contrast between the situation of German social medicine (*soziale
Medizin*) and that of Soviet social hygiene (*sotsial'naia gigiena*) was
striking. By 1922, only five years after the Bolshevik Revolution, Soviet
social hygiene was in the process of being established as an independent
discipline in the medical schools. Here the new discipline, whose chief
patron was the Commissariat of Public Health, became part of the
curriculum required of all Russian medical students.

What sort of field was Soviet social hygiene in the 1920s? According
to its earliest official definition, social hygiene was 'the science of the
influence of economic and social factors on the health of the population
and on the means to improve that health.' To the contemporary ear, this
definition may sound awkward, but to the enlightened Soviet reader of
the time, it resonated with deeply-held tenets about health and disease.
First, like most of their colleagues teaching public health, Soviet social
hygienists began from the assumption that disease was a biosocial phenomenon. But in contrast to those who concentrated on the biological
aspects of disease, social hygienists believed that disease was first and
foremost a social phenomenon, best understood in its societal context.
In the words of A.V. Molkov, the prerevolutionary specialist on school
hygiene and sanitary education who became the leading intellectual
spokesman for Soviet social hygiene, 'Medicine ... while not tearing
itself away from its biological grounding and its natural science foundation, is in its essence and its goals a sociological problem.' The social
hygienists' view of disease as a primarily social phenomenon drew
strength from the nurturist premises which were broadly accepted in
Soviet society at the time. Second, for Soviet social hygienists, health
was not simply the absence of disease; it was the positive promotion of
well-being in every area of social life through the adoption of reforms
aimed at preventing disease. While other public health physicians who
identified themselves as 'general hygienists' emphasized sanitary and
hygienic reforms, social hygienists consistently stressed the importance
of social reforms aimed at preventing disease. Third, as a science, social
hygiene aimed both to describe (by examining the social conditions

191

in which disease occurred) and to prescribe (by proposing social measures which would contribute to the prevention of disease).

Soviet social hygiene did not spring full-grown after the Revolution; it had important roots in both foreign and indigenous fields of public health. In demarcating the scope of their field, Soviet social hygienists borrowed extensively from German social medicine of the first two decades of the twentieth century: thus, the courses they taught in the medical schools, like those taught by their German counterparts, embraced such problems as demography and migration, housing and nutrition, occupational hygiene, addiction (alcoholism, narcotics), prostitution, and sexual hygiene. In their emphasis on the importance of preventing disease, Soviet social hygienists drew upon the tradition of pre-Revolutionary Russian 'community medicine' (*obshchesteven-naia meditsina*) whose spokesmen discussed the impact of sanitary and social factors on the health of such territorial or administrative entities as cities, zemstvos[9], rural settlements, and railways.

While Soviet social hygienists acknowledged (with differential enthusiasm) their intellectual debts to German social medicine and Russian community medicine, they consistently maintained that theirs was a distinctive field. In a postrevolutionary setting in which there was a widely-shared premium on novelty, that insistence had its ideological uses. But ideology aside, in my view there was some validity to the claim to distinctiveness advanced by Soviet social hygienists. For their descriptive work was animated by a strong social thrust or 'sting' (in the words of its chief patron) which by the early 1920s was being phased out of the German work. Moreover, in their prescriptive work on public health, Soviet social hygienists looked to the state as the appropriate agent of social reform, whereas proponents of Russian 'community medicine' had consistently looked to the local community as the source of change.

For a fledgling field, the attainment of an institutional niche generally marks the coming of age. In the case of Soviet social hygiene, however, institutionalization in the medical schools marked the beginning rather than the culmination of the struggle for legitimacy. Soviet social hygiene was established hastily, by government fiat, leaving to its intellectual spokesmen the daunting tasks of defining the field's content, specifying its roots, negotiating its position within the teaching of public health, and gaining acceptance for it in the medical school at large.

The attempt by social hygienists to accomplish these tasks was complicated by a variety of factors. First, since the late 1860s, the teaching of public health in Russia had been dominated by the broad umbrella

[9] *zemstvos*: local government.

field of general hygiene. To legitimate their discipline within public health, social hygienists had to argue for its differentiation from general hygiene. In making that case, social hygienists became enmeshed in a bitter rivalry with general hygienists for academic terrain, a rivalry which consumed their energies and shaped their agenda. Second, their patron, the Commissariat of Public Health of the Russian Federated Republic had its own conception of the role that social hygiene was to play in the medical school at large, as social hygienists strove to make a case for importance of their enterprise, they had to integrate their intellectual goals for social hygiene with those set by their patron. This notwithstanding the fact that between 1922–30, it was the Commissariat of Education, not the Commissariat of Public Health, that was directly responsible for the administration of and allocation of funds for medical education. Thus, for most of the 1920s, social hygienists found themselves in the uncomfortable position of being structurally linked to a patron whose ability to assist them in their quest for legitimacy in the medical schools was circumscribed. Finally, the attempt by social hygienists to gain acceptance for their discipline was made more difficult by the socioeconomic conditions of Russia in the immediate postrevolutionary decade. In their effort to persuade their colleagues of the advantages of their 'social prophylactic' approach to public health, Soviet social hygienists would have benefitted significantly from the introduction of social reforms directed at preventing the spread of such scourges as tuberculosis and venereal disease. But the combination of a world war, revolution, and civil war had wreaked havoc with the Soviet economy and therefore such social reforms ranked low on the priority list of a regime preoccupied with rebuilding its shattered economy. The possibility that social hygienists would be able to avail themselves of the 'demonstration effect' decreased markedly at the end of the 1920s, when the regime adopted the policy of rapid industrialization, triggering a near crisis in urban public health. The enormous influx of workers into the cities strained to the breaking point existing facilities for housing, sanitation, and nutrition, creating a morass of health problems (epidemics, contagious diseases, malnutrition, industrial harms, and accidents) that required emergency attention. The urgency of the health situation argued against the wholesale reorientation of the medical system toward prevention, the goal with which social hygienists had identified themselves since the beginning of the decade.

The attempt by Soviet social hygienists to gain acceptance for their discipline in the medical schools in the 1920s is the subject of this paper. The story of that attempt is at one and the same time a tale of academic politics, of patron–client relations in science, and of the role of science in a postrevolutionary society committed in the short run to economic recovery and in the long run to far-reaching social change.

Soviet social hygiene emerged as a distinct discipline in the medical schools as a result of its differentiation from the field of general hygiene which had been the core of public health teaching in Russia for a half century. The process of differentiation was accompanied by consider-able acrimony.

In fact, the challenge by social hygienists to the hegemony of general hygiene was but one in a series of challenges that punctuated the period 1880–1920. In the first half of the nineteenth century, public health was regarded primarily as an administrative (read 'medical police') concern, the rudiments of which were communicated to medical students in courses on legal medicine.[15] As a separate subject of study in Russian medical schools, public health dates back to the late 1860s when the first independent departments of 'general hygiene' were founded. Within less than two decades, such departments had proliferated throughout the country. Until the Revolution of 1917, it was in these departments that medical students learned the fundamentals of public health.

The establishment of independent departments of general hygiene in the late 1860s coincided with the growing view of public health as a science which could, and should, be taught using the experimental method. Indeed, between the late 1860s and 1890s, the field of general hygiene effectively became 'experimental hygiene.' Relying on the methods of physics, chemistry, and biology, general hygienists exam-ined the effect on human health of such environmental factors as soil, climate, air, and water, and made proposals for sanitary reform.

Such was the prominence of the laboratory in the teaching of public health in this period that, at the 1887 Congress of the Pirogov Society of Russian Physicians, bacteriologists made bold to take over the teaching of general hygiene. Speaking as the advocates of the purely biological approach to public health, they argued that the successes of bacteriol-ogy had rendered obsolete the traditional focus of general hygiene on sanitary (and social) reform. The claims of the bacteriologists upon the teaching of general hygiene were firmly turned aside at this Congress, but before the turn of the century, baeriology was successfully institu-tionalized as a separate department in the medical schools.

Soon after the challenge by the bacteriologists had been deflected, the scope of the field of general hygiene was attacked by spokesmen for a sociologically-oriented 'community medicine.' In 1899, at the VII

Congress of the Pirogov Society in Kazan, a proposal was made to include in the course on general hygiene a segment on 'community medicine' which would acquaint students 'with the range of existing community institutions in public health.' The Congress gave its executive a mandate to explore the proposal, but apparently nothing came of the suggestion. After the turn of the century, calls to broaden the concept of the environment to include social as well as natural factors resurfaced. In 1910 at the XI Pirogov Congress, there was a proposal to mount a separate course on 'social medicine' for medical students. As it was discussed in the Congress's subsection for theoretical subjects in the reform of medical education, the proposed course would devote some attention to institutions, but would also include such topics as medical geography, migration, epidemiology, factory hygiene, school hygiene, sanitary legislation, and urban hygiene. In part because of World War I very little came of this proposal. The champions of community medicine had some success in introducing courses in their subject into economic and technical institutes, but with a few notable exceptions they were unable to penetrate the hide-bound medical faculties.

In 1920, therefore, general hygiene—still the core of public health training in the medical schools—looked much the way it had a decade earlier. As A.V. Molkov, hardly a disinterested observer, put it dramatically in 1923, 'The departments of general hygiene did not develop or grow in their scope and content beyond the gloomy 1890s.'

In the wake of the Revolution, the right of general hygienists to speak authoritatively on behalf of all of public health was contested once again, this time by spokesmen for the field of social hygiene. The thrust of this challenge differed in fundamental ways from earlier challenges. For the proponents of social hygiene were not interested in taking over general hygiene or in injecting their social focus into its courses; instead, their aim was to differentiate themselves from general hygiene and to establish a new discipline.

The social hygienists' challenge to general hygiene took place in the context of serious discussions of the content of medical education. In the wake of the Bolshevik Revolution, proposals for educational reform were rife: a few of these were aimed at reducing the requirements for student physicians; most urged a more stringent course of study—increasing the scientific content of medical training, introducing more practical work, and incorporating some of the approaches of the social sciences. To be sure, the topic of educational reform had been on the agenda of the Pirogov Society of Russian Physicians at least as early as the 1890s, but the accession to power of the Bolsheviks added new impetus to the discussions. Now, educational reform assumed importance not only for those who taught medicine, but for the leaders of the newly-formed Commissariat of Public Health who believed that the success of the system of health care they had designed depended upon the type of doctor who delivered that care.

The Soviet system of health care created after the Revolution was to be free of charge, universally accessible, and oriented to the prevention as well as the cure of illness. The first Commissar of Public Health, N.A. Semashko, declared as early as 1922 that such a system demanded a physician who would be 'as much at home in sociology as biology, as much interested in preventing illness as in curing it.' By 1924 that vision was extended in an official call to the medical schools to produce doctors with:

(1) a serious natural science preparation, as familiar with physical-chemical and biological sciences as with the laws underlying the biological processes;
(2) enough social science background to comprehend the social environment;
(3) materialist thinking without which it is impossible to understand the relationship of an organism to its environment;
(4) the ability to examine the patient in relationship to his work life and life-style;
(5) the ability to study the occupational and social conditions which give rise to illness and not only to cure the illness, but to suggest ways to prevent it.

9.5

Sex education in Germany

Lutz D.H. Sauerteig, 'Sex Education in Germany from the Eighteenth to the Twentieth Centuries', in Franz X. Eder, Lesley A. Hall and Gert Hekma (eds), *Sexual Cultures in Europe: Themes in Sexuality* (Manchester and New York, Manchester University Press, 1999), pp. 16–17, 21 [pp. 9–33].

Lutz Sauerteig's work has focused on medical and moral issues concerning sexual ethics and sex education, including approaches to sexually transmitted diseases. This article concerns sex education in Germany and the changes in approach between the eighteenth and twentieth centuries. It deals with questions about who should educate the public on sexual matters, where this should take place, and what messages should be conveyed about sex. Here Sauerteig focuses on the views of the church, the early twentieth-century women's movement, and orthodox medical practitioners regarding sex education and ethics.

Altogether, sex education had become a topic of public debate by the turn of the century. One of the first highlights was the third congress of the DGBG[10] held in May of 1907, devoted solely to the topic of sex education. In the same year Sigmund Freud published a short article in which he pointed out the necessity of providing children and young people with adequate sex education. Because the DGBG combined fear of the spread of VD with demands for more detailed sex education for the young, it succeeded in gradually persuading the Ministries of Culture of the German states and the municipal school authorities to collaborate. Hence, in 1908 the Imperial Health Council (Reichsge-sundheitsrat), the most important committee of medical and public health experts consulted by the Imperial Office of the Interior (Reichs-amt des Innern), emphasised the importance of sex education. The great majority of the experts demanded more intensive instruction of the young: however, they found they were not in a position to set up uniform and universal principles.

[. . .]

The DGBG's programme for sexual ethics was a dietetic educational regimen with the motto 'a sound soul can live only in a sound body'. Since sexual drive in most humans was 'so tremendous', according to Blaschko, it 'could not always be led to that which is right by means of rational instruction and insight'. For this reason, he declared the 'strengthening of will-power' to be the foremost goal of sex education. Therefore, the entire organism would have to be strengthened and become accustomed to exhausting physical activity. Being pampered, leading a dissolute way of life, drinking alcohol and being mentally strained, on the other hand, were to be avoided.

The novel entitled *Helmut Harringa* (1910) by the teetotaller Hermann Popert, a bestseller in the youth movement, contributed to the glorifica-tion of this chastity cult. Popert furnished the prewar generation with the

[10] *DGBG*: Deutsche Gesellschaft zur Bekämpfung der Geschlechtskrankheiten, the German Society for Combating Venereal Disease.

ideal of a Germanic youth looking into the future with purity, asceticism and strength. In his novel Popert made alcohol the culprit involved in all evil. Alcohol obfuscates[11] the mind of the hero's brother, Friedrich Harringa, a member of a *Burschenschaft* (students' society), and leads him to a brothel. Afflicted with syphilis, Friedrich finally drowns himself in the Baltic Sea. His brother, Helmut, who is a judge in Hamburg, thereupon becomes an ardent supporter of the temperance movement.

At the aforementioned session of the Imperial Health Council in 1908 the leading Prussian medical officer, Martin Kirchner, took up the idea of strengthening will-power by means of dietetics. The young must be rendered capable of sexual chastity by educating them in self-restraint and self-control. They should be raised to respect women and should view the founding of a 'happy family' and the 'production of healthy offspring' as a 'marvellous and worthwhile task for every citizen'. On the other hand they should loathe prostitutes. According to Kirchner, a youth must learn 'to look at naked people without becoming physically aroused'. For this reason, Kirchner wished that schools would place more value on physical education and sports, so that young people could become 'physically toughened'.

Very detailed explanation of human sexuality, the sexual organs and sexual intercourse was, however, not planned for the schools. Alfred Blaschko insisted that the biological principles of sexuality should be explained in terms of gradually progressing educational instruction. False impressions about sexuality (which occurred particularly among urban youth) and ensuing systematic ignorance were to be eliminated as early as the primary school level. For Blaschko it was 'a grievous error to believe that young people, because these things had been passed over in total silence, would grow in purity and chastity, untouched by all things sensual'. A more detailed sex education could then be integrated into the lessons on general hygiene in the vocational schools (*Fortbildungsschulen*) and at the upper levels of higher education.

But there was still strong opposition to any form of biological sex education. In particular the Protestant and Catholic churches, as well as social purity organisations, propagated a strictly moral ethical education without touching on biological questions of sexuality. Instead, will-power training was at the core of the Catholic church's educational concept. Around the turn of the century, however, the taboo placed on sexual issues was cautiously criticised from within the Catholic church. Various Catholic pedagogues were in favour of sex education for children and teenagers which, however, should be done very cautiously

---

[11] *obfuscates*: confuses, bewilders.

and in keeping with their age while maintaining the maxims of modesty and purity. The official church line still rejected, however, any sex education that went into the physical aspects of reproduction, calling it highly dangerous, especially since thereby Darwinistic teachings would be introduced into school instruction. Therefore the Catholic church continued to warn about the negative consequences of general sex education. And in the pastoral letter of the Fulda Bishops' Conference of 1908 the German bishops called for having children strictly educated towards decency and chastity.

[. . .]

It was the sex reform movement of the 1920s which became the spearhead of sex education. The sex reform movement created an infrastructure for sex education not only with its magazines, brochures and lecture evenings, which were sometimes attended by as many as two thousand listeners, but above all with its counselling centres. Through these centres they probably reached more people than their members, whom they claimed numbered over 150,000. The advocates of sex reform came from the radical wing of the women's movement, the political left, from science and the medical profession, and from the homosexual movement. They all were convinced that it was better to regulate the sexual conduct of humans than to suppress it. While non-medical sex reformers kept on defending the principle of self-help, the influence of female and male doctors on the sex reform movement increased from the mid-1920s . . . Although the principal aims of the sex reform movement were to provide its adherents with instruction about birth control, to supply contraceptive devices and to fight against the ban on abortion, it did discuss important aspects of sex education as well: education towards a fulfilling sex life for both partners, but especially for the woman. From the mid-1920s, a number of marriage guides promoted eroticism in marriage. With its activities and publications the sex reform movement transmitted the necessary anatomical and physiological knowledge about sexuality and reproduction. Thus the sex reform movement, with its various branches and directions, was concerned with both eroticism in marriage and rationalisation of sexuality. It believed that a more fulfilled sex life in marriage would produce a better marriage and healthier children.

9.6

The Rockefeller campaign against tuberculosis

Jean-François Picard and William H. Schneider, 'The
Rockefeller Foundation and the Development of Biomedical
Research in Europe', in Giulana Gemelli, Jean-François Picard
and William H. Schneider (eds), *Managing Medical Research
in Europe. The Role of the Rockefeller Foundation
(1920s–1950s)* (Bologna, CLUEB, 1999), pp. 19–21
[pp. 13–50].

The Rockfeller Foundation was established in 1913, and since then
has been an important source of funding for scientific and medical
research and teaching. It also famously funded public health work,
such as the programme to eradicate hookworm in the southern
United States. Recently historians have explored how, through the
disbursement of funds, the Rockefeller Foundation has shaped the
course of medical research. Although much of the Rockefeller
Foundation's funding has gone to American institutions, it also
became involved in medicine in Europe. This book, edited by three
scholars working on the history of the biomedical sciences in the
twentieth century, explores how Rockefeller money influenced the
course of medical education and practice in Europe. This extract
examines one of the first initiatives, a campaign against tuberculosis in France after the First World War.

The first concerted health effort in Europe by the Rockefeller Foundation was a tuberculosis program begun in France in 1917. Until then,
plans for the International Health Division had to wait, because with the
outbreak of fighting in 1914, requests poured into the Rockefeller Foundation for war relief. Although by this time American missionary and
philanthropic organizations had some experience in sending aid to war
and disaster victims around the world, they were ill-prepared to
respond to the magnitude of needs of this European war. Neither the
charter of the Rockefeller Foundation nor the funding principles of its
new Secretary Jerome Greene made provisions for such requests. If
ever there was a case for the 'relief of suffering,' however, this was it.
Accordingly, the Foundation appointed a War Relief Commission in
October 1914 with Rose as its chairman. Ultimately, over $22 million
was given by the Foundation for various war relief projects. This began

immediately with emergency food shipments to Belgium after the Germans marched through the country in the autumn of 1914. The Foundation also modified its practice of thorough planning by creating 'commissions of inquiry' for more rapid responses to conditions in such places as Serbia, Poland, and Armenia, where supplies were also sent.

For these and various other projects, such as with prisoners of war, the Foundation often worked closely with the Red Cross, the organization with the most experience in such relief efforts. In fact, during the spring of 1915, they funded a group of 50 doctors and public health workers under the direction of Richard P. Strong, a Professor of Tropical Medicine at Harvard, to combat a typhus epidemic in Serbia. Thus, the developments of the following year which set in motion the chain of events that began the Rockefeller tuberculosis program in France, were not without precedent.

The story of the Rockefeller Foundation's campaign against tuberculosis during the First World War has been told before, but not in the context of the Foundation's wider goals for France and Europe or from the viewpoint of the development of scientific medicine in France. The decision to support a tuberculosis program was not intended, according to Foundation records, to be anything more than a limited response to an immediate wartime exigency. With the creation of the International Health Commission in 1913, Rose was certainly eager to export his American public health successes, but the board was clearly looking to countries and lands with climates and diseases similar to the American South. In fact, the tropical latitudes were explicitly identified by Rockefeller studies as the areas of expanded activity. Eventually Rose and the Foundation saw they could have an impact on European medicine; and, after Germany and England, the land of Pasteur was the most respected country in the medical world.

The Rockefeller tuberculosis program in France immediately pointed up one of the most important problems of extending American philanthropy to Europe: delicate sensibilities. This was nowhere more evident than in relations with the French. As the 1918 *Annual Report* of the Foundation acknowledged, it may well be asked 'whether it was not presumptuous for Americans to go crusading against tuberculosis in the land of Louis Pasteur.' In answer to its own question, the report admitted, '[T]he Americans had nothing to teach the French about the organization and administration of a tuberculosis dispensary.' Moreover, as to the role of sanatoria, '[T]he French had little if anything to learn.' What was lacking, however, was an 'efficient, cooperative, centralized organization among French agencies for a united, comprehensive attack on tuberculosis.'

The Rockefeller program was divided into two distinct parts. First, there was a national publicity campaign to educate the French populace about the causes and means of preventing tuberculosis. This included the latest techniques utilizing motion pictures, posters, brochures, lectures, and, for the first time in France, tuberculosis stamps.[12] The other part of the Rockefeller program focused both on treatment and what the Americans called 'teamplay against tuberculosis.' As Linsley Williams, director of the program, described it to a French audience:

> Hygienists in the United States have recognized for years the need in a given district to have a complete organization which permits the tracking down of tuberculosis cases as early as possible, to be able to observe and treat them for the entire life of the individual either until he is well or until the illness ends in death, and after the death of the individual to continue observation of the family.[13]

Another key innovation in the treatment program was the establishment and expansion of training for visiting nurses. Between 1917 and 1922, the Rockefeller program funded 700 'bourses d'étude,'[14] and a decree of June 27, 1922 gave official status to a 'diplôme d'infirmière' with a specialization as 'visiteuse d'hygiène sociale.' When the French Office Nationale d'Hygiène Sociale was created in 1925, Juliette Delagrange was appointed to coordinate the rapidly expanding nurse training schools. By 1930, there were 67 such schools and approximately 2,400 visiting nurses in France.

The American-funded program against tuberculosis in France was no small undertaking even by Rockefeller standards. The first five years of the tuberculosis and related nursing education programs cost over $2.5 million or more than one-quarter of all the expenditures by the Foundation's International Health Commission in these postwar years. Although the tuberculosis program grew beyond initial expectation, the Rockefeller Foundation was successful in honoring its goal of avoiding the kind of indefinite commitments that could hinder it from undertaking other worthwhile projects. The French government had taken over most of the tuberculosis and social hygiene programs by 1927.

In fact, one could argue that the tuberculosis campaign in France was too successful. Thus, at the height of the program, a 1919 annual report bragged that the results obtained in the French program were even more impressive because the work against hookworm, yellow fever,

---

[12] Special postage stamps sold to raise money and educate the public.

[13] Linsley R. Williams, 'La Fondation Rockefeller dans la lutte contre le tuberculose en France', *Revue de musée social* 1922, pp. 36–7.

[14] *Bourse d'etude*: scholarships.

and malaria were simple 'compared to arresting and preventing the insidious and well-nigh universal ravages of tuberculosis ... against which so many vigorous agencies, public and private, are enlisted.' Soon, however, many of those other agencies eagerly requested similar Rockefeller aid. As a result, the Foundation's annual report two years later found it necessary to temper the glowing reports of the tuberculosis program in France. 'This project represents the only effort of the International Health Board in the field of tuberculosis. It was undertaken as a form of wartime emergency aid. There is no intention of doing similar work in other countries.'

The warnings of the 1921 President's report were not simply a knee-jerk reaction against opening the coffers of the Foundation to an unending demand for help. In hindsight, the French tuberculosis program proved to be the beginning of a large and continuing funding effort championed by Rose and other Rockefeller officers during the 1920s and 30s. Rather than combating individual diseases, the strategy was for broader improvement of health and 'the spread of knowledge of scientific medicine' to France, Europe, and the whole world. As early as 1919, Rose and the director of the new Medical Education Division, Richard Pearce, visited England and Belgium. The culmination of the trip was the announcement of $8.5 million in support for construction and reorganization of medical schools in London and Brussels.

Part ten
The fortunes of eugenics

10.1
Natural selection in human populations

Charles Darwin, *The Descent of Man, and Selection in Relation to Sex* (London, John Murray, 1883 (originally published 1874)), pp. 133–40, 143, 617–18.

In *The Origin of Species* (1859) Darwin developed the theory of natural selection as the main mechanism of evolution. *The Descent of Man*, published 12 years later, confronts the issue of evolution in humans. Darwin claimed that man had descended from lower forms and continues to evolve. The problem was that due to man's noble qualities, he is sympathetic to the needs of the weak and inferior and this inhibits natural selection. Here he debates ways in which this problem could be addressed and includes references to the work of Francis Galton, his cousin and the founder of eugenics. Unlike Galton, Darwin believed that cultural influence was important and that some characteristics could be acquired.

With savages, the weak in body or mind are soon eliminated; and those that survive commonly exhibit a vigorous state of health. We civilised men, on the other hand, do our utmost to check the process of elimination; we build asylums for the imbecile, the maimed, and the sick; we institute poor-laws; and our medical men exert their utmost skill to save the life of every one to the last moment. There is reason to believe that vaccination has preserved thousands, who from a weak constitution would formerly have succumbed to small-pox. Thus the weak members of civilised societies propagate their kind. No one who has attended to the breeding of domestic animals will doubt that this must be highly

204

injurious to the race of man. It is surprising how soon a want of care, or care wrongly directed, leads to the degeneration of a domestic race; but excepting in the case of man himself, hardly any one is so ignorant as to allow his worst animals to breed.

The aid which we feel impelled to give to the helpless is mainly an incidental result of the instinct of sympathy, which was originally acquired as part of the social instincts, but subsequently rendered . . . more tender and more widely diffused. Nor could we check our sympathy, even at the urging of hard reason, without deterioration in the noblest part of our nature. The surgeon may harden himself whilst performing an operation, for he knows that he is acting for the good of his patient; but if we were intentionally to neglect the weak and helpless, it could only be for a contingent benefit, with an overwhelming present evil. We must therefore bear the undoubtedly bad effects of the weak surviving and propagating their kind; but there appears to be at least one check in steady action, namely that the weaker and inferior members of society do not marry so freely as the sound; and this check might be indefinitely increased by the weak in body or mind refraining from marriage, though this is more to be hoped for than expected.

In every country in which a large standing army is kept up, the finest young men are taken by the conscription or are enlisted. They are thus exposed to early death during war, are often tempted into vice, and are prevented from marrying during the prime of life. On the other hand the shorter and feebler men, with poor constitutions, are left at home, and consequently have a much better chance of marrying and propagating their kind.

Man accumulates property and bequeaths it to his children, so that the children of the rich have an advantage over the poor in the race for success, independently of bodily or mental superiority. On the other hand, the children of parents who are short-lived, and are therefore on an average deficient in health and vigour, come into their property sooner than other children, and will be likely to marry earlier, and leave a larger number of offspring to inherit their inferior constitutions . . .

Primogeniture[1] with entailed estates is a more direct evil, though it may formerly have been a great advantage by the creation of a dominant class, and any government is better than none. Most eldest sons, though they may be weak in body or mind, marry, whilst the younger sons, however superior in these respects, do not so generally marry.

[. . .]

---

[1] *primogeniture*: the practice of leaving the whole estate to the eldest son.

We will now look to the intellectual faculties. If in each grade of society the members were divided into two equal bodies, the one including the intellectually superior and the other the inferior, there can be little doubt that the former would succeed best in all occupations, and rear a greater number of children. Even in the lowest walks of life, skill and ability must be of some advantage; though in many occupations, owing to the great division of labour, a very small one. Hence in civilised nations there will be some tendency to an increase both in the number and in the standard of the intellectually able. But I do not wish to assert that this tendency may not be more than counterbalanced in other ways, as by the multiplication of the reckless and improvident; but even to such as these, ability must be some advantage.

[. . .]

In regard to the moral qualities, some elimination of the worst dispositions is always in progress even in the most civilised nations. Malefactors[2] are executed, or imprisoned for long periods, so that they cannot freely transmit their bad qualities. Melancholic and insane persons are confined, or commit suicide. Violent and quarrelsome men often come to a bloody end. The restless who will not follow any steady occupation—and this relic of barbarism is a great check to civilisation—emigrate to newly-settled countries, where they prove useful pioneers. Intemperance[3] is so highly destructive, that the expectation of life of the intemperate, at the age of thirty for instance, is only 13.8 years; whilst for the rural labourers of England at the same age it is 40.59 years. Profligate[4] women bear few children, and profligate men rarely marry; both suffer from disease. In the breeding of domestic animals, the elimination of those individuals, though few in number, which are in any marked manner inferior, is by no means an unimportant element towards success. This especially holds good with injurious characters which tend to reappear through reversion, such as blackness in sheep; and with mankind some of the worst dispositions, which occasionally without any assignable cause make their appearance in families, may perhaps be reversions to a savage state, from which we are not removed by very many generations. This view seems indeed recognised in the common expression that such men are the black sheep of the family.

---

[2] *malefactors*: wrongdoers, criminals.

[3] *intemperance*: excessive consumption of alcohol. In the late nineteenth century, middle-class social reformers were deeply concerned that the working classes drank too much.

[4] *profligate*: shamelessly immoral.

With civilised nations, as far as an advanced standard of morality, and an increased number of fairly good men are concerned, natural selection apparently effects but little.

[. . .]

A most important obstacle in civilised countries to an increase in the number of men of a superior class has been strongly insisted on by Mr. Greg and Mr. Galton, namely, the fact that the very poor and reckless, who are often degraded by vice, almost invariably marry early, whilst the careful and frugal, who are generally otherwise virtuous, marry late in life, so that they may be able to support themselves and their children in comfort. Those who marry early produce within a given period not only a greater number of generations, but, as shewn by Dr. Duncan, they produce many more children. The children, moreover, that are born by mothers during the prime of life are heavier and larger, and therefore probably more vigorous, than those born at other periods. Thus the reckless, degraded, and often vicious members of society, tend to increase at a quicker rate than the provident and generally virtuous members. . . .

There are, however, some checks to this downward tendency. We have seen that the intemperate suffer from a high rate of mortality, and the extremely profligate leave few offspring. The poorest classes crowd into towns, and it has been proved . . . from the statistics of ten years in Scotland, that at all ages the death-rate is higher in towns than in rural districts; 'and during the first five years of life the town death-rate is 'almost exactly double that of the rural districts.' As these returns include both the rich and the poor, no doubt more than twice the number of births would be requisite to keep up the number of the very poor inhabitants in the towns, relatively to those in the country. With women, marriage at too early an age is highly injurious; for it has been found in France that, 'twice as many wives under twenty die in the year, as died out of the same number of the unmarried.' The mortality, also, of husbands under twenty is 'excessively high,' but what the cause of this may be, seems doubtful. Lastly, if the men who prudently delay marrying until they can bring up their families in comfort, were to select, as they often do, women in the prime of life, the rate of increase in the better class would be only slightly lessened.

[. . .]

If the various checks specified . . . and perhaps others as yet unknown, do not prevent the reckless, the vicious and otherwise inferior members of society from increasing at a quicker rate than the better class of men, the nation will retrograde,[5] as has too often occurred in the history of the world. We must remember that progress is no invariable rule. It is very difficult to say why one civilised nation rises, becomes more powerful, and spreads more widely, than another; or why the same nation progresses more quickly at one time than at another.

[. . .]

With highly civilised nations continued progress depends in a subordinate degree on natural selection; for such nations do not supplant and exterminate one another as do savage tribes. Nevertheless the more intelligent members within the same community will succeed better in the long run than the inferior, and leave a more numerous progeny, and this is a form of natural selection. The more efficient causes of progress seem to consist of a good education during youth whilst the brain is impressible; and of a high standard of excellence, inculcated by the ablest and best men, embodied in the laws, customs and traditions of the nation, and enforced by public opinion. It should, however, be borne in mind, that the enforcement of public opinion depends on our appreciation of the approbation and disapprobation of others; and this appreciation is founded on our sympathy, which it can hardly be doubted was originally developed through natural selection as one of the most important elements of the social instincts.

[. . .]

Man scans with scrupulous care the character and pedigree of his horses, cattle, and dogs before he matches them; but when he comes to his own marriage he rarely, or never, takes any such care. He is impelled by nearly the same motives as the lower animals, when they are left to their own free choice, though he is in so far superior to them that he highly values mental charms and virtues. On the other hand he is strongly attracted by mere wealth or rank. Yet he might by selection do something not only for the bodily constitution and frame of his offspring, but for their intellectual and moral qualities. Both sexes ought to refrain from marriage if they are in any marked degree inferior in body or mind; but such hopes are Utopian and will never be even partially realised until the laws of inheritance are thoroughly known. Everyone does good service, who aids towards this end. When the principles of breeding and inheritance are better understood, we shall not hear ignorant members of our legislature rejecting with scorn a

---

[5] *retrograde*: take a backward step.

plan for ascertaining whether or not consanguineous marriages[6] are injurious to man.

The advancement of the welfare of mankind is a most intricate problem: all ought to refrain from marriage who cannot avoid abject poverty for their children; for poverty is not only a great evil, but tends to its own increase by leading to recklessness in marriage. On the other hand, as Mr. Galton has remarked, if the prudent avoid marriage, whilst the reckless marry, the inferior members tend to supplant the better members of society. Man, like every other animal, has no doubt advanced to his present high condition through a struggle for existence consequent on his rapid multiplication; and if he is to advance still higher, it is to be feared that he must remain subject to a severe struggle. Otherwise he would sink into indolence, and the more gifted men would not be more successful in the battle of life than the less gifted. Hence our natural rate of increase, though leading to many and obvious evils, must not be greatly diminished by any means. There should be open competition for all men; and the most able should not be prevented by laws or customs from succeeding best and rearing the largest number of offspring. Important as the struggle for existence has been and even still is, yet as far as the highest part of man's nature is concerned there are other agencies more important. For the moral qualities are advanced, either directly or indirectly, much more through the effects of habit, the reasoning powers, instruction, religion, &c., than through natural selection; though to this latter agency may be safely attributed the social instincts, which afforded the basis for the development of the moral sense.

10.2

The aims and scope of eugenics

Francis Galton, 'Eugenics: Its Definition, Scope and Aims', in his *Essays in Eugenics* (London, Eugenics Education Society, 1909), pp. 35–43.

Francis Galton, a cousin of Charles Darwin, spent his early years as a traveller and explorer. He began his studies into heredity in the

---

[6] *consanguineous*: marriages between blood relatives.

1860s, coining the word eugenics, and suggesting that human qualities could be improved through the scientific study of heredity and state intervention. He published *Hereditary Genius* in 1869, in which he discussed the inheritance of intellectual capacity, providing family pedigrees to prove his point. Galton's project consisted mostly of positive eugenic proposals – the expansion of families in the 'better' classes. This extract is from a collection of essays on eugenics, published in 1909 by the Eugenics Education Society; the original lecture was given in 1904.

Eugenics is the science which deals with all influences that improve the inborn qualities of a race; also with those that develop them to the utmost advantage. The improvement of the inborn qualities, or stock, of some one human population, will alone be discussed here.

[. . .]

A considerable list of qualities can be easily compiled that nearly every one except 'cranks' would take into account when picking out the best specimens of his class. It would include health, energy, ability, manliness and courteous disposition. Recollect that the natural differences between dogs are highly marked in all these respects, and that men are quite as variable by nature as other animals in their respective species. Special aptitudes would be assessed highly by those who possessed them, as the artistic faculties by artists, fearlessness of inquiry and veracity by scientists, religious absorption by mystics, and so on. There would be self-sacrificers, self-tormentors and other exceptional idealists, but the representatives of these would be better members of a community than the body of their electors. They would have more of those qualities that are needed in a State, more vigour, more ability, and more consistency of purpose. The community might be trusted to refuse representatives of criminals, and of others whom it rates as undesirable.

Let us for a moment suppose that the practice of Eugenics should hereafter raise the average quality of our nation to that of its better moiety[7] at the present day and consider the gain. The general tone of domestic, social and political life would be higher. The race as a whole would be less foolish, less frivolous, less excitable and politically more provident than now. Its demagogues[8] who 'played to the gallery' would play to a more sensible gallery than at present. We should be better fitted to fulfil our vast imperial opportunities. Lastly, men of an order of

[7] *moiety*: half, of two parts.
[8] *demagogues*: leaders who win support by appealing to the emotions.

ability which is now very rare, would become more frequent, because the level out of which they rose would itself have risen.

The aim of Eugenics is to bring as many influences as can be reasonably employed, to cause the useful classes in the community to contribute *more* than their proportion to the next generation.

The course of procedure . . . would be somewhat as follows:—

1. Dissemination of a knowledge of the laws of heredity so far as they are surely known, and promotion of their farther study. Few seem to be aware how greatly the knowledge of what may be termed the *actuarial*[9] side of heredity has advanced in recent years. The *average* closeness of kinship in each degree now admits of exact definition and of being treated mathematically, like birth and death-rates, and the other topics with which actuaries are concerned.

2. Historical inquiry into the rates with which the various classes of society (classified according to civic usefulness) have contributed to the population at various times, in ancient and modern nations. There is strong reason for believing that national rise and decline is closely connected with this influence. It seems to be the tendency of high civilisation to check fertility in the upper classes, through numerous causes, some of which are well known, others are inferred, and others again are wholly obscure. . . .

3. Systematic collection of facts showing the circumstances under which large and thriving families have most frequently originated; in other words, the *conditions* of Eugenics. The names of the thriving families in England have yet to be learnt, and the conditions under which they have arisen. We cannot hope to make much advance in the science of Eugenics without a careful study of facts that are now accessible with difficulty, if at all. The definition of a thriving family, such as will pass muster for the moment at least is one in which the children have gained distinctly superior positions to those who were their class-mates in early life. Families may be considered 'large' that contain not less than three adult male children. It would be no great burden . . . to initiate and to preserve a large collection of such records for the use of statistical students . . . The point to be ascertained is the *status* of the two parents at the time of their marriage, whence its more or less eugenic character might have been predicted, if the larger knowledge that we now hope to obtain had then existed. Some account would, of course, be wanted of their race, profession, and residence; also of their own respective parentages, and of their brothers and sisters. Finally, the reasons would be required

[9] *actuarial*: statistical calculation.

211

why the children deserved to be entitled a 'thriving' family, to distinguish worthy from unworthy success. This manuscript collection might here-after develop into a 'golden book' of thriving families. The Chinese, whose customs have often much sound sense, make their honours ret-rospective. We might learn from them to show that respect to the par-ents of noteworthy children, which the contributors of such valuable assets to the national wealth richly deserve. The act of systematically collecting records of thriving families would have the further advantage of familiarising the public with the fact that Eugenics had at length become a subject of serious scientific study by an energetic Society.

4. Influences affecting Marriage. The remarks of Lord Bacon in his essay on Death may appropriately be quoted here. He says with the view of minimising its terrors:

> There is no passion in the mind òf men so weak but it mates and masters the fear of death. Revenge triumphs over death; love slights it; honour aspireth to it; grief flyeth to it; fear pre-occupateth it.

Exactly the same kind of considerations apply to marriage. The passion of love seems so overpowering that it may be thought folly to try to direct its course. But plain facts do not confirm this view. Social influences of all kinds have immense power in the end, and they are very various. If unsuitable marriages from the Eugenic point of view were banned socially, or even regarded with the unreasonable disfavour which some attach to cousin-marriages, very few would be made. The multitude of marriage restrictions that have proved prohibi-tive among uncivilised people would require a volume to describe.

5. Persistence in setting forth the national importance of Eugenics. There are three stages to be passed through. *Firstly* it must be made familiar as an academic question, until its exact importance has been understood and accepted as a fact; *Secondly* it must be recognised as a subject whose practical development deserves serious consideration; and *Thirdly* it must be introduced into the national conscience, like a new religion. It has, indeed, strong claims to become an orthodox reli-gious tenet of the future, for Eugenics co-operates with the workings of Nature by securing that humanity shall be represented by the fittest races. What Nature does blindly, slowly, and ruthlessly, man may do providently, quickly, and kindly. As it lies within his power, so it becomes his duty to work in that direction; just as it is his duty to suc-cour neighbours who suffer misfortune. The improvement of our stock seems to me one of the highest objects that we can reasonably attempt. We are ignorant of the ultimate destinies of humanity, but feel perfectly sure that it is as noble a work to raise its level in the sense already

explained, as it would be disgraceful to abase it. I see no impossibility in Eugenics becoming a religious dogma among mankind, but its details must first be worked out sedulously in the study. Over-zeal leading to hasty action would do harm, by holding out expectations of a near golden age, which will certainly be falsified and cause the science to be discredited. The first and main point is to secure the general intellectual acceptance of Eugenics as a hopeful and most important study. Then let its principles work into the heart of the nation, who will gradually give practical effect to them in ways that we may not wholly foresee.

10.3
National socialist racial and social policy

M. Burleigh and W. Wippermann, *The Racial State: Germany,*
1933–1945 (Cambridge, Cambridge University Press, 1991),
pp. 304–7.

Both Burleigh and Wippermann have researched into the history of National Socialist Germany. In this book, they take as their starting point historians' debate over whether the Nazi era should be seen as a period of modernity or a return to an idealised past. This debate portrays Nazi social policy as modern while Nazi racial policy is seen as reactionary and anti-modern. The authors criticise the nature of this debate showing, for example, how racial utopias of the past were used to propagandise a racially pure future. They resist all attempts to relativise the issue; Nazi policies and solutions were unique with respect to time and place. In this passage from the conclusion, Burleigh and Wippermann summarise their stance: that social policy was absolutely integral to the building of a racially-based and economically sound state. The body politic was seen as dependent on the hereditary health of its constituents – that is, the racial purity of the individual and the family.

Racial ideologies were not solely concerned with a return to some imagined past social order. They also reflected the desire to create a future society based upon the alleged verities of race. Hitler took over existing ideas and converted them into a comprehensive programme for a racial new order. Without doubt, racial anti-Semitism was the key element in a programme designed to achieve the 'recovery' of the 'Aryan Germanic race'. Various racial-hygienic measures were designed to achieve this goal. These ranged from compulsory sterilisation to murdering the sick, the 'asocial', and those designated as being of 'alien race'. The extermination of the Jews was crucial to these policies. In Hitler's mind they were not only 'racial aliens', but also a threat to his plans for the 'racial recovery' of the German people. They were both a 'lesser race' and one bent upon destroying the 'racial properties' of Hitler's 'Aryans'.

Under the Third Reich, this racial-ideological programme became the official dogma and policy of the State. Racism replaced the Weimar Republic's imperfect experiment in political pluralism. Along with the political parties and trade unions, the Nazis also endeavoured to destroy the existing social structure. Although there were undoubtedly social classes in Nazi Germany, it was a society organised increasingly upon racial rather than class lines. The regime's racial policies struck at people whether they were rich or poor, bourgeois, peasants, or workers.

. . . [T]his racial new order was based upon the 'purification of the body of the nation' of all those categorised as being 'alien', 'hereditarily ill', or 'asocial'. That meant Jews, Sinti and Roma,[10] the mentally and physically handicapped, 'community aliens', and homosexuals. Obviously there were major quantitative and qualitative differences in the degree of persecution to which these groups were subjected. Jews, as the racial group whom the Nazis regarded as the greatest threat, undoubtedly constituted the largest single group of victims and were persecuted in the most intensive and brutal manner. Persecution undoubtedly had different specificities. This should not result in attempts either to relativise or to overlook the sufferings of others, let alone a ghoulish and profoundly inhuman competition to claim the right to having been most persecuted. All of these people were persecuted for the same reasons, although the degree of persecution was bound up with how threatening the regime perceived them to be.

The regime's 'national community' was based upon the exclusion and extermination of all those deemed to be 'alien', 'hereditarily ill', or 'asocial'. These 'elements' were subject to constant and escalating forms of selection. The 'national community' itself was categorised in accordance with racial criteria. The criteria included not merely 'racial purity' but also biological health and socio-economic performance. Members of the 'national community' were also compelled to reproduce through a series of measures ranging from financial inducements

---

[10] *Sinti and Roma*: two tribes of gypsies.

to criminal sanctions. The inducements contained in the regime's social legislation were also conditional upon an individual's racial 'value', health, and performance.

For biological reasons, women were particularly affected by the regime's attempts at racial selective breeding. Women's worth was assessed in terms of their ability to produce as many Aryan, healthy, and capable children as possible. Women were therefore reduced to the status of mere 'reproductive machines'. Racially-motivated anti-feminism represented a significant departure from traditional Christian–Conservative anti-feminism. The Nazis' hierarchically organised, racist society, with healthy, 'Aryan' German man at the apex, began to rival the existing social order. . . .

The main object of social policy remained the creation of a hierarchical racial new order. Everything else was subordinate to this goal, including the regime's conduct of foreign affairs and the war. In the eyes of the regime's racial politicians, the Second World War was above all a racial war, to be pursued with immense brutality until the end, that is until the concentration camps were liberated by invading Allied armies. All of these points draw attention to the specific and singular character of the Third Reich. It was not a form of regression to past times, although the regime frequently instrumentalised various ahistorical myths to convey the idea of historical normalcy. Its objects were novel and *sui generis*:[11] to realise an ideal future world, without 'lesser races', without the sick, and without those who they decreed had no place in the 'national community'. The Third Reich was intended to be a racial rather than a class society. . . .

10.4

The portrayal of the fit and the unfit

M. Burleigh, *Death and Deliverance: 'Euthanasia' in Germany, c. 1900–1945* (London, Pan Books, 1994), pp. 183–5.

Burleigh has written widely on political, ideological and social aspects of National Socialism. This book examines the relationship between reforms in psychiatry, eugenics and government

---

[11] *sui generis*: unique, of its own type.

cost-cutting in the Weimar Republic and Nazi era. It shows the unique nature of the Nazi euthanasia programme founded in notions of 'hard' inheritance and in the creation of a racially pure nation. Burleigh reflects on the victims and 'bystanders' as well as the perpetrators, attempting to explain how the social and ideological climate enabled so many people (the bystanders) to eschew the rights of the individual for the good of the race and nation and how many relatives and parents colluded in the euthanasia programme.

Selling murder: the killing films of the Third Reich

'Victims of the Past' (*Opfer der Vergangenheit*) . . . begins with shots of lowering clouds, mountains, stormy seas and fast-flowing rivers. Lumberjacks, ferrymen and labourers are shown battling against the hostile elements to the accompaniment of a sub-Wagnerian musical score, which shifts from the darkly swirling to the lightly stirring. The film moves in the space of a few seconds from clouds, waves and the sweaty torsos of labourers, via a wild deer in a clearing, to the courtyard of a 'luxury', 'palatial' psychiatric asylum. The commentary smoothes these inherently ridiculous transitions:

> All living things on this earth are engaged in a permanent struggle with the forces of nature. Only mankind subordinates the elements to his own ends and purposes. Wherever fate puts us, whatever station we must occupy, only the strong will prevail in the end. Everything in the natural world that is weak for life will ineluctably be destroyed. In the last few decades, mankind has sinned terribly against the law of natural selection. We haven't just maintained life unworthy of life; we have even allowed it to multiply. The descendants of these sick people look like this!

Drawing upon the propaganda of the Weimar psychiatric tabby, the film placed far greater emphasis upon therapy than was the case with its exemplar:

> A modern psychiatric asylum is not a prison. The buildings are usually situated in large, sunny gardens. Non-acute and harmless patients are kept occupied working in the fields and gardens, naturally under the constant supervision of trained warders. They are even entrusted with tools, naturally after prolonged observation. Every day the patients are escorted into the fresh, sunny air of the asylum grounds. Excitable patients are allowed to let off steam quietly in the open air. The patient cannot do any harm, since he is constantly observed by an orderly who can intervene at any given moment . . . Twice a day the asylum doctor convinces himself of the

wellbeing of his charges. There is one orderly for every five patients, and one doctor for every two hundred patients. Many of these patients will live to an old age because of this care and attention, which needs strong, healthy people to administer it. Their longevity costs thousands and thousands from the nation's resources. Healthy people have to perform arduous, often disgusting tasks, to ease the lives of these innocent victims wherever it is possible . . . The Jewish race is particularly heavily represented among the insane, and provision is made for their care too. Healthy German national comrades have to work to feed and clean up after them. Anyone who visits one of the larger asylums can establish this fact.

[. . .]

Doctors, described as 'the guardians of national hereditary health', are shown in their preventive role, through cameo scenes showing one of them advising a young couple about their genetic suitability. A general chat about the responsibilities of marriage leads on to the question of responsibilities to the hereditary collective:

DOCTOR: Therefore it is important to have one's physical constitution and hereditary health tested, so that one may discover whether the hereditary disposition of one's forebears is worth passing on.
BRIDE: Yes, that's why I've come to see you with my fiancé.
DOCTOR: You see, in cases like this, the doctor is not just a healer, but a friend, an advisor, who will protect you and will prevent you making a mistake, even an unconscious one.
BRIDE: Herr Doktor, you have a wonderful profession!
DOCTOR: Yes. Do you think so?
BRIDE: Yes.
DOCTOR: Well, now we understand one another. Now let's take a look at your file.

. . . Yet further scenes of human suffering prepare the way for the film's final message:

In future these poor creatures will no longer live alongside our healthy children. Sterilisation is a simple surgical operation. It is a humane method designed to spare the nation endless misery. The innocent should never suffer on account of the sins of the past. However, every honest and proud person will understand if we prevent these sins from becoming an endless chain. In the last seventy years our population has increased by 50%, while over the same period the number of hereditarily ill has risen by 450%. If this development continues, in fifty years there would be one hereditarily ill person for every four healthy people. An endless column of horror would march into the nation. Limitless despair would come upon a valuable population which would march towards its doom with giant steps. The Law for the Prevention of Hereditarily Diseased Progeny is not interference in divine law, but rather the restoration of a natural order which mankind has disrupted because of a false sense of humanity.

So as not to leave audiences too depressed by these issues, the film ends with a rousing overview of a strong and healthy national community, showing the Hitler Youth and League of German Maidens, athletes and gymnasts, the various branches of the armed forces, the SS, and a beaming Hitler amidst his people at the 1936 Nuremberg Party rally.

10.5
An alternative programme

Dorothy Porter, 'Enemies of the Race: Biologism, Environmentalism, and Public Health in Edwardian England', *Victorian Studies* 34 (1991), pp. 164–74 [pp. 159–79].

Dorothy Porter has written extensively on public health in the late nineteenth and early twentieth century. This article explores the extent to which eugenic notions were important in designing public health policy in the Edwardian era, and the debates between eugenists and public health medical officials concerning the cause of, and solutions to ill-health and poverty. She contrasts the situation in England with that in Germany, where medical practitioners promoted and carried out eugenic policies, and shows that in England, medical officers sought to extend legislation and policy-making that focused on the preventative and environmental aspects of public health. Eugenists believed that public health policies themselves were responsible for continuing ill-health as humanitarian concern and effort conflicted with natural selection. While eugenics did have tremendous popular appeal and eugenists did attempt to influence policy, as Porter shows, this had very limited influence with regard to policy-making or legislation.

[T]here is ... a striking contrast between the impact of eugenics in Britain and its impact in other Western, Protestant societies. How is this contrast to be explained? The answer lies in the history of British health policy and the professionalisation of a public health service.

The persistence of widespread ill health amongst the Edwardian work-ing classes, frequently revealed in the annual reports of medical officers of health, was a depressing verdict upon the achievements of nine-teenth-century state medicine. Eugenists felt vindicated: this sorry state of affairs was, they were sure, the result of past policies being directed by humanitarian rather than scientific considerations. This view was historically quite fallacious, for public health had been one policy field in which expertise and scientific specialism had been incorporated into the administrative state during the Victorian era.

By 1900 the social policies that eugenists so despised had born fruit in a swelling public health administration. From 1856 in London, and from 1872 throughout England and Wales, every sanitary district was compelled to employ a medical officer of health. His duties were the inspection and recording of the health conditions of his district and the enforcement of sanitary regulations. The establishment of this office opened up new career opportunities in salaried, state service for med-ical practitioners. Operating in small districts, the majority were part-time and remained in private medical practice. There was a growing core of officers in the larger urban and metropolitan districts, however, who were full-time, possessed specialist qualifications in preventive medicine, and whose sense of *Beruf*[12] lay in the public health.

By 1889 this occupational group consisted of 1500 officers. They had a professional organisation, the Society of Medical Officers of Health (hereafter S.M.O.H.), which published its own journal, *Public Health*. The Society spearheaded a campaign for enhanced professional status and the progressive expansion of the administrative and executive powers of medical officers of health. As a pressure group, they ener-getically lobbied the Local Government Board, which oversaw public health both in Whitehall and Parliament itself.

The members of this public health service naturally felt no intellectual rapport with, or professional investment in, a social Darwinist rhetoric which contended that their activities were fatal to biological progress and racial purity. Edward Hope, Medical Officer of Health (hereafter M.O.H.) for Liverpool and one-time president of the S.M.O.H., expressed the general mood of the public health profession in 1912: 'Today we hear a great deal of eugenics and genetics and the impairment of the race, and the mischief which is wrought by the indiscriminate sanitarian who pre-serves the lives of the weakly and the degenerate.' Yet, he suggested, those itching to dismantle the existing edifice of public health adminis-tration and the social policies on which it was built were just Malthusian

---

[12] *Beruf*: vocation or profession.

cranks. 'The Eugenists would be well advised to leave alone the criticisms upon sanitation,' he judged; they should concentrate not upon selective breeding but rather upon eliminating the slum housing that endangered health.

By the turn of the century, in other words, medical officers of health were already deeply entrenched in a structure of public policy-making, legislation, and administration which gave them a massive identification with a professional ideology of preventive medicine. Preventive medicine has been described by the health historian, René Sand, as an ideology of medicine and the state particular to late Victorian England. Many professional and educational institutions were established dedicated to its promotion, most notably the Royal Institute of Health and the Royal Sanitary Institute. Not least, the pages of *Public Health* promoted preventive medicine amongst its membership as a professional ideology.

Late-Victorian preventive medicine launched its own energetic critique of the deficiencies of earlier sanitarianism. With its focus upon drains, sewers, and nuisances, crude sanitarianism had failed to move beyond a partial, myopic[13] understanding of community health; hence it had achieved nothing but piecemeal gains. In the eyes of late-Victorian preventive medicine, responsibility for the scandalous continuation of chronic ill health amongst the Edwardian poor was to be laid at the door of Parliament for failing to pass more comprehensive legislation. Neither Parliament nor the sanitarians had grasped the relationship between urbanism, poverty, and disease.

What did this charge entail? There is no denying, of course, that the reciprocal relationship between poverty and disease had long been acknowledged by public health reformers. From early Victorian times, public health had developed as one of a variety of social initiatives directed toward solving the problem of poverty. Edwin Chadwick had sought to prevent what he saw as the diseases of 'filth' in order to reduce the burden of destitution upon the rates. After Chadwick, John Simon, first M.O.H. to the Medical Department at the Privy Council and Local Government Board, noted that, as a result of the operation of the iron law of wages in the free market, labourers' incomes often fell below adequate subsistence levels. Classical laissez-faire political economy debarred the state from intervening to raise wages. But, Simon contended, it was legitimate for the state to regulate the physical conditions of existence, so as to alleviate the plight of the labouring poor. Herein lay the role of what he called 'state medicine.' Its mission was to ensure that housing was fit for habitation, food was free of adul-

---

[13] *myopic*: short-sighted.

teration, dangerous trades were regulated, industrial pollution controlled, environmental cleanliness maintained through proper sewage and drainage, and, not least, the spread of epidemic diseases checked through vaccination and quarantine.

These policies were targeted at improving the physical welfare of industrial workers, the central focus of public health reform from Chadwick to Simon. Both men acknowledged, however, the existence of a social 'residuum,' willfully idle and habitually criminal. Chadwick had identified them as the itinerant inhabitants of 'common lodging houses,' scavenging and scrounging, moving from one town to another. He developed specific legislation for the regulation of common lodging houses to prevent this vagrant population spreading filth and disease. Simon likewise believed that health reform was limited, in the last resort, by the residuum produced by 'the aboriginal struggle of existence.' The strictest measures were needed to break the cycle—to break, in other words, what sociologists would later call 'the culture of poverty.' For instance, Simon believed the state should 'treat as parentless' and take into care children whose 'natural parents or guardians cannot, or will not, bring them up otherwise than into pauperism, or presumably into crime.'

Edwardian medical officers of health recognised that poverty was still the main challenge of preventive medicine. In 1909 James Niven, M.O.H. for Manchester for over forty years and one-time president of the S.M.O.H., pointed out, however, that poverty was a complex and protean entity. In one area at one time, there might be high levels of unemployed labour temporarily thrown out of work by the trade cycle. Elsewhere, the poor might mainly comprise orphans, widows, and the aged. Other areas might have a large itinerant population. Sometimes the causes lay beyond the control of the individual; old age and chronic sickness, for example. Yet alcoholism and deliberate idleness were also to blame, leading to the vagrant lifestyles of the common lodging house, public house, and the brothel.

[. . .]

The Victorian 'residuum' was thus still seen as a special problem for Edwardian public health reformers. But they continued to insist that the relationship between poverty and sickness could best be addressed by measures to prevent disease amongst the labouring industrial classes . . .

The response of Edwardian preventive medicine to the dilemma posed by poverty and disease was to expand its vision of what Simon had identified as the environmental influences upon the 'physical conditions of existence.' For example, Simon had urged that the housing of the working classes should be the primary target of public health reform. In the event, however, Victorian legislation to reduce urban slums and overcrowding had been piecemeal and lacking in coherence. Recognition of this provided new stimulus from the 1890s for the formulation of a more holistic understanding of the urban system. New proposals were floated for decentralising the city, redistributing industry, and taking industrial workers, metaphorically and even literally 'back to the land.'

In a significant new alliance, preventive medicine began around 1907 to join forces with the aspirations of town planners for housing reform. Town planners began to contribute to the preventive medicine journals, especially *Public Health*, and to participate in the annual congresses of the professional preventive medicine community. Thus in 1908 such leading members of the planning movement as Henry Vivian (a Liberal M.P. who led the national Tenant Co-Partnership movement), Raymond Unwin, and Barry Parker (joint architects of the first Garden City, Letchworth) directed the housing debate at an annual congress of the Royal Institute of Health in 1908. [. . .] Vivian suggested that new settlements could be planned that would regenerate health and create among the inhabitants a spirit of social and economic investment in the environment. From the viewpoint of this new civic consciousness, the 'people responsible for the abominations in estate development which deface the suburbs of our big cities and ruin the health of our people,' Vivian declared, 'will be looked upon as enemies of the race.'

I have been arguing that the spokesmen of Edwardian preventive medicine criticised earlier generations of sanitarians for failing to tackle the structural relationship governing urbanism and health. Older campaigns for housing reform needed to be transformed into forward-looking concepts of town planning. In so doing, environmentalist ideologies co-opted the *language* of degenerationism into arguments for comprehensive, holistic social planning . . . [T]he emphasis was on regeneration through nurture rather than nature. The fundamental assumption was that overcrowding spread infections and caused chronic weaknesses in each generation, whether or not these were subsequently transmitted genetically. Health levels could be raised only by a holistic approach to environmental development.

Just as the Victorian housing debate was broadened into the Edwardian ideology of urban planning, so concerns with malnutrition also acquired a new focus, a broader programme . . . Legislation was passed establishing free school meals and setting up a medical inspection service for school children. The statutory introduction of antenatal care and stricter regulation of midwifery were similarly aimed at preventing underfed mothers from producing constitutional weakness in their offspring [. . .] The introduction of health visiting extended the old 'inspection' principle into a mission to instruct the working classes about domestic mismanagement. Yet the emphasis in this educational programme was upon habit, not heredity.

[. . .]

Just as town planners vested their faith in creating a new civic consciousness, public health reformers believed they could eradicate habits of hygienic inefficiency and forge citizens who would safeguard health. Between 1900 and 1910 *Public Health* and the *Journal of State Medicine* recorded campaigns that were launched early in the twentieth century by medical officers of health for compulsory education of school children in hygiene, to indoctrinate them in the creed of personal responsibility for community health.

The individual was thus sociologically redefined as the bearer of the relations of health and illness within a refashioned concept of the environment that included not only the physical milieu but also the world of social behaviour. This new perspective validated the Edwardian philosophy of preventive medicine as the panoptic overseer of communal life. In his 1910 report to the Local Government Board, its M.O.H., Arthur Newsholme thus emphasised that infant mortality was not a 'weeding out' process of eugenic value, but simply represented the 'preventable wastage of child life.' The phrase Newsholme chose echoed the calls of William Farr and other nineteenth-century sanitarians for the reduction of preventable mortality. A new philosophy of prevention, Newsholme pointed out, had, however, to be implemented to achieve it.

[. . .]

What, then, was the significance of the role of eugenics and socio-economic planning in the politics of health care before the First World War? Social Darwinists blamed misguided environmental health policies for the continuing abysmal levels of chronic sickness in Edwardian society. The public health profession responded by mounting its own critique of the failure of earlier sanitarianism to tackle community health needs holistically. The critique adumbrated a new philosophy of preventive medicine, proposing to replace sanitarianism with rational-comprehensive health planning. Comprehensive planning encompassed an expanded environmentalist programme dedicated to regulating the social, economic, and physical conditions of existence. This new public health ideology co-opted social Darwinian rhetoric into a political programme that represented collectivist cooperation as the highest form of human evolution.

[. . .]

Why did eugenics enjoy such limited influence in British policy-making? I have shown that the answer lies, in part, in the power of an entrenched public health structure, run by a large, organised occupational group for whom a biologistic social Darwinism had no appeal. This professional group continued its ideological commitment to environmentalism, and combated biologistic determinism.

But it must also be emphasised that the comparative failure of eugenics also resulted from the continued sway of laissez-faire in practical politics. The philosophies and policies of Campbell-Bannerman's and Asquith's Liberal administrations resisted what others hailed as the inevitable march toward bureaucratisation and greater government interference in the economic and social life of the nation. Of course, the Liberals made concessions to the new electoral appeal of collectivist politics, as in the establishment of National Insurance and Old Age Pensions. Nevertheless, Asquith held out against the corporatist implications of both comprehensive planning and eugenic health policies.

Unlike elsewhere, hereditarianism subsequently exercised scant influence over British health policy. By contrast, as Charles Webster has recently pointed out in *The Health Services*, the architects of the National Health Service recognised the roots of their system in the plans and politics of late-Victorian and Edwardian public health professionals, even though some of the policy makers of the 1940s and '50s thought that the new Service they had created fell short of the comprehensive planning ideals of the pre-1911 public health reformers.

10.6
Population improvement

F.A.E. Crew *et al.*, 'Social Biology and Population Improvement', *Nature* 14 (16 September 1939), pp. 521–2.

By the 1930s, natural selection was seen as the accepted mechanism of genetic transmission. However, in England there was a growing recognition that the way in which characteristics were inherited was much complex than hitherto thought. The group of scientists who signed this article in *Nature* – a prestigious scientific journal – discussed the effect of social conditions on genetic improvement and called for more scientific research into the context and complexities of human inheritance. Some would refer to themselves as 'reform eugenists' (Crew and Huxley were active members of the Eugenic Society), and all saw themselves as scientific progressives. Crew edited the new *British Journal of Experimental Biology*, which sought to transform biology into an exact science, using mathematical and physical techniques. The group was part of the political 'Popular Front' of the 1930s of left/liberal inclination. Needham and Hogben were socialists, and Haldane joined the British Communist Party. In this paper the scientists implicitly criticised fascist racial politics, seeing science as perverted and militarised under this regime. Science should not be used for war aims but for the furtherance and benefit of all humanity. Despite this last comment, most of the scientists did use their scientific expertise in the British war effort, especially once Germany had invaded the Soviet Union – their anti-fascist stance won out over the anti-war one.

In response to a request from Science Service, of Washington, D.C., for a reply to the question 'How could the world's population be improved most effectively genetically?', addressed to a number of scientific workers, the subjoined statement was prepared, and signed by those whose names appear at the end.

The question 'How could the world's population be improved most effectively genetically?' raises far broader problems than the purely biological ones, problems which the biologist unavoidably encounters as soon as he tries to get the principles of his own special field put into practice. For the effective genetic improvement of mankind is dependent upon major changes in social conditions, and correlative changes in human attitudes. In the first place, there can be no valid basis for estimating and comparing the intrinsic worth of different individuals, without economic and social conditions which provide approximately equal opportunities for all members of society instead of stratifying them from birth into classes with widely different privileges.

The second major hindrance to genetic improvement lies in the economic and political conditions which foster antagonism between different peoples, nations and 'races'. The removal of race prejudices and of the unscientific doctrine that good or bad genes are the monopoly of particular peoples or of persons with features of a given kind will not be possible, however, before the conditions which make for war and economic exploitation have been eliminated. This requires some effective sort of federation of the whole world, based on the common interests of all its peoples.

Thirdly, it cannot be expected that the raising of children will be influenced actively by considerations of the worth of future generations unless parents in general have a very considerable economic security and unless they are extended such adequate economic, medical, educational and other aids in the bearing and rearing of each additional child that the having of more children does not overburden either of them. As the woman is more especially affected by child-bearing and rearing, she must be given special protection to ensure that her reproductive duties do not interfere too greatly with her opportunities to participate in the life and work of the community at large. These objects cannot be achieved unless there is an organization of production primarily for the benefit of consumer and worker, unless the conditions of employment are adapted to the needs of parents and especially of mothers, and unless dwellings, towns and community services generally are reshaped with the good of children as one of their main objectives.

A fourth prerequisite for effective genetic improvement is the legalization, the universal dissemination, and the further development through scientific investigation, of ever more efficacious means of birth control, both negative and positive, that can be put into effect at all stages of the reproductive process—as by voluntary temporary or permanent sterilization, contraception, abortion (as a third line of defence), control of fertility and of the sexual cycle, artificial insemination, etc. Along with all this the development of social consciousness and responsibility in regard to the production of children is required, and this cannot be expected to be operative unless the above-mentioned economic and social conditions for its fulfilment are present, and unless the superstitious attitude towards sex and reproduction now prevalent has been replaced by a scientific and social attitude. This will result in its being regarded as an honour and a privilege, if not a duty, for a mother, married or unmarried, or for a couple, to have the best children possible, both in respect of their upbringing and of their genetic endowment, even where the latter would mean an artificial—though always voluntary—control over the process of parenthood.

Before people in general, or the State which is supposed to represent them, can be relied upon to adopt rational policies for the guidance of their reproduction, there will have to be, fifthly, a far wider spread of knowledge of biological principles and of recognition of the truth that both environment and heredity constitute dominating and inescapable complementary factors in human wellbeing, but factors both of which are under the potential control of man and admit of unlimited but inter-dependent progress. Betterment of environmental conditions enhances the opportunities for genetic betterment in the ways above indicated. But it must also be understood that the effect of the bettered environ-ment is not a direct one on the germ cells and that the Lamarckian doc-trine is fallacious, according to which the children of parents who have had better opportunities for physical and mental development inherit these improvements biologically, and according to which, in conse-quence, the dominant classes and peoples would have become geneti-cally superior to the under-privileged ones. The intrinsic (genetic) characteristics of any generation can be better than those of the pre-ceding generation only as a result of some kind of *selection*, that is, by those persons of the preceding generation who had a better genetic equipment having produced more offspring, on the whole, than the rest, either through conscious choice, or as an automatic result of the way in which they lived. Under modern civilized conditions such selection is far less likely to be automatic than under primitive conditions, hence some kind of conscious guidance of selection is called for. To make this possible, however, the population must first appreciate the force of the above principles, and the social value which a wisely guided selection would have.

Sixthly, conscious selection requires, in addition, an agreed direction or directions for selection to take, and these directions cannot be social ones, that is, for the good of mankind at large, unless social motives predominate in society. This in turn implies its socialized organization. The most important genetic objectives, from a social point of view, are the improvement of those genetic characteristics which make (*a*) for health, (*b*) for the complex called intelligence, and (*c*) for those tem-peramental qualities which favour fellow-feeling and social behaviour rather than those (to-day most esteemed by many) which make for personal 'success', as success is usually understood at present.

A more widespread understanding of biological principles will bring with it the realization that much more than the prevention of genetic deterioration is to be sought for, and that the raising of the level of the average of the population nearly to that of the highest now existing in isolated individuals, in regard to physical wellbeing, intelligence and temperamental qualities, is an achievement that would—so far as purely genetic considerations are concerned—be physically possible within a comparatively small number of generations. Thus everyone might look upon 'genius', combined of course with stability, as his birthright. As the course of evolution shows, this would represent no final stage at all, but only an earnest of still further progress in the future.

The effectiveness of such progress, however, would demand increasingly extensive and intensive research in human genetics and in the numerous fields of investigation correlated therewith. This would involve the co-operation of specialists in various branches of medicine, psychology, chemistry and, not least, the social sciences, with the improvement of the inner constitution of man himself as their central theme. The organization of the human body is marvellously intricate, and the study of its genetics is beset with special difficulties which require the prosecution of research in this field to be on a much vaster scale, as well as more exact and analytical, than hitherto contemplated. This can, however, come about when men's minds are turned from war and hate and the struggle for the elementary means of subsistence to larger aims, pursued in common.

The day when economic reconstruction will reach the stage where such human forces will be released is not yet, but it is the task of this generation to prepare for it, and all steps along the way will represent a gain, not only for the possibilities of the ultimate genetic improvement of man, to a degree seldom dreamed of hitherto, but at the same time, more directly, for human mastery over those more immediate evils which are so threatening our modern civilization.

F.A.E. CREW	G.P. CHILD	P.C. KOLLER
C.D. DARLINGTON	P.R. DAVID	W. LANDAUER
J.B.S. HALDANE	G. DAHLBERG	H.H. PLOUGH
S.C. HARLAND	TH. DOBZHANSKY	B. PRICE
L.T. HOGBEN	R.A. EMERSON	J. SCHULTZ
J.S. HUXLEY	C. GORDON	A.G. STEINBERG
H.J. MULLER	J. HAMMOND	C.H. WADDINGTON
J. NEEDHAM	C.L. HUSKINS	

Part eleven

The growth of the asylum

11.1

Contemporary accounts of the increase of insanity

(i) James Coxe, 'On the causes of insanity, and the means of checking its growth', *Journal of Mental Science* 18 (1872), pp. 312–13, 315–16, 320 [pp. 311–33].

(ii) John Carswell, 'Contribution to the inquiry into the increase in pauper lunacy in Scotland', *Glasgow Medical Journal* 5 (1892), pp. 263–7 [pp. 262–70].

(iii) Ethelinda Hawden, 'On the supposed increase in insanity. A plea for prevention', *Poor Law Magazine and Local Government Journal* 11 (1901), pp. 349–58 [pp. 349–59].

These three extracts reveal the late nineteenth-century concern over the growth in the numbers of patients (especially paupers) in Scottish asylums, and the confusion as to what might be the cause of the apparent growth in insanity. The authors all had direct experience of the asylum system. James Coxe was one of the Commissioners in Lunacy for Scotland, responsible for inspecting conditions in asylums, and president of the Medico-Psychological Association. John Carswell was the Lecturer on Mental Diseases at Anderson's College, Glasgow. Ethelinda Hawden, as member of the Edinburgh Parish Council, had experience of the asylum system from the perspective of the Poor Law authorities, responsible for paying for the care of pauper lunatics.

(i)

[T]o what is this increase in the proportion of lunatics to be ascribed?...
[It] is to a considerable extent the result of the operation of the statutes.[1]
... When the present lunacy system was inaugurated, many parts of the
country were totally unprovided with asylum accommodation. The erection of asylums ... increased the list of the insane brought under official
cognisance, without, however, adding to their actual number. There was
merely a transfer of patients from private dwellings, where their existence was not officially known, to public establishments where they
were registered and reported. But the statistics of every asylum show
that the tendency of such establishments is to foster a continuous
increase in the number of their inmates. The admissions exceed the discharges and deaths, and from this cause alone there results a steady and
persistent increase in the number of patients....

Still, that the sole cause of the growth in lunacy lies in the mere tendency of patients to accumulate in asylums, is a theory which cannot be
accepted. ... There must be taken into consideration all the different
influences which in modern society lead to persons being reckoned as
lunatics, and removed as such from home. Chief among these are the
facilities afforded by the poor-law for the gratuitous disposal of indigent
patients in asylums; and next to these the opportunities which asylums
afford of getting quit of persons who from temper, disease, vice, intemperance, or old age, have become troublesome or expensive inmates at
home. Under such influences the definition of lunacy has expanded, and
many a one is accordingly now treated as a lunatic who formerly would
not have been regarded as coming within the meaning of the term ...

[W]e must come to the conclusion that during the last twenty years
medical science has not succeeded in effecting any increase in the proportion of recoveries, or any decrease in the rate of mortality, among
insane patients in asylums. What, then, is the object sought to be
attained by the establishment and constant enlargement of asylums for
the insane? ... When the Lunacy Acts were passed, a belief was extensively prevalent that the establishment of asylums would powerfully
contribute to check the growth of lunacy. ... We have seen that this
hope has not been realised, but that, on the contrary, the number of
lunatics has been greatly increased. ... Of course, it is impossible to
call in question the fact that a large proportion of the patients admitted
into asylums are restored to sanity. But this fact, nevertheless, leaves
totally unsolved the problem, how far recovery is due to any special

[1] laws.

influence of asylum treatment, or simply to the recuperative powers which nature displays . . .

The great increase in the numbers of the insane has not taken place among the upper and educated classes, but mainly among the lower orders. It is for pauper lunatics that the constant demand for increased accommodation is raised. . . . [I]t may be assumed that . . . [what] mainly tends to produce insanity . . . [are] those causes of physical disease to which the lower orders are chiefly exposed. Such are dissipation[2] in its various forms, over-work of body, insufficient food, the respiration of a corrupted air, and the neglect of intellectual and moral culture. . . . [M]any of the upper classes also suffer from insanity . . . It may be, that emotional excitement is with them a more frequent cause of insanity than with the lower orders, but it will generally be manifest, that debasing practices, dissipation, bodily disease, hereditary predisposition, sunstroke, accidents, or thorough neglect of the most common rules of health are here also at the root of the evil.

(ii)

[T]he increase in the number of lunatic patients maintained from private sources keeps well within the limits of the natural increase of the population, instead of being, as in the case of pauper patients, much beyond it. . . . Insanity is mainly the product of bad heredity and unhealthy conditions of physical existence, and both of these elements in the etiology[3] of insanity are more likely to be found among the ignorant and depraved than in better social circles . . . The population has increased most in the direction of that class of the population from which pauper lunacy is derived, and least among the well-to-do classes. . . . There is . . . a larger population in Scotland who have to seek parochial assistance on account of insanity, and who are also more amenable to the influences which produce insanity, than was the case twenty or thirty years ago . . . [N]ot only is there a larger constituency for pauper lunacy, but when we consider certain social changes that have been gradually occurring in this country during recent years, other elements in the causation of the increase will appear . . . [T]he provision meant for the cure of insanity is being taken advantage of by the public as comfortable homes for troublesome or burdensome relatives at the public expense. The tendency to seek relief from personal

[2] The unrestrained pursuit of pleasure, debauchery.
[3] Causes.

and family obligations, on account of insanity, is only one manifestation of a general movement in many directions that characterises the social ideas of the present time. . . . [M]edical opinion and public policy in this matter must make common cause. The Lunacy Commissioners,[4] in their last report, state their opinion that 'the remedy for the increasing burden of pauper lunacy, in so far as a remedy is desirable or possible, lies primarily in the hands of Parochial Boards.' But Parochial Boards are in the hands of their medical officers in regard to what constitutes certifiable mental unsoundness, and neither the General Board of Lunacy, medical men, nor Parochial Boards will or can ignore the element of public sentiment in relation to the provision necessary for persons afflicted, whether temporarily or permanently, with mental unsoundness. . . . Patients suffering from delirium tremens, hysteria, and various states of excitement and stupor are reported to the inspector of poor. . . . They are troublesome at home, and general hospitals will not receive them, or immediate removal there is not possible owing to admission being dependent upon a subscriber's order.[5] It is an open question whether transient disturbances of the nervous system . . . are increasing in the frequency of their occurrence, but there can be no doubt that there is a greater readiness on the part of the public to avail themselves of the advantages of public institutions, and I incline to the opinion that the latter consideration may be held to account for the increasing number of lunacy applications made to the inspector of poor.

There is no reason for supposing that insanity is increasing, but . . . it might easily happen that the number of persons sent to asylums would increase if medical opinion regarding the certification of lunatics should become conformed to the pressure of public sentiment and ideas of social necessity, instead of being guided by a rigid regard to the diagnosis of definite forms of nervous and mental diseases. Opinion regarding the nature or degree of mental disturbance that may be considered to require asylum treatment has shown a tendency to expand. . . . [I]t has come about chiefly as a part of a general social movement towards relieving individual persons of unusual or special burdens at the public expense. The pressure . . . of public opinion will have the effect of further widening the limits of what may be considered certifiable mental disorder, whereas medical opinion on that point ought to be free from considerations of that nature; . . . there is a general desire on

---

[4] The government body for inspecting and ensuring proper standards of care in asylums.

[5] A letter from one of the donors to the hospital, recommending the patient as a suitable case for admission.

the part of the profession for some provision whereby temporary care may be secured for the kind of cases we are now referring to, and the certification of lunatics be placed upon a better basis.

(iii)

Registered Pauper Insanity in Scotland has, as shown by the Reports of the Commissioners of Lunacy in Scotland, steadily increased . . . to an enormous extent within the last 40 years. . . . There are . . . many factors involved in the production of this increase . . .

Since 1860, there has been a steady growth in the numbers of insane paupers in Scotland, both absolutely and relatively to the population. In other countries . . . there has been nothing to compare with this increase. . . . In Prussia in 1880 the number of insane of all classes, including idiots,[6] was 243 per 100,000, and the corresponding figure for France in 1879 was 252. Including idiots there were in the United States in 1890, 323 insane persons per 100,000 of the general population; in England and Wales 1891, 336; in Scotland 1891, 384; in Ireland 1891, 450; in Austria in 1890, 217 . . .

Since 1858 the ratio of ordinary paupers to the general population has fallen considerably. In 1858 it was 2,630 per 100,000 of the population . . . at the present time it is 1507. Since 1858 the number of lunatics of all classes has risen from 5,824 to 15,399 on 1st January, 1899, an increase of 164 per cent., the increase of population being only 41 per cent. . . . [T]he major portion of this increase is in pauper lunatics. . . . [E]ven if we assume . . . that only one-half of the private patients are registered, . . . the number of first admissions is twice as great in pauper lunatics as in private lunatics. . . . [T]he increase has been much more marked in country than in urban districts, and still is so to a large extent, with the single exception of Haddington. . . . In general the more sparsely populated and least civilised counties have suffered most. . . . [T]he highest proportions of lunatics are to be found in such counties as Argyllshire, Bute, Caithness, Elgin, Inverness, Ross, Shetland, Sutherland, Perth, Kinross, Nairn, Orkney. It is precisely these counties that were most backward in civilisation until railways came . . .

Is it not extremely probable that the greatly increased prosperity of the country, resulting in luxury unheard of before, may have affected the sanity of the people? . . . In . . . counties where the prosperity of the

---

[6] In the nineteenth century this was the usual term for people suffering from some sort of learning difficulty.

people has increased by leaps and bounds, insanity has increased enormously. . . . It would be instructive to know how many of the enormous
number of pauper lunatics now chargeable in the northern counties
have been returned to their parishes insane after having transferred
their residence to large towns. . . . [I]n 1875 . . . many lunatics who had
become insane in towns where they had not acquired a settlement[7] . . .
had been returned to their native parishes which they had left long
years ago . . .

Prosperity also brings in its train increased power to purchase harmful luxuries, such as excessive stimulants.[8]

There is another element in the growth of pauper lunacy which is of
great importance. It is in the parts of the country which have been
longest supplied with lunatic asylums that the increase is least. Insanity
is emphatically a hereditary disease. In places where the insane have
been for a considerable time placed under restraint the hereditary cases
should naturally be fewer. . . . [B]efore the days of systematic registration of lunatics, hundreds of these poor creatures were allowed to
wander about the country . . . looked upon merely as weak-minded or
eccentric in the past generation — and who were allowed to go free and
to perpetuate their kind, but who would now be properly regarded as
persons requiring supervision and care — whose descendants are now
increasingly crowding our lunatic asylums . . .

Drunkenness and immorality have been for generations the favourite
sins of the Scottish people, and both are fertile causes of insanity, both
in the parents who commit them, and their children who suffer for the
sins of the parents. . . . [A] high rate of insanity accompanies a high rate
of illegitimacy in many counties . . .

There is another reason for the increase of pauper lunatics, and that
is the tendency of chronic cases to accumulate in asylums. . . . [U]nless
Parish Councils are alive to their duties, and exercise vigilance over
their officials, cases are allowed to remain in asylums, at a heavy cost
to the ratepayers, who might be boarded out in the country[9] as invalids
at very much less expense, and to the benefit of the patients . . .

It is becoming the rule among working people to refuse to retain moderately insane relatives in their houses. Parents who have become
childish and troublesome, and children who are, as it is called, 'wanting',

---

[7] i.e. had lived in town long enough to become the responsibility of the poor law there, and
not in the parish of their birth.

[8] i.e. alcohol.

[9] A system of having lunatics stay with families in the countryside, which was popular in
Scotland. The families were given a small allowance for their support.

are brought to the parish authorities without scruple, where formerly they would have been allowed to go in and out of the house or sit by the fire, and share the family meals. There are various reasons for this. One of the most important is undoubtedly the expense of house accommodation in towns, and the narrow space in which families are condemned to live from this cause. . . . [T]he rate of board in asylums having become far too high for any ordinary working man to meet, still less a working wife, the patient becomes chargeable[10] to the ratepayers in whole or in part. Pauper insanity has increased, while ordinary pauperism has decreased. This is owing to the fact that many persons, who would not allow ordinary infirm or old relatives to become chargeable, are unable to pay the lowest rate of private board — *i.e.*, £40— for an insane relative, and consequently have to allow him to be put on the pauper roll . . .

The conditions of life in Scotland are now changing. The incomplete census returns already show us that the population is leaving the country and collecting in the towns. The towns are becoming overcrowded, and the struggle of the poor intensified . . . [L]ives in towns are very much more unhealthy . . . The children of the slums grow up with impaired constitutions, and in their turn bring children into the world who are more degenerate than they are themselves . . .

On the whole, country life produces less insanity than town life, where the question is not complicated with other considerations, as in parts of Scotland. It would seem reasonable therefore in view of the very large proportion of insanity in cities, that measures should be enforced to minimise the evils of town life, as far as that can be done, in the interests of our city ratepayers.

There will always be a much larger proportion of insane people among the poor than among the well-to-do, however. Bad conditions of life, working at monotonous occupations where there is a continual strain on the attention, as in the case of railway servants, dangerous trades . . . alcoholic excess, dyspepsia from bad food, anaemia from want of food, poisoning from drains and bad air, lack of mental control from defective training acting on inherited nervous instability, and in women the insanities due to sex conditions,[11] or to defective nutrition and bad sanitary conditions, are naturally much commoner among the poor.

Relapses are more likely to occur among the poor owing to difficulty in obtaining work after discharge from an asylum. . . . [W]hen a rich man shows signs of nervous breakdown he is sent away for a sea

---

[10] To require the support of the poor law, which was regarded as a severe social stigma.

[11] i.e. to forms of insanity particular to women. Among the most serious was puerperal insanity, episodes of madness following childbirth.

voyage, or to some quiet country place where he can vegetate till his jarred nerves can regain tone. The poor must continue where they are, and struggle on under all sorts of trying conditions till they actually cross the borderland and go to find the rest and peace in an asylum.

11.2
The impact of industrialisation

Andrew Scull, *The Most Solitary of Afflictions. Madness and Society in Britain, 1700–1900* (New Haven and London, Yale University Press, 1993), pp. 26–33.

Andrew Scull is one of the most prolific and influential writers on the history of insanity in the nineteenth century. Scull's work serves as a criticism of self-congratulatory Whiggish accounts of the rise of psychiatry and the mental hospitals as situated within a moral and humane enlightenment project. He puts forward critical accounts which focus on control and coercion within the institutional system, thus raising historical debate concerning the tension between actors' claims to moral, humane approaches and the asylum practices themselves that show increasing regulation and control as necessary to produce and manage 'docile bodies'. This particular book is a re-exploration and expansion of an earlier study – *Museums of Madness: The Social Organisation of Insanity in Nineteenth Century England* (London, Allen Lane, 1979). Scull discusses the transformation in practices and notions of madness that underlay the change from the domestic care of insanity to an institutionalised system. He also demonstrates how the institutional system ratified the legitimacy of the new psychiatric profession, and that, as the asylums became more overcrowded, the doctors' stated aims of treatment and cure became impossible to achieve.

. . . [T]he limited growth of the private trade in lunacy, and the parallel creation of a number of charity asylums, serve to demonstrate that the traditional, family-based response to insanity (and indeed to all forms of dependency) was beginning to be questioned and abandoned, a process which gathered steam as the eighteenth century drew to a close. Those who see this process, and the asylum's ultimate triumph in the nineteenth century, as a relatively direct and uncomplicated consequence of

236

the rise of an urban-industrial society argue that the rise of segregative forms of social control represented a 'natural' response to the inability of a community – and household-based relief system to cope with the vastly greater problems created by this new form of social organization. In Mechanic's words, 'Industrialization and technological change . . . , coupled with increasing urbanization brought decreasing tolerance for bizarre and disruptive behavior and less ability to contain deviant behavior within the existing social structure.[12] The increased geographical mobility of the population and the anonymity of existence in the urban slums were combined with the destruction of the old paternal relationships which went with a stable, hierarchically organized rural society. Furthermore, the situation of the poor and dependent classes, huddled together in the grossly overcrowded conditions which accompanied the explosive, unplanned growth of urban and industrial centres became simultaneously more visible and more desperate . . .

The suggestion is that families in these conditions were much less capable of sustaining a non-productive member, and that both the scale of the problems and the anonymity of urban existence threatened the easy and uncomplicated system of relief which had sufficed in earlier times. Though for a long time the implications of these developments were evaded, and 'the whole frame of historical and economic reference remained agrarian in an economy undergoing an industrial revolution', eventually the new problems posed by poverty and dependence in an urban environment had to be faced. . . . [D]espite their growing conviction that many of the poor were 'underserving', the new class of entrepreneurs could not wholly avoid making some provision for them, if only because of the revolutionary threat they posed to the social order. The asylum – and analogous institutions such as the workhouse – allegedly constituted their response to this situation.

But there are serious problems with this line of argument. While the proportion of town dwellers in England rose sharply from the late eighteenth century onwards, the process of urbanization was simply not as far advanced as this account necessarily implies when pressures developed to differentiate and institutionalize the deviant population . . . [A]lthough large towns absorbed an increasing proportion of the English population, city dwellers remained a distinct minority during the first decades of the nineteenth century, by which time powerful pressures were already being exerted to secure the establishment of lunatic asylums (and other segregative forms of social control) on a compulsory

[12] David Mechanic, *Mental Health and Social Policy* (Englewood Cliffs, New Jersey, Prentice-Hall, 1969), p. 54.

basis. London, it is true, already had a population of 840,000 in 1801, and grew to contain more than a million people by 1811 – but it remained unique. In 1801, there were only six other cities with a population of more than 50,000; by 1811, there were eight; by 1821, there were twelve, including three which had passed the 100,000 mark. More significantly, at the turn of the century, 'only one third [of the English population] lived in a town of any size, only one in six in a town over 20,000.'

By themselves, these figures suggest that the notion that it was *urban* poverty which forced the adoption of an institutional response to deviance is by no means as self-evident as is commonly assumed. And when one looks for direct, concrete evidence of such a connection, one's faith in the traditional wisdom is still further diminished. During the initial growth of the private madhouse trade in the eighteenth century, the 'regions most conspicuous for asylum building were not the industrial boom-towns. Georgian private asylums commonly sprang up away from dense population centres, in Kent, Sussex, Wiltshire, Gloucestershire, etc; and their catchments [*sic*] areas were quite restricted.' The pattern is not altered much, as we shall see, even in the opening decades of the nineteenth century: in 1808 local magistrates were given discretionary power to provide asylum accommodation for pauper lunatics. Whether any given county adopted this solution to the problem of the dependent insane bore little or no relationship to the degree of urbanization of its population. While Lancashire and the West Riding of Yorkshire, two of the most heavily populated counties in England, were among the first to plan and open county asylums, Middlesex, the most densely populated county in the country, made no effort to do so until 1827, and then acted only under the spur of direct Parliamentary pressure. None of the counties in the West Midlands, along with the North the most industrialized and urbanized region of England, built an asylum until 1845, when they were compelled to do so. At the other end of the scale, the second county to open an asylum under the 1808 Act (in 1812) was small, rural Bedfordshire. Other rural counties exhibited a similar enthusiasm for the institutional solution at a comparatively early date. Indeed, the majority of the asylums built on the basis of the permissive act were situated in rural counties: Norfolk (1814), Lincolnshire (1820), Cornwall (1820), Gloucestershire (1823), Suffolk (1829), Dorset (1832), Kent (1833).

No clear-cut connection exists, therefore, between the rise of large asylums and the growth of large cities. Instead, I suggest that the main driving force behind the rise of a segregative response to madness (and to other forms of deviance) can much more plausibly be asserted to lie in the effects of a mature capitalist market economy and the associated ever more thoroughgoing commercialization of existence. While the urban conditions produced by industrialization had a direct impact which was originally limited in geographical scope, the market system observed few such restrictions, and had increasingly subversive effects on the whole traditional rural and urban social structure. These changes in turn prompted the abandonment of long-established techniques for coping with the poor and troublesome . . .

Some may object that these contentions rest upon a chronological confusion: that the rise of capitalism in England occurred too early to be plausibly invoked as the explanation for events occurring in the late eighteenth and the first half of the nineteenth century. But such criticism is itself confused and misplaced, for I am concerned here not simply with the initial moves towards commercialized production and the rise of a market of national reach and scope, but with the massive reorganization of an entire society along market principles . . . And this takes place only in the late eighteenth and early nineteenth century.

[. . .]

The changing structure of the English economy from the second half of the eighteenth century onwards undermined and then destroyed the old order. An ever more robust and abrasive commercialism established itself in every realm of social existence, scurrying around in search of opportunities for profit, and remorselessly broadening the geographical scope of the market. Profound shifts occurred in the relationships between the superordinate and the subordinate classes, and in upper-class perceptions of their responsibilities towards the less fortunate – changes which can be summarized as the transition from a master-servant to an employer-employee relationship; from a social order dominated by rank, order, and degree, to one based on class. There emerged a 'general sense of betrayal of paternal responsibilities by the naked exercise of the power of property'. As part of the general change from regulated to self-regulating markets, centuries-old legislation protecting workers' standard of living and conditions of work was abolished. Increasingly, 'the process of acquisition set the terms on which other social processes were allowed to operate'. Capitalism broke the social bonds which had formerly held it in check, and a modern commercial consumer society was born.

[. . .]

The economy as a whole came under the sway of the notion that '[the employer] owed his employees wages, and once these were paid, the men had no further claim on him'.

239

Thus, just as surely as urbanization, the market when given its head destroyed the traditional links between rich and poor which had characterized the old order. The 'great transformation' wrought by the advent of a thoroughly market-oriented society sharply reduced the *capacity* of the lower orders to cope with economic reverses. Wage-earners, whether they were agricultural labourers or the early representatives of an urban proletariat, shared a similar incapacity to make adequate provision for periods of economic depression. Quite apart from the centres of urbanization and industrialization, and to a much greater degree than the geographically limited scope of these processes would indicate, the burgeoning market economy was rendering anachronistic the idealized conception of a population living amidst 'the ever-sustaining resources of an uncomplicated rural parish'. To make matters worse, along with the closing off of alternatives other than wage work as a means of providing for subsistence went the tendency of the primitive capitalist economy to oscillate wildly and unpredictably between conditions of boom and slump.

All in all, among the lower classes in this period, family members unable to contribute effectively towards their own maintenance must have constituted a serious drain on family resources. In the situation which they faced, 'any interruption of the ability to work or the availability of a job spelt dire want . . . The aged and children became a greater burden . . .', as, of course, did the insane. Consequently, while a family-based system of caring for the mad may never have worked especially well, one suspects that by the turn of the century it was likely to have been functioning particularly badly.

11.3
Getting rid of 'inconvenient people'?

J.K. Walton, 'Casting Out and Bringing Back in Victorian
England: Pauper Lunatics, 1840–70', in W.F. Bynum, Roy
Porter and Michael Shepherd (eds), *The Anatomy of Madness.
Essays in the History of Psychiatry*, vol. II, Institutions and
Society (London, Tavistock Press, 1985), pp. 137–41
[pp. 135–46].

John Walton has published widely on British social history, including local studies in Lancashire. The 'casting out' of the article title refers to the process of isolating the mad from society into the asylum; 'bringing back' describes the process of return to the community. As Walton points out there was very little of the latter, demonstrating a disastrous failure of the promises held out for moral treatment. This article reconsiders Scull's argument concerning the institutionalisation of 'inconvenient' people by working-class families. Walton sets out to discover the route by which people became defined as insane and whether the family or outsiders were the instigators of the process, using local records from the Lancaster Asylum.

Who stuck the label 'pauper lunatic' on an individual? To what extent did the initiative come from those in authority, from workhouse masters, police, justices of the peace, medical practitioners, employers? To what extent did it come from the lunatics' own families, in response to behaviour that was so intolerable that it overrode the usual antipathy to the Poor Law system in general and the workhouse, through which most lunatics passed, in particular.

The short answer is that we do not know. We can identify a range of influences and possibilities, but we cannot yet quantify a pattern. The basic administrative procedure is clear enough. A deposition[13] had to be sworn before two JPs[14] to the effect that the individual in question was 'a Lunatic or Insane person'. Usually, no doubt, this was initiated by the overseers of the parish or township,[15] who then had to bring the candidate along for examination by the JPs, after which, if satisfied that he or she was mad and chargeable to the parish in question, the JPs caused a 'medical person' to conduct a further examination. If all were agreed, a certificate of lunacy was duly signed, and the new patient was supposed to be conveyed to the asylum. But we cannot reconstruct the circumstances leading up to the involvement of the officials in any regular or systematic way. We do not usually know what social processes lay behind the initiation of the administrative procedures. Sometimes the route to the asylum is traceable back to the workhouse, the prison or the magistrates' court. . . . We can take matters a little further by looking at some evidence from Lancaster Asylum.

Some asylum admissions clearly did originate with people in authority, anxious to dispose of the difficult and dissolute. Workhouses, especially, sent their quota of the hard-to-manage, many of whom

[13] *deposition*: sworn evidence.

[14] *JPs*: justices of the peace.

[15] *Overseers of the parish and township*: administrators responsible for distributing relief to paupers under the Poor Law.

might not have been regarded as insane on initial admission . . . The courts also brought the attention of JPs to bear on habitual drunkards and petty offenders . . . Vagrants, too, were often passed on to asylums through the courts, and of course there was the numerically small but controversial and difficult category of criminal lunatics as such, 'homicidal maniacs' and the like. But it is difficult to show, despite the vagrants and the occasional prostitute, and a disproportionate representation of unskilled labourers and domestic servants among asylum admissions, that the asylum population was dominated by a subculture of the disorderly poor, chosen for the threat they posed to property, decorum, and the social order . . .

Any such repression did not extend to the systematic persecution of political or religious deviants, although political or religious delusions, and delusions about property, are frequently noted by asylum officials. We cannot recreate the context or nature of these utterances, however, and it is highly likely that they were usually, if not always, the garbled and distorted products of more generally disordered minds. Admissions deemed to be politically related form a very thin trickle from the early 1820s through to the 1870s. In 1821 Henry Whittaker 'appears to have been deranged by the constant, petty vexations together with great violence attempted, and partly effected on his person by several radicals who were his fellow workmen in a manufactory', so here our causal mechanisms are inverted; but in the early 1840s we find odd cases ascribed to *'politics'* and to excitement occasioned by attending a meeting of the Anti-Corn Law League.[16]

[. . .]

[It] should be stressed that even Lancaster Asylum, large and close to centres of unrest as it was, generated no more than a handful of suspicious-looking cases in the sample years I have studied . . . After all, why bother to use the complicated and controversial machinery of certification for insanity when, as the events of 1839–42 made abundantly clear, straightforward physical and legal coercion could do the job of repression admirably without compromising the appearance of ruling-class legitimacy? In any case, the roots of most asylum committals clearly lay in domestic troubles, as families at the end of their tether sought succour even though it meant the Poor Law and the asylum. The typical case . . . was nearer to the experience of Eliza Hartley's family, who told the relieving officer that she was 'constantly rambling about

---

[16] *Anti-Corn Law League*: major society formed to protest against the tariffs on the import of corn.

the house and removing furniture, and bringing it downstairs as if the family were going to remove. Constantly blowing kisses to everyone she meets.' A more severe level of stress is epitomized by a case from Staffordshire in which 'the Lunatic was constantly attacking his mother, as well as his brothers and sisters'. The mother, too, was eventually certified insane. The invocation of the asylum brought relief from impossible circumstances to many families, and at this stage and under these conditions its availability and use became an unalloyed benefit, not least to those patients who were rescued from squalid confinement in locked rooms and filthy workhouse wards.[17] . . . Scull is probably right about the growing acceptability of the asylum for desperate working-class families, but the evidence is more problematic than he allows, and the causal mechanisms he suggests are sometimes simplistic and out of line with empirical evidence and recent historiography.

The analysis of case-registers may provide some clues as to the kinds of behaviour families found intolerable and those in authority frowned upon: categories which remain analytically impossible to separate in studying the vast majority of asylum admissions . . . [A] sample of 400 admissions, evenly divided between the sexes and between the years 1842 and 1843, produced the results shown in [the] Table.

. . . Drink and violence (especially intra-familial violence, usually of husbands towards wives, or involving a wife's rejection of her husband), bulk largest in the table, along with the threat of suicide, which was at once crime, sin, and evidence of derangement in contemporary eyes. Drink and sexual misdemeanour . . . are more in evidence among

Table Aspects of behaviour of patients admitted to Lancaster Asylum, 1842–43, as recorded in the medical registers

characteristics of admissions	*men* %	*women* %	*all* %
1 violence or threat of violence	22.5	17.0	19.75
2 suicidal	12.5	14.5	13.5
3 'intemperance', 'irregularity', 'dissipation', etc.	24.0	12.0	18.0
4 religious delusions	6.0	5.0	5.5
5 problems involving family and sexual relationships	2.5	11.5	7.0
6 physical feebleness	2.5	5.5	4.0

[17] A large proportion of the insane continued to be confined in homes and in workhouses without special care.

men than women, perhaps surprisingly in the light of contemporary attitudes; and among women the patriarchal family and the behavioural expectations which surrounded it were probably more important than the figures suggest. Physical debility was noted in only a small minority of cases, even in the economically depressed year of 1842, although the stresses of unemployment and the poverty cycle are regularly mentioned in the registers as contributory factors, and must have reduced families' ability to cope with, and to survive without, psychologically ailing members. Many female patients were discharged from Lancaster Asylum 'not improved', at the request of husbands who were presumably desperate for whatever help and comfort they could get; and this is itself an eloquent commentary on the problems faced by the families of pauper lunatics.

The most misleading aspect of [the] Table, and of the source on which it is based, is probably the lack of weight given to passive depression and withdrawal, which tends to attract a diagnosis of 'melancholia' in the register, and little other comment. When this neglected form of quiescent desperation is added to the violence, delusions, and bizarre behaviour that lie behind the categories analysed in the Table, it becomes apparent that the asylum was not resorted to lightly by families and Poor Law authorities. It was the final resource when all else had failed, in the vast majority of cases; and most of those who were admitted and remained within its walls were not so much 'inconvenient people', in Scull's terminology, as impossible people in the eyes of families, neighbours, and authorities. Attitudes may have changed in late Victorian times, but in the middle decades of the nineteenth century the county asylum provided relief for desperate families rather than an easy option for the uncaring or irresponsible.

11.4

The effects of the whirling chair

Extracts from Case Notes of the use of Rotary Chair at
Glasgow Asylum, 1820–21, from the Greater Glasgow Health
Board Archives, 13/5/2–6.

In the early nineteenth century, patients in asylums were occasionally subjected to all sorts of physical therapy – they were suddenly drenched in water, swung violently in suspended seats or, as here, rotated rapidly in rotary or whirling chairs. Such treatments were justified on the grounds that they jolted the body and helped to expel corrupted matter, or shocked the body back into normal physiological function. Such treatments also had the effect of intimidating patients into good behaviour. These very brief notes from the Glasgow Asylum give a snapshot of the sorts of patients who were subjected to these physical therapies.

Margaret Gibson, private case.
3rd admission 19/7/1820.
August 18 1820. She is very unsettled. Let her be put in the rotary chair for a few minutes.
August 19. The chair seemed to produce no effect.
Discharged relieved 2/10/1820.

Georgina Ferguson, private case.
1st admission 20/7/1822.
Sept. 21 1822. Refuses to sew or amuse herself in any way. To use the rumbling chair.
Sept. 23. Still refuses to do any thing. Let her be put on the whirling chair.
Sept. 24. Was in the chair for an hour would not promise to sew, or do any thing. Was very sick & vomited several times.

Mary McKindlay, pauper case.
29 Dec. 1819. She was in the Circular chair for five minutes yesterday morning. She is more composed since.

Isabella Rankin, pauper case.
1st adm 12/12/1814 (Died 8/1/1827)
Sept. 4 1819. She was this day fastened in the Circular chair which was then put in motion for a quarter of an hour. It seemed to produce but little effect during the time she was in the chair but she became sick & vomited after she was removed from the chair.

John Reid, age 18, pauper case.
Single, weaver.
2nd admission 1/11/1816 (Died 4/12/1843)
4 Oct. 1819. Continues very mischievous.
4 Nov. No alteration.
27 Nov. He was in the circular chair for a few minutes this morning.
11 Dec. No amendment.

James Rankin, age 40, private.
Weaver
Admitted 2 Jan. 1819.
4 Sept. 1819. He was in the Circular Chair 20 minutes without it
producing . . .
8 Sept. Not the least degree of improvement.
Discharged relieved 14/7/1821.

Daniel Hall, age 38, pauper case.
Weaver.
2nd admission 22/3/1819.
14 August 1819. Is gradually becoming worse in mind.
26 August. Is occasionally very troublesome.
3 Nov. Has not worked at all since last report.
8 Dec. Was in the circular chair this morning for ten minutes.
13 Dec. He vomited several times while in the chair, and after he came
out. He is less obstinate.
24 Dec. Continues less obstinate.
Discharged relieved by his own desire 22/9/1825.

David Rowan, age 40, pauper case.
Single, weaver.
1st admission 7/4/1819 (Died 18/11/1820)
13 Nov. 1819. Not the least amendment. Let him have the warm bath
with the shower bath.
3 Dec. He was yesterday put for ten minutes into the circular chair. No
change was . . .
7 Dec. Continues in every respect the same.

John Dunclair, age 34, pauper case.
1st admission 11/8/1819.
14 Nov. 1819. Is becoming gradually worse in every respect.
24 Dec. Was in the circular chair for a quarter of an hour. No effect.
5 Sept. He was in the circular Chair for a quarter of an hour, without its
producing any effect.
Discharged unfit 25/2/1823.

John McNair, age 18, private case.
Single, clerk.
1st admission 6/10/1819.
8 Nov. 1819 . . . constantly confined with the Jacket.[18]

---

[18] i.e. straitjacket, used to restrain violent patients and prevent them from harming themselves or others.

11 Nov. Is very incoherent & sleepless. Let his head be shaved.

23 Nov. No amendment in mind.

29 Nov. He was ten minutes in the circular chair without any effect.

Discharged cured 25/3/1820.

James Nichol, age 40, pauper case.

Single, wireworker.

1st admission 9/10/1819 (from Towns Hospital, Glasgow[19]).

10 Nov. 1819 Let him have the shower bath twice a week.

27 Nov. He is very sullen and morose.

7 Dec. Continues sullen. Let him be put in the Circular Chair for 5 minutes.

15 Dec. He was not sick, but complained of head ache for some hours after he was in the chair. Next day he became more lively, and has continued better ever since.

Dismissed cured 10/1/1820.

William Turner, age 21, pauper case.

Single, discharged soldier.

2nd admission 12/10/1819.

19 Nov. 1819. He is very obstinate and indolent.

3 Dec. Let him be put into the chair for five minutes.

7 Dec. The chair seemed to produce no effect beyond a slight degree of alarm.

27 Dec. Is continually teazing the servants to let him out.

20 Jan. 1820 No alteration.

21 Feb. Was in the circular chair yesterday for twenty minutes.

18 April. He is become much addicted to self pollution.[20]

Dismissed by his own desire.

Alexander McTavish, age 30, private case.

Single, fisherman.

1st admission 15/9/1819.

19 Dec. 1819. He was in the warm bath yesterday.

25 Dec. He yesterday mixed his faeces in his porridge and supped them. Let him be put in the Circular chair for a few minutes.

26 Dec. Was in the bath yesterday and was much the better of it.

Discharged relieved 3/7/1821.

[19] A general hospital.

[20] Masturbation.

11.5
The power of medical men?

David Wright, 'The Certification of Insanity in Nineteenth-
Century England and Wales', *History of Psychiatry* 9 (1998),
pp. 271–6, 288 [pp. 267–90].

David Wright is one of the younger generation of researchers
working on the history of psychiatry, of people with learning
disabilities and community care. This paper aims to fill a gap in our
understanding of the processes of certification of the insane, an
act of crucial importance in admission to asylums for most of
the nineteenth century. The picture is, as Wright suggests, more
complex than a straightforward assumption that power for certification was held by the asylum experts. The role of the doctor in the
certification process was gradually changed over the course of the
century. Legislation gradually curtailed the power of the asylum
expert and also began to prohibit collaboration between families
and individual practitioners and proprietors.

In 1774, Parliament responded to 'many great and dangerous abuses' in
the detention of persons in private madhouses for the rich by institut-
ing the practice of licensing and regulating these institutions. The
resultant Private Madhouses Act laid down several principles which
were to continue throughout the next century. Protection against
wrongful confinement was to be ensured by inspection and certification. . . . The principle of certification was enshrined in section twenty-
one, which stated that every keeper of a licensed house had to have an
'Order, in Writing, under the Hand and Seal of some Physician, Surgeon,
or Apothecary, that such Person is proper to be received in to such
House or Place as a Lunatick'. . . .

The Madhouses Act enshrined the principles of inspection and of
medical certification, but shortcomings of the legislation were soon
apparent. The Act did not stipulate what was to be done with uncertified
admissions. Moreover, many provincial justices did not comply with the
licensing laws out of ignorance or deception. . . . There were no
requirements that the medical men certifying the lunatic be unconnected to the receiving licensed home, thereby allowing for the possibility of collusion between medical practitioners and the asylum
proprietors, though it did state that members of the commission could
not be keepers themselves. . . .

Certification of pauper patients dates from amendments to the 1808 County Asylums Act, . . . and an Amendment Act of 1811. Overseers of the Poor[21] were to send to the county magistrate an application for the 'conveyance' of a 'Lunatic, insane Person, or dangerous Idiot' to the county asylum with a certificate in writing from one 'Medical Person'. The magistrate would then issue a 'Warrant' for the conveyance if he was satisfied with the application. He could also order his own medical examination, or he could refuse the application if the insane person was not dangerous. . . .

Three amendment acts between 1811 and 1819 extended this system and put into place the building blocks for the later Victorian asylum system. The 1811 Act arranged for regular visits of a county asylum by a visiting committee of justices which included a 'Medical Person', and required annual returns of the general condition of insane persons to the county magistrates. . . . A brief Amendment Act in 1819 extended the powers of magistrates to summon any allegedly insane person for examination by him, with the assistance of a 'medical man'. If insane and dangerous, the magistrate could send this person to the county asylum upon certification. The form of the pauper certificate was, for the first time, formalized in the statute:

I Do hereby certify, That by the Directions of *L.M.* and *N.O.* Esquires, Justices of the Peace for the County of *H.*, I have personally examined *C.D.* and that the said *C.D.* appears to be of Insane Mind.
Dated this   Day of
A.B. (Physician, Surgeon or Apothecary, *as the case may be*) resident at *R.*

The certificate is interesting in many respects, not least in its explicit reference that the medical man is acting under the directions of the magistrates. Further, it did not inquire as to the reasons why the medical practitioner deemed the person to be 'lunatic, or insane, or a mischievous idiot' . . .

Thus by 1819 many of the basic elements of the nineteenth-century asylum system had been put in place. Rate-aided county asylums were legally permitted and run by magistrates through a visiting committee; licenses for private homes were granted by the permission of the magistrates (with the exception of Middlesex); certification was the province of a licensed medical practitioner and was a prerequisite for admissions to all licensed homes, voluntary hospitals or county pauper asylums. Annual returns of admissions, deaths and discharges were

---

[21] *overseers of the poor*: official responsible for overseeing the distribution of relief to paupers under the Old Poor Law.

sent to the magistrates, generating statistics on institutional confinement. One also sees the origins of the tension between magistrates and Overseers of the Poor: the magistrates were given powers of ordering certification and confinement; the Overseers (later Guardians) of the Poor had responsibility for paying the bills.

Once again, legislation strengthened the hand of magistrates against local Overseers by making the censuses of insane persons in the county parishes obligatory under the 1828 County Asylums Act. Once Overseers had returned lists to the county magistrates, the magistrates could demand a medical examination of an insane person, though it is clear that this process was still intended for dangerous cases. Any person, whether summoned by the justice of the peace, sent by the Overseers of the parish, or apprehended as a vagrant, needed a medical certificate before being admitted to the county asylum. Certificates were to be kept by the medical superintendent, with duplicates being sent to the Committee of Visitors. The Madhouses Act of the same year outlined the form for non-pauper insane persons accepted into private licensed homes. The Act required medical certificates signed by *two* medical men, which included the date of certification, the person by whose authority the insane person was sent (and his place of abode, and degree of relationship to the insane person), the place of residence of the insane person, his/her former occupation, and 'time spent previously in asylum'. . . . This Act also introduced the first statutory safeguard against collusion by stipulating that neither one of the two signing medical practitioners could have an interest in the asylum to which the private insane person would be sent.

Seen in the light of previous legislation, the Lunatics Act of 1845 was not a watershed in the process of certification, and can be perceived partly as a consolidation of 'lunacy reform'. It continued, for instance, the tradition of the testimony of a single medical practitioner for pauper patients and that of two medical practitioners for private patients. Although a national Lunacy Commission was created out of the now defunct Metropolitan Lunacy Commission, magistrates retained control over licensed homes in the provinces and the running and visitation of county pauper asylums. In one respect, however, the Lunatics Act (1845) changed the nature of certificates for private patients, by stipulating that 'facts' had to be given to verify the 'insanity' of all (non-pauper) persons:

> I _____ being a Physician or Surgeon or an Apothecary, duly authorised to practise as such, hereby certify that I have this Day, separately from any other medical practitioner, visited and personally examined A.B. a Person named in the accompanying Statement and Order,

and that the said A.B. is a Lunatic [or an insane Person, or an Idiot, or a Person of unsound Mind], and a proper Person to be confined, and that I have formed this Opinion from the following Fact or Facts; viz.

Signed   *Name*
           Place of Abode

Dated this _____ Day of _____ One thousand eight hundred and _____

Those patients admitted without certificates or with incomplete certificates were liable to be immediately released; in the case of private homes, the license to receive immates could be revoked. The Asylums Act of 1845 also had a direct impact on the *number* of people liable to be certified by obliging all counties and boroughs who had not done so, to erect alone, or combine to erect, asylums for their pauper insane within three years of the Act. It also extended certification to any single insane persons kept at a charge.

There were early teething troubles concerning who should and should not be certified which added to the headaches of an understaffed and overstretched Lunacy Commission. These troubles included confusion over whether those already in licensed institutions needed to be certified, whether certificates of insanity were needed for pauper lunatics admitted to workhouses, whether certification continued to be applied only to 'dangerous' lunatics, and whether patients transferred from one asylum to another needed to be (re)certified. Many of these issues were ironed out in the following years: swamped with responsibilities beyond their resources, and faced with continued hostility from poor law Guardians, the Lunacy Commission decided not to pursue the issue of workhouse lunatics and idiots by not requiring certificates for those remaining within the Guardians' responsibility. Furthermore, they tolerated the emergence of idiot and lunatic workhouse wards. The 1853 Lunatics (Amendment) Act obviated the need for certification for those transferred from one institution to another, creating in its place a transfer order. Under this system, medical officers of the discharging asylum were obliged to send duplicates of the original certificate to the medical officer of the receiving asylum. In addition to the section of certificates which asked for the 'indications of insanity' given by medical practitioners, this Act added a section on 'indications of insanity' given by others. This addition of other testimonies had operated informally for decades at the York Retreat, which in 1818 formalized its certificates to include sections for both a medical practitioner *and* the patients' family members.

Regardless of the route whence the insane person came, admission to any asylum was still dependent upon the certification by qualified medical practitioners. Thus the certificates originally stated that only those persons licensed as 'physicians, surgeons or apothecaries' were eligible to fill in the details. After the medical profession created a unified registration system in 1858, the next Lunatic Amendment Act, in 1862, substituted 'those licensed under the 1858 Act' for 'physician, surgeon or apothecary'. Several measures were written into the Lunacy Acts to safeguard against possible collusion, either between families and medical practitioners, or between medical practitioners and operators of private licensed homes. Thus, any medical practitioner with an interest, or with a close relative with a direct interest, in a private licensed home could not legally sign a document for a patient to be taken into that same home, nor could a medical officer of any institution sign a certificate for an admission to his own asylum. In cases of non-pauper certificates, the two medical men could not be in practice together, nor could they examine the person at the same time. For pauper patients the signing medical practitioner (before 1853) could not even be the official medical officer of the inmates' parish or union of settlement. Certificates had to be signed within seven days of confinement or they were invalid. In an emergency, a patient could be admitted with only one signature, provided a second *and third* signature were added within three days. Lastly, any signing medical practitioner showed to have deliberately falsified a statement was guilty of a misdemeanour. Not surprisingly, some confusion, or avoidance, persisted. . . . Occasional letters to the editors of medical journals reveal that the system was not foolproof.

The revised Certificates of Insanity for pauper and private patients, and Reception Orders (for all admissions) created by the 1853 Act were relatively successful, remaining for thirty-three years until the Idiots Act came into effect in 1887 and changed the law regarding the certification of idiots.

[. . .]

In conclusion, certification evolved in a piecemeal fashion, repeatedly extended and revised during the six decades following the Madhouses Act of 1774. Legislation enshrined the centrality in, rather than monopoly over, the certification of insanity by the medical profession, but this role was circumscribed and mediated by a number of influences, not least of which were the wishes of the families and the financial considerations of statutory authorities. The survey of legislation concerning the certification of insanity highlights two themes. First, that contrary to general historical interpretation, the nineteenth century did not witness the slow capture of the mad by a medical élite. Rather, the evolution of legislative provision, at first investing medical men with virtually unmediated authority, gradually curtailed the power of doctors, and especially the power of medical superintendents, over the process of certification and confinement. Certification increasingly devolved to non-expert medical men, in collaboration with lay informants. Secondly, legislation progressively erected barriers to the abuse of certification by prohibiting the collaboration of medical men and asylum proprietors, and between individual medical doctors and families.

Part twelve
War and medicine

12.1
Military medicine in the Crimea

Edward M. Wrench, F.R.C.S., V.D., 'The Lessons of the
Crimean War', *British Medical Journal* 1899, II, pp. 205–8.

The Crimean War 1853–56 was fought between England and
France on one side and Russia on the other. The Anglo-French
troops were poorly equipped and suffered from disease and insufficient medical support. Wrench had been an army medical officer
in the Crimea and at the time of this account in 1899 he was
Surgeon Lt. Colonel to the Volunteer Battalion, the Sherwood
Foresters. He was prompted to write this account by the first Boer
War, which began in 1899; there were increasing reports in the
medical journals expressing concern about the medical provision
for the troops in South Africa from late September onwards.

The Crimean campaign was described by the pioneer of war correspon-
dents (Dr. Russell)[1] as 'the most ruinous, most cruel, and least justifiable
of all modern campaigns.' Of the vast host of over a million men that for
nearly two years fought for the occupation of the beautiful harbour of
Sebastopol, I possess the qualification of being one of the now comparatively few survivors, and I trust that the narrative of some of my personal
experiences may be interesting, and, though egotistical, help to explain
why the Crimean war has left such an indelible mark on the minds of

---

[1] William Howard Russell, war correspondent at *The Times* newspaper brought the
appalling conditions in the Crimea to public attention as well as the work of Florence Nightingale and Mary Seacole.

those who were youths in the Fifties. Although the medical establishment of the army was considerably increased when the war was declared in the spring of 1854, the mortality from battle (nine surgeons were killed in the campaign), and disease from overwork, was so alarming that in the autumn surgeons were hurried to the East as rapidly as possible.

I obtained my nomination on Monday, was examined on Tuesday, and started for the Crimea on Friday. I arrived there a few days after the hurricane in November to find the harbour of Balaclava strewn with the wrecks of 17 ships, and was immediately placed in charge of a ward in the hospital located in the Russian Military School, a substantial building, but quite devoid of hospital conveniences, and with every window destroyed by the recent hurricane.

I had charge of from 20 to 30 patients, wounded from Inkermann,[2] mixed with cases of cholera, dysentery and fever. There were no bedsteads or proper bedding. The patients lay in their clothes on the floor, which from the rain blown in through the open windows, and the traffic to and from the open-air latrines, was as muddy as a country road.

There were no nurses, no washing conveniences, either personal or for clothing. Two old soldiers, called orderlies, did their ignorant best to attend to the wants of the patients, but were chiefly occupied in rude cooking and burying the dead.

There was no bread except hard ship's biscuit – of course no milk. I cannot remember if there was any tea, but I believe not, only the famous green coffee. There was certainly no beef tea. Liebeg's extract,[3] and the substitutes of the present day, had not then been invented, and tinned meat was not procurable . . .

Notwithstanding all these shortcomings . . . each surgeon had to make out a daily diet roll with the pretentious headings – Milk, Fish, or Full Diet – to satisfy the red-tape system, and prevent the purveyor being surcharged for the scanty food he was able to supply.

We were practically without medicines; the supply landed at the commencement of the campaign was exhausted, and the reserve had gone to the bottom of the sea, with the winter clothing (and several surgeons) in the wreck of the large steamer (the *Prince*) so that in November, 1854, even the base hospital at Balaclava was devoid of opium, quinine, ammonia, and indeed of all important drugs. Sanitary

[2] The battle of Inkerman was fought in 1854. The Russians were defeated.

[3] Justus von Liebig made an extract of meat by low-pressure evaporation of soup made from lean meat. In 1860s with the help of Giebert (a Brazilian, who worked for Fray Bentos in Uruguay) Liebig marketed 'Liebig's Extract of Beef' as invalid food.

science was then in its infancy, and sanitary precautions were not capable of being carried out, when the living were so hard pressed to live, and dead men were floating about among the ships at Balaclava harbour like dead cats in a canal. You will not be surprised to hear that many of our patients died, but even they were more lucky than the wounded Russians in another building in the town, where hospital gangrene[4] carried off, I believe, every one, which sad termination to his devoted labours young Hervey Ludlow – the surgeon in charge – took so deeply to heart that he died from overwork and exhaustion.

He was, however, the exception, for most of the young surgeons possessed the secret of health – light hearts and good digestion – and instead of being depressed or miserable, indulged when off duty in practical jokes on one another, and believed that each week that Sebastopol would be captured in the next; an opinion, I may remark, shared by the rank and file all through that terrible winter. We should have had better reason for our belief had we known that the Russians (except that they had roofs over their heads) were suffering from scanty food and disease as badly as ourselves. But, as Napoleon remarked . . . 'in war you can see your own troubles: those of the enemy you cannot see.'

Wars always have been and always will be cruel. It is, however, the pride of our profession that, while sharing the fatigues and dangers of the campaign, our sole duty will always be the protection of the soldier from what after all is his most deadly enemy – disease, and the alleviation of the sufferings of the wounded.

The Crimean campaign taught a lesson that I trust will never be forgotten by the nation, that unless the medical department of the army is made efficient, and supplied with its proper compliment of officers and ambulance during peace, it cannot be expected to do its duty efficiently during war.

---

[4] Gangrene is a bacterial infection caused by *Clostridium welchii*, a bacteria common in surgery before antisepsis and on battlefields.

12.2

Nursing in the Crimea

Mary Seacole, *Wonderful Adventures of Mrs. Seacole in Many
Lands* (Oxford, Oxford University Press, 1988 (originally
published in 1857)), pp. 124–6, 143–4, 166.

Mary Seacole (1805–81) was born in Kingston, Jamaica. Her father
was a Scottish soldier and her mother a free-born black woman
who was a doctress. Mary learnt her medical skills from her
mother whose own practice was based in traditional Caribbean
medicine. She had a love of travelling and this took her to Central
America and the Caribbean and to England in 1854. Seacole had no
formal connection to the military, and was refused government
permission to travel to the Crimea, so she financed the journey herself. Her work there made her famous; William Russell, the *Times*
correspondent she refers to in this extract, testified to her skill and
perseverance. After the war, she published this autobiography
which became a best seller.

I hope the reader will give me credit for the assertion that I am about
to make, viz., that I enter upon the particulars of this chapter with
great reluctance; but I cannot omit them, for the simple reason that
they strengthen my one and only claim to interest the public, viz., my
services to the brave British army in the Crimea.

I have never been long in any place before I have found my practical
experience in the science of medicine useful. Even in London I have
found it of service to others. And in the Crimea, where the doctors were
so overworked, and sickness was so prevalent, I could not be long idle;
for I never forgot that my intention of seeking the army was to help the
kind-hearted doctors, to be useful to whom I have ever looked upon and
still regard as so high a privilege.

But before very long I found myself surrounded with patients of my
own, and this for two simple reasons. In the first place, the men (I am
speaking of the 'ranks' now) had a very serious objection for going into
hospital for any but urgent reasons, and the regimental doctors were
rather fond of sending them there; and, in the second place, they could
and did get at my store sick-comforts and nourishing food, which the
heads of the medical staff would sometimes find it difficult to procure.
These reasons, with the additional one that I was very familiar with the

diseases which they suffered most from, and successful in their treatment (I say this in no spirit of vanity), were quite sufficient to account for the numbers who came daily to the British Hotel[5] for medical treatment.

That the officers were glad of me as a doctress and nurse may be easily understood. When a poor fellow lay sickening in his cheerless hut and sent down to me, he knew very well that I should not ride up in answer to his message empty-handed. And although I did not hesitate to charge him with the value of the necessaries I took him, still he was thankful enough to be able to *purchase* them. When we lie ill at home surrounded with comfort, we never think of feeling any special gratitude for the sick-room delicacies which we accept as a consequence of our illness; but the poor officer lying ill and weary in his crazy[6] hut, dependent for the merest necessaries of existence upon a clumsy, ignorant soldier-cook, who would almost prefer eating his meat raw to having the trouble of cooking it (our English soldiers are bad campaigners), often finds his greatest troubles in the want of those little delicacies with which a weak stomach must be humoured into retaining nourishment.

[. . .]

Before I bring this chapter to a close, I should like, with the reader's permission, to describe one day of my life in the Crimea. They are all pretty much alike, except when there was fighting upon a large scale going on, and duty called me to the field. I was generally up and busy by daybreak, sometimes earlier, for in the summer my bed had no attractions strong enough to bind me to it after four. There was plenty to do before the work of the day began. There was the poultry to pluck and prepare for cooking, which had been killed on the previous night; the joints to be cut up and got ready for the same purpose; the medicines to be mixed; the store to be swept and cleaned. Of very great importance, with all these things to see after, were the few hours of quiet before the road became alive with travellers. By seven o'clock in the morning coffee would be ready, hot and refreshing, and eagerly sought for by the officers of the Army Works Corps engaged upon making the great highroad to the front, and the Commissariat and Land Transport men carrying stores from Balaclava to the heights . . . about half-past nine my sick patients began to show themselves. In the following hour they came thickly, and sometimes it was past twelve before I had got through

---

[5] The British hotel was set up by Seacole, two miles from Balaclava; it provided food and provisions, and also the space for an officer's club.

[6] i.e. ramshackle.

this duty. They came with every variety of suffering and disease; the cases I most disliked were the frostbitten fingers and feet in the winter. That over, there was the hospital to visit across the way, which was sometimes overcrowded with patients ... By this time the day's news had come from the front, and perhaps among the casualties over night there would be some one wounded or sick, who would be glad to see me ride up with some comforts he stood most in need of; and during the day, if any accident occurred in the neighbourhood or on the road near the British Hotel, the men generally brought the sufferer there, whence, if the hurt was serious, he would be transferred to the hospital of the Land Transport opposite. I used not always to stand upon too much ceremony when I heard of sick or wounded officers at the front. Sometimes their friends would ask me to go to them, though very often I waited for no hint, but took the chance of meeting with a kind reception. I used to think of their relatives at home, who would have given so much to possess my knowledge; and more than one officer have I startled by appearing before him, and telling him abruptly that he must have a mother, wife, or sister at home whom he missed, and that he must therefore be glad of some woman to take their place.

[. . .]

I attended to the wounds of many French and Sardinians, and helped to lift them into the ambulances, which came tearing up to the scene of action. I derived no little gratification of being able to dress the wounds of several Russians; indeed, they were as kindly treated as the others.

[. . .]

The *Times* correspondent ... noticed me, and his mind, albeit engrossed with far more important memories, found room to remember me. I may well be proud of his testimony, borne so generously only the other day, and may well be excused for transcribing it from the columns of the *Times*:– 'I have seen her go down, under fire, with her little store of creature comforts for our wounded men; and a more tender or skilful hand about a wound or a broken limb could not be found among our best surgeons. I saw her at the assault on the Redan, at the Tchernaya, at the fall of Sebastopol, laden, not with plunder, good old soul! but with wine, bandages, and food for the wounded or the prisoners.'

12.3

Civilian health in the First World War

J. Winter, *The Great War and the British People* (London,
Macmillan, 1985), pp. 117, 120–1, 123–4, 134–5, 138–40.

The historian J.M. Winter has published widely on the First World
War, especially on family work and welfare. *The Great War and the
British People* was one of the first books to examine in detail the
effect of the war on civilian life. Up to this point, it had been
assumed that the health of the civilian population had suffered
during the war due to food and fuel shortages. Winter argued that
civilian health, especially that of the poorer classes, actually
improved during the war as the result of better nutrition.

**Mortality decline among civilians in wartime Britain: the
female population of England and Wales, 1912–21**

We can broaden our discussion of the impact of the First World War on
civilian health by considering evidence on mortality decline among the
female population. These data are a better guide to demographic
trends, since they do not have the drawback of statistics concerning
men, which inevitably reflect a highly unusual age structure among non-
combatants in wartime. The female population of Britain was more
stable and therefore a better subject for analysis over time.

[. . .]

[A]part from providing additional reasons to discard the view that civilian health deteriorated in wartime Britain, these data also permit us to
explore many features of public health in this period. These suggest
possible ways in which to account for the unanticipated gains in survival chances registered during the 1914–18 war. In particular, they
indicate that an important factor in maintaining and improving public
health in wartime was better nutrition. This was particularly important
in the case of infants, whose death rates dropped more dramatically
than was the case for any other age group in this period.

. . . These data [Table 1] show the extent and components of female
mortality decline in England and Wales in the war decade. First let us
deal with variations over time, and then turn to variations by cause of

TABLE 1 *STANDARDIZED ANNUAL FEMALE DEATH RATES, BY GROUPS OF CAUSES, AT ALL AGES, TO A MILLION LIVING, ENGLAND AND WALES, 1912–21*[a]

Cause	1912–14	1915	1916	1917	1918	1919–21
1. All	12,263	13,368	11,999	11,702	15,135	10,992
(without flu epidemic)					11,893	10,694
2. Respiratory tuberculosis	850	864	928	982	1,082	795
3. Other infectious and parasitic infections	1,291	1,525	1,087	1,121	1,402	902
4. Neoplasms	1,027	1,064	1,063	1,039	1,029	1,039
5. Cardiovascular diseases	2,374	2,470	2,338	2,277	2,129	2,084
6. Influenza, bronchitis, and pneumonia	2,006	2,587	2,113	2,092	5,498	2,228
(without flu epidemic)					2,264[b]	1,943[b]
7. Diarrhoeal diseases	519	508	472	367	357	335
8. Certain degenerative diseases[c]	568	567	502	446	405	392
9. Complications of pregnancy	181	174	164	131	125	176
10. Certain diseases of infancy	795	718	719	686	759	788
11. Accidents and violence	308	323	316	312	286	264
12. Other and unknown causes	2,344	2,568	2,297	2,249	2,063	1,989

[a] Crude death rates were standardized by the direct method, using the age structure of the female population of England and Wales in 1901. (Rounding errors account for the difference between the totals and the sum of the 12 categories.)

[b] The average death rate in 1915–17 was used to approximate non-epidemic mortality levels in 1918 and 1919.

[c] Nephritis, Bright's disease, stomach ulcer, diabetes, and cirrhosis of the liver.

SOURCES: Preston, *et al.*, *Causes of Death*, Table 1–2, and p. 242; *Registrar-General's Annual Report, 1912–1919*, and *Statistical Review, 1920–21.*

261

death. Taking standardized annual female death rates in 1912–14 as our basis of comparison, index figures show that 1915 was a year of high mortality due both to influenza, bronchitis, and pneumonia and to the general category of 'other infectious and parasitic diseases', incorporating common diseases of childhood, such as whooping cough, diphtheria, and measles, as well as more general ailments such as non-respiratory tuberculosis and meningitis. Some of this increase was probably due to the normal periodicity of infectious diseases, a point to which we shall return below. After 1915, though, mortality rates for most categories clearly declined.

This is most emphatically the case with diarrhoeal diseases, which afflicted the very young and the very old, and which are a very sensitive indicator of nutritional levels. Death rates due to this one cause declined by 35 per cent between 1912–14 and 1919–21. A similarly impressive decline of over 30 per cent over the war period was also registered by certain degenerative diseases (such as nephritis[7] and cirrhosis of the liver[8], which kill older people. Between 1912–14 and 1918, mortality due to complications of pregnancy also dropped by 30 per cent, although some of these gains were reversed in the immediate post-war period. This was probably a reflection of the high incidence of influenza among young women in 1918–19, a point to which we shall return below.

These data also show which diseases did not contribute to the overall pattern of declining mortality in wartime . . . [I]t is apparent that the only category which moved unambiguously against the general trend was respiratory tuberculosis.

In Table 2, which lists index figures of age-specific female death rates, we can see which age groups' death rates declined most sharply during the war. Taking age-specific death rates in 1912–14 as 100, these data show that after 1915, children below the age of 5 and adults between ages 30 and 60 registered clear gains in survival chances. The very elderly and those in the age group 10–30 were not so fortunate, largely because of an increase in their death rates due to respiratory tuberculosis and other infectious diseases. The first conclusion we can draw from this analysis, therefore, is that a number of nutrition-related diseases, affecting in particular, young children, older adults, and (with some qualifications) women in childbirth, led the overall decline in wartime mortality rates.

[. . .]

---

[7] *nephritis*: inflammation of the kidneys.
[8] *cirrhosis of the liver*: serious damage to liver cells.

TABLE 2 AN INDEX OF AGE-SPECIFIC FEMALE DEATH RATES, ENGLAND AND WALES,
1912–21 (1912–14 = 100)[a]

Age	1912–14	1915	1916	1917	1918	1919–21
0–1	100	99	87	85	92	71
1–4	100	122	85	92	103	68
5–9	100	119	99	99	109	81
10–14	100	114	108	109	113	84
15–19	100	113	111	119	125	93
20–24	100	108	107	108	119	94
25–29	100	106	105	101	112	94
30–34	100	103	97	94	84	84
35–39	100	111	105	99	101	83
40–44	100	103	95	93	90	73
45–49	100	105	96	92	90	74
50–54	100	111	101	94	94	76
55–59	100	104	95	92	87	75
60–64	100	108	94	93	88	77
65–69	100	108	103	98	97	82
70–74	100	111	102	95	90	76
75–79	100	115	108	107	101	81
80–84	100	111	106	100	95	75
85+	100	114	111	104	97	68

[a] Age-specific death rates for pneumonia and influenza in 1915–17 have been used to approximate non-epidemic mortality trends.

SOURCES: Totals of causes of death were found in the *Registrar-General's Annual Reports* (later *Statistical Reviews*) *for England and Wales*, 1912–21; age-specific populations were taken from *Decennial Supplement to the Registrar-General's Report for England and Wales, 1911–20*, (1933) Pt 1, Table 1.

[R]isks of pregnancy and childbirth in the war years were no worse but not much better than in either the pre-war or post-war periods. In 1917, for example, total puerperal mortality[9] rates were almost identical to those registered in 1911; associated mortality rates were also indistinguishable from the 1912 levels. As we shall note below with respect to infant mortality, 1915 was a relatively bad year, but taken as a whole, the pre-war trend was not significantly altered during the war. If anything stands out . . . it is that the post-war decade was a period of greater risk for women in childbirth than were the years of the 1914–18 conflict.

[. . .]

[9] *puerperal mortality*: deaths associated with childbirth.

The material we have presented above does suggest other ways in which the 1914–18 war effort set in motion contradictory forces affecting the health and survival chances of the civilian population. The war economy created some conditions which helped reduce mortality rates. Indeed, the substantial fall in deaths due to diarrhoeal disease and to complications of pregnancy and childbirth would not have been possible had there been a major deterioration in levels of nutrition during the war. The same is true in the case of common infectious diseases, as well as in diseases of maternity and early childhood. We shall present substantial evidence as to the unintentional effects of the war in raising family incomes and thereby nutritional levels especially among the worst-off sections of the community. Despite (or as we shall argue, because of) the fact that a sizeable number of married women joined the workforce during the war, mortality rates among women during childbirth and among their offspring dropped substantially. This was in flat contradiction of the views of many who argued before 1914 that high female workforce participation rates were responsible for high infant and maternal mortality . . .

The evidence concerning respiratory diseases seems to point in the opposite direction and suggests countervailing aspects of the impact of war. The Registrar-General of England and Wales, in the Decennial Supplement for 1911–20, concluded that undernutrition was responsible for the increase in tuberculosis mortality during the war. Other scholars have followed this lead. But it is surprising that relatively little attention has been directed to two other aspects of the war experience which may account for the recrudescence[10] of respiratory tuberculosis and other respiratory diseases during and after the war. The first is the transfer of large populations, many from rural or suburban areas, to urban centres of war production and their concentration in munitions factories. The second is the deterioration in housing conditions and the postponement of necessary demolition and sanitary work by local authorities during the war. Together these adverse effects of the war probably provided ideal conditions for the spread of respiratory infections, and helped tip the balance between latent and active cases of tuberculosis. The stress of overwork and anxiety over the fate of family and friends in the army may also have undermined the resistance of those (especially among the elderly) suffering from this and other diseases. It is important to note that similar, if not worse, housing conditions during the 1939–45 war produced very similar results. There was a recrudescence of tuberculosis mortality in 1940–2 which paralleled

---

[10] *recrudescence*: return after a period of abatement.

that of 1914–16, and in Hitler's war it was clear that nutritional levels had improved.

It is always dangerous to isolate any one environmental variable and to declare that it was the key element influencing trends in vital statistics . . . But the link between tuberculosis and other respiratory diseases on the one hand and inadequate housing on the other is well enough established to permit us to advance an argument about the likely effects of this aspect of war conditions on public health.

The view that working and housing conditions rather than increasingly inadequate levels of nutrition were responsible for the rise in tuberculosis death rates in wartime is reinforced by a glance at the post-war history of the cohort which evidenced the most substantial increase in tuberculosis death rates – young people aged 10–25. Had this cohort suffered undernutrition at a critical period of their development, we would expect to see higher than normal death rates among this group ten years later, that is, at ages 20–35 in 1925–28, or 20 years later, at ages 30–34 in 1935–8. But such was not the case. The most likely reason is that most recruits to munitions production returned home after the war, and that by the mid-1920s and certainly by the end of the 1930s, deferred housing improvements had finally been carried out.

The overall interpretation that emerges from this analysis of female mortality rates is that the war period was one of major gains in the survival chances of the civilian population. Again we find substantial corroboration for the results of our analyses of life tables and occupational mortality statistics. It is important to note, though, that some causes of death (especially tuberculosis) did rise, and some age groups (especially the very elderly) did not share in the general improvement.

But the general picture seems clear. The Great War created the conditions which helped eliminate some of the worst features of urban poverty which lay behind the appallingly high death rates of late-Victorian and Edwardian Britain. Long-term trends towards improving life expectancy were no doubt of importance, but special features of the war economy underlay the increasing survival chances of civilians . . .

In sum the evidence presented in this chapter suggests that one of the most important demographic effects of the First World War in Britain was to compress the class structure in such a way as to reduce the distance between the survival chances of different classes and between different strata within classes. It would have surprised many of those who took the decision to go to war in 1914 to know that they were unleashing forces leading not only to unprecedented slaughter but also to an improvement in the conditions under which large sections of the urban and rural population lived. But unbeknownst to them, that may have been precisely where their action led.

12.4

The causes of shell-shock

Report of the War Office Committee of Enquiry into 'Shell-Shock' (London, His Majesty's Stationery Office, 1922), pp. 17, 55–7.

Between 1920 and 1922, this committee of enquiry investigated the nature and treatment of shell-shock in the Great War. During and after the war, practitioners and administrators debated whether shell shock was 'malingering' or cowardice, or a functional neurosis. This debate was further complicated by investigations into the execution of soldiers during the war; popular opinion and the Labour Party demanded answers as to whether these soldiers had in fact been suffering from shell-shock. Furthermore, the worsening state of the economy in 1921 provoked cuts in various services including war pensions; in 1920 there had been 65,000 ex-serviceman drawing disability pensions on the basis of neurasthenia.

William John Adie was an Australian who trained at Edinburgh and joined the 1st Northamptonshire Regiment as a medical officer on the outbreak of war. He worked throughout the war on the Western Front, including acting as consultant to the army centre for head wounds. On demobilisation he took up medical positions in London, and published on neurological subjects. In 1922, he was acting as neurologist for the Ministry of Pensions in addition to his clinical duties.

William Halse Rivers Rivers was an anthropologist, neurophysiologist and psychologist. His anthropology had taken him to the Torres Strait in 1898 and to India in the early twentieth century. He later worked as a physician in several London hospitals, and was University lecturer in psychology at Cambridge. During the First World War he worked as a psychiatrist with the Royal Army Medical Corps. Part of this time was spent at Craiglockhart Hospital in Scotland where he worked with patients with a diagnosis of shell-shock, including Siegfried Sassoon.

Major W.J. Adie, M.D., M.R.C.P., R.A.M.C. (Special Reserve); Physician, Great Northern Central Hospital; Neurologist Min. of Pensions.

Another witness (Major Adie), who was asked to tell the Committee what he thought 'shell-shock' was, answered in these terms:-

'It seemed to me to cover all the various conditions which have been described as "shell shock" in the late war. I should say any state of mind or body engendered or perpetuated by fear, which renders the soldier less efficient or enables him to evade his duty with impunity. I have thought about that, and I think we must admit that all these conditions are either engendered by fear, or having been engendered by something else, such as concussion, are perpetuated by fear. I say "renders the soldier less efficient" as many of us were suffering more or less from "shell shock," which made us not so efficient, and yet we remained in the line; "or enabled him to evade his duty with impunity" – I mean by that that all sorts of people got out of the line with so-called "shell shock", and the result was that they evaded their full duty and yet were not punished'.

When the witness was asked whether he considered that 'shell shock' would arise not only in the individual from some strong commotion or emotion, but also in a body of men, he answered that that was certainly so. He instanced two battalions side by side in . . . France. In one the morale was good – it had a good colonel and officers and a good medical officer – and they had practically no men going down with 'shell shock'. The other battalion was sending ten men away at a time. 'You could have foretold that it would be so by looking to the men's appearance. In the good battalion the men were always smart, but the others were bad soldiers with bad officers. That is the crux of the matter. Keep up the morale of the troops and you will not have emotional "shell shock", at least you will reduce it tremendously.'

The late W.H.R. Rivers, Esq., M.D., F.R.C.P., LL.D.; late Consultant in Psychological Medicine to Royal Air Force; Praelector in Natural Science, St. John's College, Cambridge.

Dr. Rivers, asked what he thought of the term 'shell shock', said he objected to it root and branch. The reason why he objected to the term was that so far as he could see the main factor had been stress, and the shock in most cases was merely the last straw. Any disturbance might have produced the same result. Stress, in his opinion, was really the important factor. Although one could not make a division accurately one ought to distinguish between two varieties of case.

One is the officer who breaks down soon after going to the front because he is unfitted for the position in which he finds himself, and the other is the officer who breaks down after long and continued strain. It is doubtful whether the cases of the first class ought to be called cases of neurosis. In his experience they were not very severe as a rule and got well easily, unless they were mismanaged when sent home. The other class of case, which is much more important, is the man who breaks down after long and continued strain. These were the men who, especially in the early stages of the war, after some shell explosion or something else had knocked them out badly, went on struggling to do their duty until they finally collapsed entirely. Cases of that kind presented especially severe symptoms. All these cases were much of the same order, only people who broke down before they went over to France did not want stress to cause them to break down; they were ready to break down immediately. The man who got to France had stress. There is no question of that; perhaps, for him, a very big stress indeed. The case of the man totally unfitted for warfare finding himself in the trenches meant a very big stress for him. Stress is relative. He had not immediate experience of men who broke down shortly after joining the army, but he was doubtful whether they ought to be called cases of war neurosis.

A man should not develop a real neurosis unless he had strain; it depends on the man. There are cases intermediate between the two classes. Men whom a small shock would knock out. If a patient was asked to compare the shock which knocked him out with his previous experience of shell explosion, the answer usually was that the shell explosion which knocked him out finally was trivial compared with his previous experiences. He had had much severer shocks after which he had picked himself up and perhaps laughed at the experience . . .

That was the kind of experience which lead the witness to lay so much weight on the fact of stress, using stress as a wide term, including sleeplessness, anxiety, fatigue, responsibility.

Asked whether there was any doubt in his mind as to the existence of a mental wound arising from emotional shock in contradistinction to any concussion, the witness said he should be inclined to put it in this way, that when the man began to have a number of disturbances of different kinds, such as loss of sleep, etc., he either consciously or more or less unconsciously looked for an explanation, and this tended to centre around some particular experience, in many cases a comparatively trivial experience. Asked whether it would be fair to say that there is such a thing as a mental wound arising under these conditions, the witness answered in the affirmative, adding that he had got into the habit of calling it trauma rather than wound . . .

Asked as to morale, the witness said, 'My experience is that the whole object of military training is to produce *esprit de corps* and other factors which give good morale, and that the lack of them is a very strong factor in the production of neurosis of certain kinds. It would tend to diminish these varieties of neurosis in which the soldier breaks down rapidly, if the military training were successful as it was in the regular army, where it was exceptional for a man to break down except after severe stress. One influence of this was that when the regular soldier broke down, particularly the private soldier and the regular non-commissioned officer, he suffered severely from shame; the soldier serving only for the war had not that sentiment produced by the regular training. The reason why we had such enormous numbers suffering with neurosis in this war was the incomplete training.'

[. . .]

Every animal has a natural reaction to danger, perhaps more than one, and man's is manipulation of such a kind as to get him out of the dangerous situation. Of course, the pilot [of a plane] is able to utilise that in a supreme degree. When in danger his whole mind is taken up with guiding the machine and so on. The observer,[11] on the other hand, although occupied in various ways, is not occupied to the same extent. He had periods of considerable stress, especially when going up, when he has not anything to do. He is not in charge; he has his own special work to do, but he has not the same chance of manipulative activity as the pilot. . . . If he cannot have that [manipulative activity], or if it is restricted in any way, you have a prominent condition for the occurrence of neurosis in one form or another.

[11] In a tethered observation balloon.

269

12.5
Civilian health re-examined

Linda Bryder, 'The First World War: Healthy or Hungry?',
History Workshop Journal, vol. 24, 1987, pp. 142–50.

Linda Bryder is a historian of medicine who has published extensively on the history of tuberculosis. In this article she challenges
J. Winter's thesis laid out in his book, *The Great War and the
British People* (1985), that civilian mortality declined between
1914 and 1918 as a result of improved nutrition. According to
Bryder, the causal relationships between specific diseases and specific social factors is much more complex than Winter portrays.

Winter bases his argument on health statistics as well as economic data.
His health statistics consist of an analysis of the causes and rates of death
(mortality). Data on the incidence of disease and ill-health (morbidity)
are not readily attainable, they are unreliable and difficult to quantify,
and for that reason Winter neglects them. However, death rates are
not necessarily a reliable indication of the health of the people at any
particular time and may disguise a prevalence of chronic ill-health. Thus,
the neglect of a discussion of morbidity must remain a serious short-
coming and limits the value of any conclusions reached on the topic
under discussion.

A study of health relies on epidemiology, the study of the relationship
between certain factors such as nutrition, housing, sanitation, working
conditions, and disease patterns. These relationships are complex, with
no simple straight-forward causal links. Assertions by Winter such as
that nutrition had nothing to do with tuberculosis and everything to do
with infantile gastro-enteritis must be regarded with suspicion, as will
be discussed. Moreover, Winter accepts certain assumptions, such as
that infant mortality rates are a reliable index of the health of the entire
population, which are not necessarily valid.

[. . .]

Apart from increases in 1915 and 1918, female mortality rates declined
during the First World War. That the decline in female mortality during
the war was directly related to improved nutrition was evident, according to Winter, as the decline occurred primarily in 'nutrition-related
diseases': diarrhoea, and complications in pregnancy and childbirth.

The former may indeed be indicative of an improvement in nutrition, although, as will be discussed below, diarrhoeal diseases may also be an indication of the quality of the food supply – its cleanliness – rather than of its nutritional value. The maternal mortality data show that the risks of pregnancy and childbirth in the war years were no worse, but not much better, than in either the pre-war or post-war periods (see Table I) . . . Winter concludes, therefore, that the pre-war trend was not significantly altered during the war. He writes that if anything stands out, it is that the post-war decade was a period of greater risk for women in childbirth than were the years of the war. These statistics and Winter's own interpretation of them, do not, however, support his later statement that 'the substantial fall in deaths due to diarrhoeal disease and to complications of pregnancy and childbirth would not have been possible had there been a major deterioration in levels of nutrition during the war'.

TABLE I

Maternal mortality rates in England and Wales, 1911–33 (per live births registered)

1911	3.87	1919	4.37	1927	4.11
1912	3.98	1920	4.33	1928	4.42
1913	3.96	1921	3.92	1929	4.33
1914	4.17	1922	3.81	1930	4.40
1915	4.18	1923	3.82	1931	4.11
1916	4.12	1924	3.90	1932	4.21
1917	3.89	1925	4.08	1933	4.51
1918	3.79	1926	4.12		

Source: Winter, pp. 136–7.

The role of nutrition in maternal mortality in any case has been thrown into question by the recent work of Irvine Loudon. Loudon shows that mortality rates in childbirth from 1850 to 1935 were often higher among middle-class working-class women, and concludes that there was a marked correlation between high death rates and medical intervention. If Loudon is right in pointing to medical intervention as a prime determining factor, then we may be forced to a startling conclusion about the slight (but not substantial) improvement noted by Winter during the war. The decline in mortality might actually have been a function of the depletion of the medical profession owing to wartime mobilisation; and the increase in the post-war period, which Winter notes, a result of the resumption by doctors of normal duties!

While the general trend in female mortality was one of decline during the war, significant rises occurred in mortality from respiratory diseases, an anomaly which Winter addresses. A dramatic increase in deaths from influenza occurred in 1918 owing to the influenza epidemic. . . .

While it can be accepted that the 1918 epidemic was unrelated to the war economy (although it was possibly still related to war conditions, the movement of troops helping to spread the disease), the death rates from respiratory diseases in general rose during the war before the epidemic, which requires explanation. Winter believes this to be somehow related to 'the peculiarities of the English', unconnected with the war:

> The fact that in the war period mortality due to respiratory complaints moved against the general downward trend therefore may have had as much to do with enduring features of British life, such as the climate and the degree of urbanization, as with the special circumstances of war.

This explanation sounds exceedingly familiar to anyone who has made a study of the annual reports of the Chief Medical Officer of the Ministry of Health in the inter-war years, 'the climate' and 'the degree of urbanisation' often being used to explain away undesirable lapses in improving health trends. While it is true that bronchitis was so prevalent in England compared to some other countries that it was known as the 'English disease', this does not satisfactorily explain the rise during the war.

However, it is the rise in deaths from respiratory tuberculosis which Winter has most difficulty in reconciling with his thesis. There was a 25 per cent increase in deaths from respiratory tuberculosis in England and Wales from 1913 to 1918, and a 35 per cent increase among women aged 20–25. Respiratory tuberculosis is an infectious disease, most commonly spread by droplet infection,[12] but there are also predisposing factors accounting for the susceptibility of certain persons at certain times. Winter postulates two reasons for the rise in tuberculosis death rates during the First World War: first, the transfer of large populations to urban centres of war production and their concentration in munition factories, and second, the deterioration in housing conditions, and the postponement of necessary demolition and sanitary work by local authorities during the war. He claims that virtually all observers accepted that the rise in tuberculosis death rates was 'a negative and largely unavoidable consequence of the concentration of large numbers of factory workers working under considerable stress and living in inad-

---

[12] *droplet infection*: infection spread in droplets of moisture from the upper respiratory tract by coughing or sneezing.

equate housing'. He quotes 'one observer' who stated that 'TB deaths were a direct outcome of "overcrowding, overwork, and overstrain", but not of poor nutrition'.

Housing and working conditions were undoubtedly important factors in the rise in tuberculosis death rates during the war. However, present-day epidemiologists would not dismiss malnutrition as a possible predisposing cause of tuberculosis in the way Winter does or claims contemporaries to have done. In fact, it is not true to say that contemporary observers denied the significance of nutrition . . . [Many] immediately after the war, stressed the importance of malnutrition in causing the rise in respiratory tuberculosis during the war.

In his annual report for the Ministry of Health in 1921, Newman wrote, 'The close association of poverty or lack of nutrition with a tendency to higher tuberculosis death rates is increasingly evident' . . .

It was commonly believed immediately after the war that the rise in death rates from pulmonary tuberculosis among young women was associated with their employment in the munition industries, although . . . there was no statistical evidence available to support this. In the view of F.J.H. Coutts, senior medical officer in the Ministry of Health, the overstrain associated with industrial conditions was an important factor, as well as nutrition. However, the death rate also increased in the age group 5–14; and industrial employment could not explain this rise. Stevenson suggested that these children may have suffered from a change in diet, such as deprivation of fats. A study of tuberculosis rates and female employment in 28 London boroughs in 1911–13, which Greenwood referred to in 1919, showed a negative correlation between the index of employment for women and the tuberculosis rates. Greenwood thought that this probably demonstrated that better nutrition compensated for the ill-effects of industrial environment, explaining, 'the parlous state of unemployed or casually employed widows with dependents is notorious'.

[. . .]

Thus, it is certainly not true to say, as Winter does, that most observers following the war denied or even belittled the possible role played by nutrition in causing death rates from tuberculosis to rise between 1914 and 1918. It was only much later that Sir George Newman denied the importance of malnutrition as a predisposing factor in tuberculosis. This was a response to the challenge of the nutritional studies which by the early 1930s were revealing a proportion of the population to be suffering from malnutrition. Social investigators and nutritionists were arguing that the government's social policies were responsible for widespread malnutrition. Given that Newman was now committing himself to the view that 'Though specially sought for, of evidence of widespread malnutrition there is none', and that there was 'no available evidence of any general increase in physical impairment, in sickness or in mortality, as a result of the economic depression or unemployment', it is hardly surprising that he sought the causes of the (undeniably) high tuberculosis rates in depressed areas elsewhere, most commonly in theories of 'the strain of modern living'.

[. . .]

Thus the rise of tuberculosis during the First World War is not adequately explained. Moreover, most of Winter's discussion of health deals with national statistics which disguise regional and class variations and do not support his argument that the poorest people gained most in terms of health improvement.

12.6
The soldier's view

'The Misfit Soldier', Edward Casey's War Story, 1914–1918,
ed. Joanna Bourke (Cork, Cork University Press, 1999),
pp. 52–4.

Edward Casey was born in 1898, in the East End of London to a family of Irish extraction. He left school at 14 and volunteered to join the Royal Dublin Fusiliers in late 1914. His labelling of himself as a 'misfit' began during his training in Ireland, where he saw himself as a cockney first and Irish only by descent. He was not an enthusiastic soldier. He struggled against military discipline and deserted a number of times. He suffered from shell-shock, and admits to trying to avoid duty by feigning madness. Despite this, he served throughout the war both in France and in Salonika (Greece). He survived and moved to Australia, where, in 1980, he wrote this memoir.

NB: Casey's original text is full of idiosyncratic spellings and grammar: for instance he refers to himself as both 'I' and 'he' sometimes in the same sentence. In this extract I have retained Joanna Bourke's editing which makes the sense of the text clear.

My chance came for my greatest malingering effort. There was talk of a big push, and the bombardment was raging all along the whole front, and our section (Ypres) seem[ed] to be getting more than its fair share. The village where we lived suffered a long barrage [of] shell fire. Houses tumbled. [There were] great big holes in the ground which were quickly occupied by civvies[13] and troops alike. I was in very bad shape: it was the worst shelling I had experienced. When it was over . . . I decided I had had enough and lay in the mud with my tunic covering my head. When they found me, after my black[out], the two bearers lifted me and took me to the Clearing Station[14] . . . On examining me, one of the Bearers was telling the Doctor, saying 'I don't think he got one[15] I can see no blood. The exam[ination] was very brief and [I heard the Doctor] telling [them] to take me away. [They] put the usual label on my tunic, carried [me] out to an ambulance with four other (2 lying and us sitting). It was a very rough ride, and I was very thankful [that] I was not wounded. I know I would [have] bled to death like the bloke on the bottom bunk. I was still shivering and shaking with fright, and [with a] lump on my head (how I got it, God knows). [They] carried [me] into a big tent, with stretchers lying on the floor [and] Orderlies, Nurses and Doctors [were] examining Patients, telling [them] where they were to go. My turn came, and I heard [them say], Base.

At the base hospital, I did not have a clue what Base I was in [or] what front I had come from. I heard talk of Loos, Cloth Hall Hill 60.[16] I was still in a state of shock. Now [I was] lying in the bed with clean sheets, clean body, [and] Orderlies that cleaned him. My thoughts were now on whether I can fool the Doctors . . . I had the usual tests . . . The Doctors were asking me questions while the examination went [on], and to every[thing] they asked I replied, 'I don't remember'. The Head Doctor said, 'We cannot keep him here. He requires special treatment, [and] saying something like, 'Amnesia. Shell shock.' He wrote on my card, 'Evacuate'.

Later, I was carried to the Hospital Train. It was dark. I woke to the noise of whistles blowing. The noise of seagulls made [me] think I was on a wharf, and very soon [I was] being carried on a very large Hospital Ship. Although I could not see [much, I could see] only the long wards with all beds with their white quilts in a straight line. VADs [Voluntary Aid Detachment nurses] everywhere. It must have been a rough trip, the

---

[13] Civilians.

[14] The Casualty Clearing Station – where wounded troops were taken from the battlefield. There, they received some treatment, and would be returned to their units or sent on to hospitals.

[15] A wound.

[16] These were places on the Western front.

way she rolled from side to side, and up and down. Sleepily, I noticed we were in calm water. And when we were unloaded and I was in the Hospital, I heard them say we were in the Infirmary in Bristol.

It was not very long [before] I was wondering, 'how the hell I was to get memory back'. [For a] week or so I was in my coma, being fed, taken to the toilet, being examined by various Doctors, one who (when I [was] taken to his office) [was] telling me to lay down. He was going to put me to sleep. I was telling myself, 'Oh no you don't! I won't let you! [I saw the Doctor] taking out a gold watch, swinging it by the chain, saying, 'You are now very sleepy. Just raise your arm.' I was telling myself, 'I won't raise my arm!', but I could not stop my arm rising till it was straight and rigid. I felt very angry with myself for obeying his commands. Now this happened in 1916, and mermerism[17] was then (I'm told) a medical rarity and not very often practised. Those Medical Blokes tell you nothing, for when they carried [out] all their tests, and found I was malingering, I felt certain I would be for the firing squad: it would be 'fini'. The solution came that night. The sound of anti-aircraft guns thundered in the still night, flashes were everywhere in the sky, [and I found myself] jumping out of bed, yelling at the top of his voice, 'Lay down! Dig your face in the mud! They'll be over after this!' [I was] running to the toilet and jumping into the bath. I was getting expert at putting on a shivering fit. I heard the nurse running after me, followed by a couple of Convalescents, who lifted me out and carried me back to bed. Later, the MO [medical officer] came to see me, giving me some dope saying, 'This will [help you] sleep for a while.' The Nurse [who was] stroking my head, said, 'When you wake tomorrow, everything will [be] all right. Sleep now, Dear.' This very young VAD treated me as if I were a child. Now I had obtained my objective, and was back in blighty,[18] things looked so different.

The Doctor who put me to sleep examined me again. I had to tell him everything I remembered before the barrage. [Here I was] talking and telling him lies, while he wrote every word I spoke in a book, telling me my complaint of shattered nerves was becoming very prevalent among fighting troops. [He said] 'You may suffer further attacks if frightened or [on] hearing sudden explosions. All you require now (for a while) is rest, exercise, and good food.'

[17] Casey's misspelling of 'mesmerism', now called hypnosis.
[18] Back in Britain.

Part thirteen

Access to care, 1880–1930

13.1

Self-medication

Robert Roberts, *The Classic Slum. Salford Life in the First Quarter of the Century* (Manchester, Manchester University Press, 1971), pp. 97–9.

In the early twentieth century – as in the present – most illness was diagnosed not by doctors, but by the sufferer, who also treated the problem using over-the-counter remedies. Robert Roberts's account of working-class life in the north of England, seen from the vantage point of the corner shop, gives a valuable insight into the trade in patent medicines, and the criteria by which purchasers judged the value of these remedies.

This was the heyday of quack medicines, a time when millions of the new literates were reading newspaper advertisements without the knowledge to gauge their worth. Innumerable nostrums, some harmless, some vicious, found ready sale among the ignorant. One had to be seriously ill before a household would saddle itself with the expense of calling a doctor,* in our case an elderly Irishman famous for kindness and wheezing whisky fumes. At week ends people purged themselves with great doses of black draught, senna pods, cascara sagrada, and

---

* In our district more people were sued in the county court for non-payment of doctors' bills than for any other reason. This somewhat dents the myth of the golden-hearted medico 'forgetting' the debts of his poorer patients. But in that world of private enterprise many slum doctors were hard up enough until the Health Insurance Act of 1911 (against which the BMA fought tooth and nail) put them off their bicycles and into motor cars.

their young with Gregory powder, licorice powder and California syrup of figs. For all these on Friday they came to the shop in constant procession. Through the advice of doctors and wide advertisement the working class had an awful fear of constipation, a condition brought on by the kind of food they ate.

The sick too found relief in medicaments from the corner shop, supplied by manufacturing 'chemists'. Few of these had any qualifications. One of the traders who sold to us had entered the profession via the mineral water business. His early attempts at a cough medicine (6*d* per two-ounce bottle), though attractive in colour, had run thin as ginger beer and fallen a drug on the market.[1] But he learned quickly. With such mixtures content and colouring meant little; high viscosity was all. His next concoction slid down the gullet like warm pitch. Bronchitics swore by it and sales soared.

Pills sold at a penny a box, any doubts as to their potency being quieted by the venerable image of their maker smiling from the lid. He had cause for amusement. Nearly all the pills appeared to possess a dual purpose: they 'attacked' at one and the same time the ills of two intestines—'Head and Stomach', 'Blood and Stomach', 'Back and Kidney', 'Back and Bladder', and indeed almost any pair of organs that could in decency be named. Whatever their aim, however, for ease of manufacture all pills contained the same ingredients—soap and a little aperient;[2] but they differed in colour, the 'blood and stomach' variety being red, say, and the 'back and bladder' a pea green. Some colour sense was required, it seemed, in marketing. A pink blood and digestive pill might go down famously in Leeds, only to be rejected entirely by Liverpudlians, whose stomachs would settle for nothing but a pellet in a warm brown shade.

With us a week seldom passed without somebody's baby having 'convulsions'. 'Mother's Friend', known in the district as 'Knock-out Drops', was always in demand for the fretful, especially on mid-Saturday evenings. 'It relieves your child from pains,' said the advertisement, 'and the little cherub awakes bright as a button.' This 'Soothing Mixture' (laced with tincture of opium) would guarantee to keep baby in a coma until late Sunday morning. Meanwhile mother spent two happy hours in the Snug of the 'Boilermaker's', undisturbed yet not unmarked. Tincture of opium figured too as the kick in a pricey cough cure we sold. A good dose would grip for a short while even the consumptive's spasms, to bring flickers of renewed hope that soon died.

---

[1] failed to sell.

[2] *aperient*: a laxative.

'Therapion' had a good run. This 'New French Remedy' was unique in that it claimed not only to induce venery[3] but also to heal any unfortunate consequences of it. 'Therapion', we read, 'stimulates the vitality of weak men, yet contains besides all the desiderata for curing gleet,[4] discharges, piles, blotches and premature decay.' 'French and Belgian doctors' swore by it. Floratino, too, was 'highly recommended'. At 2*s* 6*d* a bottle it 'imparted a peculiarly pearly whiteness to the teeth [before the enamel flaked] and a delightful fragrance to the breath'. With his best suit out of pawn, a dose of Therapion and a mouth washed with Floratino, a young man could feel all set for Saturday night. 'St Clair's Specific for Ladies' had more serious aims; this 'prevented', among other ailments, 'Cancer, Tumurs [*sic*] and varicose veins'.

The boldest purveyor, who took a quarter-page spread in the local newspaper, appeared to be a 'Mr W.H. Veno'. A charismatic figure, he was shown standing before a screen in a great beam of light. 'His marvellous diagnostic power', the advertisement assured us, 'borders on the superhuman. He sees a sick person at a glance, reads his disease without asking a question and with the utmost accuracy.' He could do this 'blindfold', too, and had withal a 'rare gift' which enabled him to 'cure the sick and diseased in a manner that reads like miracles'. 'Priests and ministers of every denomination' were numbered among his patients. They all took, we were informed, 'People's Strengthener and Health Giver'—Sea-Weed Tonic at 1*s* 1½*d* and 2*s* 9*d* a bottle. Doctors used it too, because 'they recognised in Sea-Weed Tonic the most successful medicine that science has yet produced for liver, kidney and blood diseases'.

The imposition of the first tax on patent medicines put their manufacturers in a dilemma. A clause in the Act appeared to imply that proprietary medicines could still be sold free of tax provided their purported curative powers were not advertised. From then on, until the Act was revised, some firms merely announced the title of their product: others paid the tax and hired professional advertising men. The pushers of one pill, in keeping with a claim to have 'the largest sale of any patent medicine in the world', made boasts of almost megalomaniac proportions. Their pellet 'Cured Biliousness, Nervous Disorders, Wind and Pain in the Stomach, Sick Headaches, Giddiness, Fulness and Swellings After Meals, Dizziness and Drowsiness, Cold Chills, Flushes of Heat, Loss of Appetite, Shortness of Breath, Costiveness,[5] Scurvy and

---

[3] *venery*: the pursuit of, or indulgence in, sexual pleasure.

[4] *gleet*: a discharge of thin, purulent matter.

[5] *costiveness*: constipation.

Blotches of the Skin, Disturbed Sleep, Frightful Dreams and All Nervous and Trembling Sensations, Etc.' 'This is no fiction,' the ad-man went on. 'These are FACTS testified continually by members of all classes of society. No Female should be without them. They will restore Females of all ages to sound health.'

And the females took his advice: we sold them at the shop in screws of paper, three for a halfpenny, in endless succession. A simple aperient had taken on magic potency.

Tucked away in corners of the local newspaper one saw other medical announcements. These offered assurances to 'Ladies', 'Women' and 'Females' of their ability to remove 'obstructions' of all kinds, 'no matter how obstinate or long-standing'.[6] The advertisers usually had foreign names and obscure London addresses. But most of our women in need of such treatment relied on prayer, massive doses of pennyroyal syrup, and the right application of hot, very soapy water. There were even those who in desperation took abortifacients sold by vets for use with domestic animals. Yet birth control continued to be looked upon as a sin against the Holy Ghost.

13.2
Services under the National Health Insurance Act

Anne Digby, *The Evolution of British General Practice 1850–1948* (Oxford, Oxford University Press, 1999), pp. 318–22.

Anne Digby's research has focused on the development of general practice in the nineteenth century, and especially on the economics of medical practice. In *The Evolution of British General Practice* she analyses the work and careers of ordinary general practitioners through a wide range of archival material and published medical journals. This extract examines the quality of state-funded primary care provided through the National Health Insurance Act of 1911.

---

[6] A euphemism for pregnancy. These advertisements were for drugs to induce abortions.

Amongst key issues posed by the NHI [National Health Insurance] was the question of whether panel patients were second-class citizens when compared to private patients. Informing discussion were implicit value judgements as to the appropriate standard to be sought in a public service catering for poorer patients. Class assumptions shaped the perceptions of bureaucrats as well as of doctors. English Insurance Committees were circulated on whether panel patients received as good a service as private patients, and the omissions and face-saving phraseology in their replies pointed to a divided system of medical care. An obvious indication of the two-tier nature of practice could be readily observed in the differentiated physical accommodation and reception of patients. Panel patients frequently queued at a back door to enter a cramped, barely furnished surgery, there to wait their turn for the doctor during fixed surgery hours. In contrast, their middle-class counterparts chose personally convenient times for appointments, were greeted by a maid at the front door, and waited in a comfortable room in the doctor's house for more extended medical interviews. Indeed, there was neither incentive for the panel doctor to improve accommodation, nor any effective coercion to do so, since although the rare insurance committee (such as Birmingham) inspected the surgery accommodation of insurance doctors several times, others (like London or Devonshire), did so only rarely or unsystematically.

The usual divide between panel and private patients was narrower in the Manchester and Salford Scheme. A local newspaper commented that 'it is to the doctor's interests to treat his panel patients with the same consideration he treats his private patients. Otherwise he would speedily find himself without any panel patients.' This local initiative was predicated on payment to doctors on the basis of patient attendance and not, as was the case elsewhere, on an annual capitation payment. Panel patients were therefore on the same footing as private ones. Running for only a dozen years, the scheme collapsed under the weight of the administrative work it had generated.

Insurance doctors had to give all proper and necessary medical services except those requiring special skill. This meant *inter alia*[7] that treatment of fractures or dislocation was expected but not an operation for piles or an operation on tubercular glands. More serious cases were referred for treatment in the outpatients departments of hospitals. Practitioners were supplied with 'Lloyd George' record cards for their NHI patients. Panel doctors recorded brief but intermittent entries for patients, usually in relation to more serious conditions, and/or those

---

[7] *inter alia*: among other things.

requiring certification in relation to employment. Diagnoses were almost entirely for physical ailments, and few clinical measurements were recorded as having been made in reaching them. Panel doctors seem to have shown little or no appreciation of the value of the NHI clinical record for their patients. The financial committee of one Scottish panel even minuted that 'the present medical record system is serving no useful purpose and in the interest of economy should be scrapped'. Patient–doctor confidentiality in relation to NHI certification was an issue raised by one NHI practitioner, who was outraged by the local insurance committee's insistence that the precise illness suffered by the panel patient be inserted on a certificate of incapacity for work. Interestingly, the point was made that 'health and character are so closely bound together that the declaration of a malady may blight the fair face of a whole family'. The doctor won his case, and the word 'illness' was deemed sufficient thereafter.

Doctors complained about the fluctuating composition of their panels, although this was usually articulated in a grouse about form filling, rather than in manifesting concern about its implications for the continuous care of patients—a defining characteristic of good general practice. Many panel patients moved on to a new doctor's list because of changes of address or of employment. Panel patients did have the right to choose their insurance practitioners, but only very small numbers (between 3 and 5 per cent) were estimated to have initiated a change in their doctor by giving notice at the end of a quarter. This finding might indicate either satisfaction with the standard of service or low patient expectation. That there was only a small trickle of panel patients' grievances about their doctors does not resolve this ambiguity. Complaints were usually about the practitioner charging for a procedure without prior warning, or charging for one which it was thought should have been in the category of insurance treatment rather than private practice. Also prominent were allegations that the doctor showed insufficient courtesy or did not respond promptly to a request for a visit. Discourtesy or incorrect charging were complaints which were far more likely to be upheld by insurance medical committees, and the patient vindicated, than were charges of medical negligence when doctors on NHI medical committees might feel impelled to salvage colleagues' professional reputations by finding facesaving rationales for their conduct. In some instances, however, a doctor was so clearly clinically negligent that he was severely censured, and a substantial fine was imposed. One Scottish doctor, for example, was fined £50. He had been sent for on a Saturday afternoon, failed to attend the panel patient until Sunday morning, when castor oil was prescribed, called subsequently on Monday morning, when the patient was sent to hospital, where death soon ensued from appendicitis. Friendly societies also criticized panel doctors for supplying inadequate certification in cases involving society members as insured patients; their allegations were well substantiated, and were usually upheld.

Standards of practice varied, not only (predictably) between individual doctors, but also in the standards laid down by insurance committees between different areas. Nottinghamshire, for example, debated the merits of a Local Formulary, such as that introduced into the City of Nottingham, by which a limited pharmaceutical range had been sanctioned for panel patients. It concluded that stock mixtures partook of club practice[8] would encourage hasty prescribing, lead to deterioration in the mixture during storage and, although producing economies, would not be in the interest of the insured person. Barrow in Furness, in contrast, was only too ready to sanction and introduce a local Formulary. Out of twenty-eight stock mixtures which the BMA and the Pharmaceutical Society of Great Britain listed as suitable for storing in bulk, the Barrow in Furness Insurance Committee selected only ten stock mixtures for use by its practitioners including cough mixtures, tonics, and digestive or laxative medicines.

If panel doctors prescribed expensive drugs they might be vulnerable to accusations of over-prescription, and liable to subsequent surcharging. The annual prescription cost of Fife panel doctors was continually singled out as having been well above the Scottish average. In 1925 nineteen local doctors there were even surcharged £100 each for their excessive prescription. The Fife insurance practitioners defended their expenditures on the grounds that they were due both to inexperienced panel doctors as well as to the prescription of new expensive drugs, such as extract of liver, which was 'of great therapeutic value'. Later, local doctors considered that this restrictive bureaucratic policy had been beneficially modified . . .

The calibre of NHI pharmaceutical practice has received little academic attention, but it is obvious that the predominance of small chemists, making up a few NHI prescriptions for a handful of doctors, was unlikely to encourage accurate dispensing. When the Nottinghamshire Insurance Committee inquired into panel prescriptions, the analyst they employed found that as many as one in three were substandard. Generally, new drugs were not sanctioned for NHI use, because it was stated that 'as a specific it is still in question', but to the

---

[8] *club practice*: practice through private insurance schemes or 'sick clubs'. Club practice had a reputation for providing low standards of care, in order to keep down costs.

historian the suspicion lingers that its cost was the material factor. Appliances which were sanctioned by the NHI authorities in each locality were listed. These might include cheaper alternatives to those which doctors were accustomed to use, and Burnley doctors protested, for example, about the cheaper grey bandages they were expected to substitute for white ones for their panel patients.

For the patient the 1911 act brought real, if heavily qualified, blessings. A panel doctor concluded that 'the Insurance Act was a boon both to the insured patient and to their medical attendant.' The doctor was no longer involved in 'balancing the value of his services against the length of his patient's purses', while the patients were not faced with bills and debts. But although access to a doctor undoubtedly improved after 1911, the quality of care given was generally mediocre. Club doctors before the NHI had reduced visits in favour of a swift throughput through the surgery, and the panel doctor continued with this. The panel system therefore institutionalized a pre-existing tension between the club doctor and his patient in that it emphasized the quantity of care delivered rather than intervening to improve its quality. Routinization linked to a low standard of patient care: with overprescription; a reluctance to treat difficult cases rather than to refer them elsewhere; and under-investment in modern equipment and premises were thereby encouraged. This trend was linked to the capitation system[9] of British insurance practice. In Germany where doctors were paid through items of service, insurance practitioners were encouraged to offer specialist as well as generalist services to their patients.

It was almost inevitable that the pressure of treating large numbers of patients should have had an adverse impact on the range and quality of patient–doctor encounters. A reluctance by panel doctors to engage in clinical work for which no remuneration was likely, meant a readiness to refer patients to hospital outpatient clinics. Even Dame Janet Campbell (formerly in the Ministry of Health), admitted that 'Panel practice does not justify the keen doctor ... Work is hard, hours are long'. At that time the doctor gave on average three-and-a-quarter minutes to each insurance patient in the surgery, and four minutes when on a visit to the patient's home. But perhaps we should not be too critical on this score: it was not very different from the five minutes that the NHS doctor later spent.

---

[9] *capitation*: payment according to the number of patients, regardless of how much treatment was provided.

13.3

Care in hospital

Bella Aronovitch, *Give it Time. An Experience of Hospital 1928–32* (London, André Deutsch, 1974), pp. 38–43, 50–2, 55–6, 60, 62–7, 71–2, 74.

In February 1928 Bella Aronovitch suffered some abdominal pain. She went to the out-patients' department of a London hospital, where she was diagnosed as suffering from appendicitis. She was operated on, but the wound would not heal. As a result, she spent the next five years being shuttled between various hospitals. Her book gives a rare patient's-eye-view of hospital care in the 1920s, and makes clear the different quality of care offered by different types of hospital.

A few days after this first operation I had a visit from the hospital almoner.[10] She came into the ward carrying a huge sheaf of papers and looked terrifyingly efficient. Following a few minutes' talk with Sister she came over to me, made herself comfortable on a chair beside my bed and for the next quarter of an hour, her conversation consisted entirely of questions. She started with questions about my family. How many of us were there at home? Who went to work and who were still at school? How much did I earn when I went to work? How much rent did we pay? What was our total income from all sources? etc., etc. Now all the questions were the preliminary skirmishes leading to the final question, which was; could my family afford to pay towards my upkeep while I was in hospital and if so, how much? Having had a major operation I was stiff and sore with numerous stitches and draining tubes. Tied under my knees was a hard, uncomfortable pillow called a 'Donkey', and I was very tightly tied round the middle with an arrangement known as a 'many tailed bandage'. I found all those questions rather trying. However, I answered them truthfully and to the best of my ability. As the almoner left, she told me to be sure to tell my mother to call at her office next mid-week visiting day. She then double checked with Mother on the answers to all questions.

---

[10] *almoner*: a hospital official who questioned patients about their financial circumstances to ascertain whether they could pay something towards the cost of their treatment.

[. . .]

I recovered fairly well after the first operation. However, the incision did not close properly though I had been in hospital over two months. There were strange murmurings by the ward sister which I did not understand, about the wound being 'slow healing' and healing by 'second intention'. I was able to walk a little but the difficulty of the wound not healing persisted and it began to be evident that I could not get beyond this stage. The specialist then suggested I should have a second operation; as he cheerfully said, 'Just to clear things up.' I hardly received this news with wild enthusiasm, but philosophically decided that something else must be attempted, since I could hardly be very mobile with an open wound. Moreover, I faithfully believed in that mystique about the medical profession which is known as 'having faith in doctors'. Like numbers of working-class people I was overawed by the fact they wrote in Latin and carried on conversations among themselves which nobody else understood. They swept into the ward in a procession akin to Royalty. First came the specialist, flanked by his first-assistant on one side and the house-surgeon on the other side: some two paces behind were a varying number of students and this group were immediately joined by the ward sister. The rest of the nursing staff also became alerted. It seemed like a ceremony – a rite – I imagined I heard the sound of trumpets heralding the arrival of the sacred and the great, for they appeared to take on a God-like aura and be segregated from ordinary mortals.

[. . .]

After two weeks' grace and some ten weeks after the first operation, I had a second. . . . In those days surgery was a much slower process and it was again six weeks before I was rid of the tubes and other paraphernalia. I sensed an air of concealment on the part of the doctor, though this was just a fleeting thought on my part and I did not worry.

When the specialist came to see me his face wore the usual sauve, calm expression which concealed the fact that anything was seriously amiss. Sister told him I was getting along fine. I regarded the fact that I was in hospital longer than anticipated as a mere nuisance. On the surface all seemed well. . . . This same specialist had . . . set habits. When he came into the ward he visited his own patients, of whom there were quite a number, and I noted that he shook hands very cordially with some of his patients. I wondered why this privilege was extended to some and not to others. Although his cases were all surgical, there was considerable variation as to the type of complaint, but I afterwards discovered that there was one thing which all the patients had in common with whom he shook hands – they had all paid him a private visit at his Harley Street surgery.

The result of the second operation was much the same as the first, that is, the incision did not heal beyond a certain stage. As part of the treatment it was decided to give me four-hourly fomentations,[11] as this was much used before the discovery of antibiotics. The fomentation started off by feeling burning hot, after which it soon became lukewarm then, for most part of the four hours between one treatment and another, I had the feeling of being wrapped round with a cold, clammy blanket. This was continued for two weeks, day and night, making no difference whatsoever. Among other treatments, I remember being prescribed iodine – a few drops on a lump of sugar.

[. . .]

A conspiracy of silence was being maintained by the doctor and the staff – if doubts existed, they were certainly not expressed either to myself or Mother. The sister on this ward rarely did any dressings though she occasionally looked on. During these viewing periods she was always sure so far as I was concerned, it was a question of time, a very short time and success was round the corner . . .

I walked slowly and with difficulty. The deadly monotony of hospital routine made it hard to keep up morale and remain cheerful. There was nothing to look at. The walls of the ward were painted dead white and were completely bare. There was no decor, no pictures or ornaments of any kind. The only splash of colour during the day, were the flowers brought in by the patients' visitors.

. . . Above all, there was nothing to do. In the days before radio was installed in all hospitals, the only communication with the outside world were newspapers, letters, books brought in by visitors and the official visiting days. There were no organized handicrafts, no library service, no mobile telephones; in short, there was nothing available to prevent people with long illnesses from sinking into depression.

[. . .]

With the exception of two or three who had been there a long time, there was a complete changeover of ward patients about every three weeks.

[. . .]

---

[11] *fomentation*: the application to the body of flannels soaked in water with or without some added medicinal substances.

There was no flexibility in the strict hospital rules laid down for visiting times. One and a half hours on Sunday afternoon and one hour on Wednesday afternoon were the official visiting times. Two and a half hours each week was considered quite sufficient, neither was there any allowance made for long-stay patients. Some of the ward sisters openly considered visiting times an unwarranted interference in the cycle of work and, as such, a nuisance. Sometimes the nurses were unable to get the ward work done in time, so that even these meagre periods were cut short by as much as twenty minutes and this time was always lost.

Officially the hospital allowed four visitors and not more than two at a time for each patient. As to how this rule was implemented depended on who was in charge. Sometimes the sister or nurse might spend the entire time policing the ward, to see that an extra visitor did not slip through the net. Other times a more tolerant nurse would be in charge and not bother to harry anybody. Both visiting periods were in the afternoon, so fewer people came on Wednesdays, since many who were working could not get away. . . . [Shortly after, Bella Aronovitch briefly went home, but was then admitted to another voluntary hospital.]

This new hospital was one of the smaller voluntary hospitals, looking grey and forbidding . . . The nurse informed me that it was a rule for all new patients to have a bath so, rather unsteadily, I followed the nurse into a small, very untidy bathroom . . .

Hospital bathrooms, invariably cluttered with all kinds of gear, were at best untidy, and at worst downright dirty. There never seemed to be enough space with the result that the ward bathroom became a general dumping ground. Neither were the bathrooms designed to provide anything like enough baths or washbasins. This ward in which I had just arrived had eighteen beds, and one small bathroom containing one very deep bath, difficult to get in and out of . . .

However, there was this curious dichotomy in the attitude towards cleanliness. On the one hand, all sterilized dressings and treatments were performed with fanatical attention to the smallest detail and on the other hand, was this antiquated Victorian bathroom equipment.

[. . .]

It was definitely more cheerful in the previous hospital; this ward was quiet, dreary, with a prison-like effect. . . .

Next morning I had the usual visit from the house surgeon who, much to my surprise, was a woman doctor. She was attractive, very feminine and had great charm. . . . Following her visit was one from the specialist, who greeted me with an expression I was to hear many times. He said, 'And how are you – none the better for my asking?' He was the only consultant I had ever seen who cultivated no bedside manner and was completely devoid of 'side'. He would help himself to anything I happened to have on top of my locker such as sweets or fruit; cut himself buttonholes from flowers in the ward – this with the help of nurses' surgical scissors, then sit on the side of the bed and talk in a perfectly natural way. . . .

After this first visit the specialist had a long talk to Sister away from my bed. Sister afterwards told me that the day of operation had been fixed for the coming Thursday. . . .

The result of this operation was absolute disaster. Within hours of it being performed the doctor had to remove the dressing because of the bleeding. There was some talk of my going up to the theatre again, which really reduced me to a state of terror, since I was vomiting badly as a result of the recent anaesthetic. The consultant came back twice to have a look at it and finally decided to leave it alone – to my great relief. About a week later when the sister was changing the dressing I plucked up enough courage to have a look at it and found it hard to believe that part of my body was also part of myself. The specialist, who was much given to puns and banter, kept up a running commentary with the house surgeon, the students and the nursing staff about this piece of surgery; somehow I found it very difficult to join in the fun.

None of the sutures held and there was a gap of some three to four inches between one side of the incision and the other. The house surgeon was very kind to me during this period. She kept reassuring me that Time was a great healer and it would all right itself . . . I do not wish to go any further into the harrowing details, except to say my chances of getting better were almost nil. I became completely bedridden. I did not realize the enormity of what had happened for some time and still thought I would get better, though it might take longer.

The behaviour of doctors and nurses towards the patient always seemed the same – that is, whatever happened to the patient was regarded as normal and in the natural order of things. They discussed treatments and conditions among themselves, but there was a united front towards the patient which might be summed up as, 'this is how it is – it cannot be otherwise'. . . .

One day the specialist made a very strange remark. In the course of the usual routine questions and answers he suddenly said to me, 'You must hate me.' I considered this surprising statement and decided there was no one to blame. In taking the decision to bring me to this hospital, Mother had intended only my good and every doctor wants his work to be successful. I have always remembered this conversation, since it was the only time any doctor had ever said a thing like that to me. He was unconventional in the whole of his approach to patients, and I was disconcerted by this remark, especially the use of the word 'hate'[. . .].

[T]he specialist came into the ward and, after gazing thoughtfully at the floor for some time, walked slowly towards my bed. . . . This was the first time for some weeks he had spoken to me, although he had been in to see his other patients. He was quite straightforward and without any preliminaries he came quickly to the purpose of his visit. He explained to me that the doctor in charge had to satisfy the governors that any patient who occupied a bed for a longer than average period, would either get better or not. . . . It seemed it was possible to stay in hospital for a long time, if the doctor could satisfy the governors to that end. However, if such an assurance was not forthcoming, the patient must be moved to another hospital where they could keep people for an indefinite period. He bluntly told me that he did not know how long I would take to get better and would therefore have to move to another hospital nearby: Sister would give me all the details. He added he was very sorry, he would like to keep me but he was being pressed by the hospital governors. . . .

[. . .]

Arriving by ambulance at this third hospital I could not see the outside of the building, though what I saw of the inside resembled a morgue. The entrance was dark with dingy yellow paintwork: there seemed to be miles of corridors and passageways. It was curiously quiet, having none of the bustle and sense of purpose one usually notices on entering a hospital. There were several old people ambling about who seemed to be dressed in a kind of uniform. . . . This was my first experience of a Poor Law hospital. It was in 1929 and the far-reaching Public Health Act of that year had only just been passed.

As I was wheeled through the door I was astounded by the size of the ward – it was simply enormous. It was not only long but exceptionally wide. There were four rows of beds very close together, with only just enough room between each row to move around . . .

I was put into a bed along one of the inner rows, far away from the light of any of the windows. My spirits sank and I felt over-whelmed as I looked round this sea of beds and faces . . .

The nurse came over, looked at me and my belongings and told Mother to take my nightdress home. She said that the hospital supplied nightwear and did not allow patients to wear their own clothes. I took off my thin nightie, gave it to Mother and I was given the hospital night-gown. This garment, made from coarse, grey flannelette, was so hard and stiff I did not have the strength to unfold it and Mother helped me to get into it. The weather was very hot, and on this summer's day I was enveloped in this monstrous garment, which dragged a full half yard over my legs, with wide, gathered sleeves almost twice as long as my arms – I felt I could scarcely breathe because of the weight. It is difficult to imagine such a scene in the twentieth century; it was more in keeping with 1829 than 1929.

[. . .]

Looking back over this period I am better able to place it in perspective. The two previous hospitals I had been in were voluntary. I now found myself in a Poor Law hospital attached to the workhouse. This explained the rules with regard to clothing and why people appeared so odd when I first saw them – they were, in fact, dressed in the workhouse regulation clothes. I was in an institution which belonged more to the London of Charles Dickens than the beginning of the nineteen-thirties. . . . [T]he Law which empowered the London County Council to take over and administer the workhouses had only just been passed. The changeover took years to have full effect and I came into this hospital before any perceptible change had taken place.

One of the arrangements made during this time was that voluntary hospitals could, by mutual consent, get rid of their long stay and chronic sick patients by sending them to the newly constituted council hospitals. It was obviously pressure of this nature that obliged the specialist to have me moved here. . . .

This hospital consisted of several very large wards. There was no Outpatients' department and, so far as I could see, few amenities in the way of specialized treatment other than an operating theatre. The ward in which I now found myself was mainly geriatric. . . .

The nursing staff were of a different background and educational level than those in the voluntary hospitals, though they were certainly not unkind and did their best in antiquated buildings with outmoded, limited equipment. There was one doctor for the entire ward, a man in his early thirties, uncommunicative and tired-looking, which was not surprising as he always seemed to be on duty. I almost expected him to be on duty for ever and was mildly surprised to see another doctor on night duty.

[. . .]

I have never, before or since, been in a hospital ward where so many people died. Almost every night someone died and occasionally there were as many as four deaths. . . . All this was not as sinister as it sounds. Then, as now, the problem of the aged sick was a very difficult one. Not to have to die in the workhouse was the unspoken prayer and greatest wish of many aged, working-class people. The family of the aged did their best, often in the face of unemployment and great poverty. Having nursed an aged person for a long time, the difficulties towards the end became more than the ordinary family could cope with, so it was that many of these old folk were finally brought into hospital, literally dying. Sometimes they would last a few weeks, whilst others died overnight.

[. . .]

Time dragged in this ward. As usual, there was nothing to do. The only break in the deadly monotony were the two visiting periods, Wednesday and Sunday. By this time, I had developed a large area of extreme soreness round the wound which most doctors who had not seen it before, thought was a burn. . . . This wound gave me years of pain and made it difficult for me to concentrate, though I did try to read every day. I was almost completely cut off from friends I had known at home, although some wrote or very occasionally paid me a visit. This ward was particularly lonely because of the number of helpess and aged people.

[. . .]

I continued to lie in bed and became progressively less able to move. For months I had experienced difficulty when trying to sit up in bed and one day I noticed with a shock that both my legs were so stiff that I was only able to bend them with great effort. Even simple exercises might have saved me some of the misery I endured later, as a result of not being helped to move about more, although this difficulty of movement certainly did not start in this hospital. I went on this way for several months.

13.4

Resistance to care – sanatorium treatment

Linda Bryder, *Below the Magic Mountain. A Social History of Tuberculosis in Twentieth-Century Britain* (Oxford, Clarendon Press, 1988), pp. 205–11.

Bryder's book is one of a number of works on tuberculosis published in the 1980s. Tuberculosis was one of the greatest killers in the nineteenth and twentieth centuries, and the factors behind its decline are complex. *Below the Magic Mountain* explores the campaign against tuberculosis in Britain, the treatment for the disease, the experience of TB sufferers, and public attitudes towards the disease. In the early twentieth century, a regime of care in sanatoria – including a rich diet, fresh air (patients even slept outside) and exercise – was the standard form of treatment. In this extract, Bryder records patients' sometimes rebellious attitudes towards the strict sanatorium regime.

Evidence suggests that the majority of patients, whether working-class or not, were not totally submissive. . . . The two greatest disciplinary problems faced by medical superintendents were familiarity with members of the opposite sex and consumption of alcohol.

Rules on socializing were generally strict. For example, at Eversfield Hospital the regulations specified that 'conversation between men and women patients is not allowed'. Similarly at the Cheshire Joint Sanatorium, female and male patients were gathered together only for Christmas dinner. Wingfield was said to be proud of the fact that not a single patient in his institution had become pregnant, suggesting that other superintendents could not make the same boast, although even at Frimley, Bignall considered it doubtful that no children were conceived in the forbidden pine-forests. In 1922, analysing instances of patients discharged irregularly, McDougall noted that in one institution for 200 patients (male and female), there occurred only 6 cases of undue familiarity between the sexes leading to dismissal over a period of 15 months—which he thought was very low. There was a large number of young people in sanatoria, not only because tuberculosis was a disease which struck the young, but also because institutions were more receptive to young cases who were more likely to recover than to older patients whose disease was often more chronic. Most sanatoria admitted both sexes although generally men outnumbered women 60 to 40. It was reputed to be not uncommon for nurses to marry patients suggesting that despite the prohibition, some socializing occurred there as well. Two nurses who still live at Papworth married patients there. One pointed out that, with the isolation of the sanatorium, there were few other social diversions. . . .

Patients were strictly forbidden to enter public houses during the Saturday or Sunday afternoon leave from the institutions which was often granted to those who were well enough. Entering a public house, or returning to the sanatorium intoxicated, often led to instant dismissal. McDougall reported in July 1929 that three men were discharged that month for returning to the sanatorium in a disorderly condition. Possession of alcohol by patients was also strictly forbidden, although W.E.

Snell, medical superintendent of Colindale Hospital appeared amused by the extreme lengths to which some patients went to acquire alcohol, suggesting that at least some medical superintendents turned a blind eye . . .

Complaints by patients in sanatoria, particularly regarding the food, were not uncommon but were generally futile, dismissed as a manifestation or symptom of the disease. Tuberculous patients were reputed to be particularly finicky about their food and therefore complaints in that direction were not taken seriously. Norman Langdon at Papworth claimed that there was no point complaining about the food; he recalled one patient who was 'sent on the bus' in 1926 for doing so. . . .

A patient at the West Wales Sanatorium in 1923 said that all the patients were objecting to the food. When asked why they did not repeat their complaints to the medical superintendent, who had received none, the witness said they were afraid. The 1923 inquiry into the administration of the West Wales Sanatorium following complaints by Maud Morris revealed once again the futility of registering discontent. Llewellyn Williams explained concerning the evidence of Maud, 'The advanced stage of the disease at the time she gave her evidence would naturally have affected her memory and perspective.' A local doctor maintained, 'It is true that here as well as in other Institutions of different kinds, carried out at very best [*sic*], there are a certain few whose pathetically hopeless physical condition reacts upon their imagination and distorts their judgement—nothing satisfies them—though deserving every pity and consideration the truth is seldom got at by listening to [them] . . .

Another frequent cause of discontent was the total absence of heating. The *South Wales Argus* reported in 1937 that all the patients in the South Wales Sanatorium were complaining of the cold and that a visitor who was wearing an overcoat also felt cold. Conditions in sanatoria were often spartan, particularly in some of the converted smallpox and isolation hospitals. Cymla Hospital in Wales was such an institution, with 20 beds in 1914 and 60 by 1924. In 1927 its two main buildings were described as very damp; the roof in one leaked. . . . At least one patient discharged herself from Harefield Sanatorium, Middlesex, in 1929 because she found it too damp. In 1922, McDougall discovered that 'the severe climatic conditions during the winter months were the immediate cause of 26 premature discharges in the West Riding County Council sanatoria, chiefly on account of rheumatism'. In 1923, a visitor to Cowley Road Sanatorium, Oxford, found that all the male patients on the verandah, with two exceptions, were soaked with the rain which had fallen during the night, and that without any exception the top blankets on the beds were wet. The water had reached the patients partly through the roof and partly by being driven in by the wind.

[. . .]

While complaints were often futile, patients did ultimately have the power to leave, although Marcus Paterson's famous remark to a patient taking his own discharge, 'Tell your widow to send us a postcard', was used more than once in the following decades by medical officers of tuberculosis institutions. . . . Peter Edwards of the Cheshire Joint Sanatorium was said to despise those who were unable to tolerate the rigorous life and left the sanatorium, 'only to come or be carried back when the disease became more progressive; of those poor unfortunates, he [was] quoted as saying "they come crawling back on their knees, after death comes knocking at the door" '. . . .

Few figures are available on self-discharges, but in 7 sanatoria in Lancashire, 127 out of a total of 305 patients leaving altogether in 1921–2, took premature discharges, that is almost half, which did not strike the Ministry of Health observers as extraordinary. In 1922, a survey of West Riding CC sanatoria showed that out of a total of 3,205 discharges from sanatoria (2,396 men and 809 women), 44 per cent of the male and 32 per cent of the female discharges were 'irregular'. This included those who discharged themselves and those who were discharged for disciplinary reasons (24 per cent came into the latter category). Similarly at Peel Hall, Lancashire, 44 out of 113 patients left for reasons other than medical, of which 39 took their own discharge and 5 were dismissed.

The high proportion of self-discharges suggests that working-class patients did not submit to the discipline and the conditions of the sanatorium regime as easily as the medical superintendents . . . hoped. Self-discharging patients were also probably primarily responsible for modifying the rigorous conditions of the institutions. Powell said in 1937 that since installing heating in some of their institutions, they had been able to keep patients longer. The number of patients in tuberculosis institutions was also higher in summer months suggesting a reluctance to remain during the cold winter months. . . .

However, 'pull factors' from home were possibly most important in causing self-discharges. At least one female patient at Eversfield Hospital discharged herself prematurely without consulting the medical superintendent because her home was 'in a dreadful pickle'. She explained that her husband was unable to cope alone with the children and a dependent father. H. Old of the Welsh Board of Health referred to the constant difficulty they had in persuading women (for whom there was little outside assistance available) to leave their domestic responsibilities and undertake institutional treatment.

13.5
The health of working-class women

Margery Spring Rice, *Working-Class Wives. Their Health and Conditions* (London, Virago, 1981, first edn, 1939), pp. 39–43.

In 1933, the Women's Health Enquiry Committee, formed of representatives from voluntary associations, launched an investigation into the health of married women, believing that illness was more widespread than was generally believed. Their concern reflected a general concern with the health of mothers and children, who were seen as crucial to the 'national health'. The 1,250 responses to the Committee's questionnaire confirmed their suspicions – few working-class women enjoyed good health. Most were worn down by large families, bad housing and poor diet. The Committee recommended the extension of maternity and child health services and of National Health Insurance cover to families, more government support for housing, and the provision of family allowances.

[W]omen show a general disinclination to fuss about themselves, which is the result partly of their exhausting work, partly of their preoccupation with the welfare of their families and partly of ignorance, or a curious failure to apply to themselves what they do know about health in general. Advice therefore is not sought as often as it should be, or if sought is not taken. . . .

The most important controlling factor in this is poverty, especially in those illnesses which the woman thinks she can fairly safely overlook, such as headaches, constipation, anæmia and bad teeth. Here is a typical example of this attitude, governed by lack of funds. . . . Mrs. F. of Sheffield. She is 47 and has had seven children, of whom two have died. Her husband is a railway drayman. She gets £2 17s. 0d. housekeeping . . . She has rheumatism, (since she had an operation for gall-stones two years ago,) toothache, headache and back-ache. For none of these does she consult anyone. She owes her private doctor for the last five years' attendance, including the last confinement, £14, which she pays off in 1/– weekly instalments . . .

Rheumatism, gynæcological troubles and bad legs being much more crippling to work, show a larger percentage of advice sought and treatment taken. Gynæcological trouble has other features in respect of treatment. The woman probably does not recognise the symptoms herself. ('Backache since birth of baby'. 'Internal trouble through confinements', are frequent complaints for which no advice and treatment have been sought,) and in the absence of a thorough post-natal examination, the trouble is not discovered till the birth of the next child, often not then if she has not been attended by a doctor. When it *is* discovered, much greater pressure is brought to bear on her by the doctor or nurse to have the matter attended to. An example of this is given by a Manchester woman of 35 who has three children. She has had very bad backache since her first confinement, and at her second confinement the doctor diagnosed a prolapse[13] and advised an operation. She could not face this then, but the condition has got worse since the birth of the third child, and she is now 'waiting for the bed in the hospital'. . . .

The comparative percentages for professional treatment in the seven specially analysed ailments are:—

Headaches	30%	are	professionally	treated.
Constipation	36%	"	"	"
Anæmia	38%	"	"	"
Bad teeth	43%	"	"	"
Rheumatism	56%	"	"	"
Gynæcological trouble	59%	"	"	"
Bad Legs	60%	"	"	"

The best of these figures shows a deplorably low percentage of treatment and it is not entirely explained by poverty, or a courageous neglect. There is also a good deal of prejudice and/or fear due to ignorance. This is apparent particularly in cases where hospital treatment, an operation or otherwise, is needed . . .

Another country woman aged 41, very poor, with four children, and a very bad house, has a 'torn lower bowel and dropped womb' and she says of both 'These could be righted in hospital, but don't like the idea.' The bowel trouble dates from her first confinement, the prolapse from her second.[. . .]

An even sadder story of the efforts to cure ill-health is given by the records of the inefficacy of treatment. Over and over again the woman is unable to continue a treatment begun, either because it involves too much expense, or a weekly visit to a hospital and hours of waiting for which she cannot spare the time. Almoners and Health Visitors who

---

[13] *prolapse*: a slipping downward of an organ (in this case, the uterus) from its normal position.

have added notes show disappointment in the woman's improvement after treatment, but the one method of treatment which seems to have a magical effect is three or four weeks convalescence at the sea.

The professional advice that the women receive appears to vary greatly in value. It is noticeable that many who have consulted their own doctor for such an ailment as bad backache or anæmia have been told to change their diet, to eat more nourishing food, to rest more, to sleep more and to get more fresh air. The changes are rung on these remedies over and over again.

A woman in Leeds who has had nine children of whom the seventh and eighth have died, has 44/– a week house-keeping money, and a poor house; she suffers from anæmia, neurasthenia and loss of appetite. She has a private doctor who 'advises rest, nourishment and not to worry'. . . . Another in London with six children says 'My Doctor before each child advised always rest and usually bed which is practically impossible.'

Index